I0091958

FUNCTIONAL REHABILITATIVE TRAINING

A PROFESSIONAL APPROACH

Ben Boulter
Training & Education Director, Clinic Director & Chiropractor

Medical Illustrations by
Victoria McCulloch

Photography by
Charlie Blewett

B2: Fitness Training Solutions
Boulter, Ben
     Functional Rehabilitative Training: *A Professional Approach*

ISBN: 978-0-9931843-0-7

© 2015, B2: Fitness Training Solutions Ltd. All rights reserved.
Company Number: 09040791

This book, or any parts thereof, may not be used or reproduced in any manner without written permission from the author.

Every effort has been made to ensure that the information provided in this book is accurate. However, due to the nature of the industry, information is constantly changing. Neither the author nor contributors assume any liability for any injury and/or damage to persons or property arising from this publication.

www.b2fitnesstraining.com

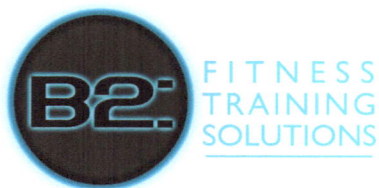

TABLE OF CONTENTS

TABLE OF CONTENTS   III

PREFACE   VII

ACKNOWLEDGMENTS   IX

INTRODUCTION   X

1. MUSCULAR & NERVOUS SYSTEM ANATOMY   1

1.1 ANATOMICAL POSITION & PLANES   2
1.2 MUSCLE CONTRACTION   5
    CONCENTRIC OR ISOTONIC CONTRACTION   7
    ECCENTRIC CONTRACTION   7
    ISOMETRIC CONTRACTION   8
1.3 BODY COMPOSITION   8
    ENDOMORPHS   9
    MESOMORPHS   10
    ECTOMORPHS   11
    MEASURING SOMATOTYPES   11
1.4 NERVOUS SYSTEM   17
    DERMATOMES   17
    MYOTOMES   18
    NEUROMUSCULAR CONTROL   18
    PROPRIOCEPTION   18
    CUTANEOUS RECEPTORS   20
1.5 SPINAL ANATOMY & JOINTS   22
    ZYGAPOPHYSIAL (FACET) JOINTS   24
    INTRA-ARTICULAR PRESSURE   25
1.6 MUSCLE ANATOMY   26
    SPLENIUS CAPITUS   27
    LEVATOR SCAPULAE   29
    TRAPEZIUS   31
    RHOMBOIDS   33
    SUPRASPINATUS   35
    ERECTOR SPINAE   37
    QUADRATUS LUMBORUM   39
    ILIOPSOAS   41
    GLUTEUS MEDIUS   43
    HAMSTRINGS   45
    VASTUS MEDIALIS OBLIQUE   47
    PERONEUS LONGUS   49
    SOLEUS   51

2. PSYCHOLOGICAL BEHAVIOUR & PAIN 55

2.1 SCHEMAS 56
2.2 LEARNING AND CONDITIONAL BEHAVIOUR 58
   CLASSICAL CONDITIONING 59
   OPERANT CONDITIONING 60
2.3 MOTIVATION 62
2.4 FEEDBACK 63
   FEEDBACK AND GOAL SETTING 65
2.5 SOCIAL LEARNING THEORY 66
2.6 PAIN AND BEHAVIOUR 67
2.7 LEARNED HELPLESSNESS 70

3. POSTURE & FUNCTION 74

3.1 POSTURE 75
   STANDING POSTURE 78
   SEATING POSTURE 84
   NEUTRAL SPINE 88
3.2 UPPER & LOWER CROSSED POSTURES 91
   UPPER-CROSSED POSTURE (UCP) 92
   LOWER-CROSSED POSTURE (LCP) 94

4. CORE STABILITY 100

4.1 CORE STRENGTH & STABILITY 101
4.2 CORE ACTIVATION & STIMULI 103
4.3 CORE & TRUNK STRENGTH 105
4.4 TRUNK ENDURANCE 108
   TRUNK ENDURANCE TEST 110
4.5 ABDOMINAL BRACE 113
4.6 ABDOMINAL HOLLOWING 115

5. TORSIONAL CONTROL 119

5.1 TORSION & CONTROL 120
5.2 BASIC BIOMECHANICAL PRINCIPLES 120
5.3 TORSIONAL CONTROL & EXERCISE 129
5.4 ISOLATING TORSIONAL CONTROL 129
5.5 TRAINING TORSIONAL CONTROL 131

6. PHYSIOLOGICAL ADAPTATIONS OF TRAINING 137

6.1 INTENSITY 139
6.2 FAILURE 140

6.3 MUSCLE FIBRES   **141**

6.4 MUSCLE HYPERTROPHY, STRENGTH & ENDURANCE   **143**

6.5 TEMPO   **147**

6.6 ADVANCED TRAINING TECHNIQUES   **151**

DROP SETS OR STRIP SETS   152

PYRAMID SETS   153

BURN-OUT SETS   154

HEAVY SINGLES   154

SUPERSETS   155

TRI-SETS   157

GIANT SETS   158

NEGATIVE SETS   160

BREAKDOWN SETS   161

7. GAIT   **165**

7.1 GAIT ANALYSIS FORM   **168**

HEAD & TRUNK   171

SHOULDER COMPLEX   172

HIPS & LEGS   173

KNEES   175

ANKLES   176

FOOT & HALLUX   178

7.2 RUNNING TECHNIQUES   **182**

HEEL STRIKE RUNNING   183

NEUTRAL STRIKE RUNNING   185

FOREFOOT STRIKE RUNNING   187

BAREFOOT RUNNING   188

8. FUNCTIONAL MOTOR PATTERNS   **193**

8.1 SHOULDER RANGE OF MOTION   **194**

8.2 APLEY SCRATCH TEST   **197**

8.3 PUSH UP TEST   **198**

8.4 WALL ANGEL TEST   **200**

8.5 PARALLEL SQUAT TEST   **201**

8.6 LUNGE TEST   **204**

8.7 ACTIVE & PASSIVE STRAIGHT LEG RAISE   **206**

8.8 HIP EXTENSION   **209**

8.9 HIP HINGE   **211**

8.10 STEP-DOWN TEST   **213**

8.11 SINGLE-LEG SQUAT   **216**

8.12 STANDING HOP TEST   **219**

8.13 MODIFIED THOMAS TEST   **221**

8.14 SOLEUS STRETCH TEST   222

8.15 HAMSTRING STRETCH TEST   223

8.16 QUAD STRETCH TEST   225

REFERENCES   229

INDEX   237

Preface

In a career fully immersed in both the healthcare and fitness industries, it has become clear that their remains a distinct gap between the two. The only bridge being provided by the well established GP Referral system.

This drove a desire to integrate the knowledge that I have accumulated in both fields, to draw the two professions of client/patient care closer together. In hope of creating a new generation of professionals focused on treating and preventing acute biomechanical pain and dysfunction with the use of exercise in conjunction with continuing professional manual care.

This textbook runs alongside the Functional Rehabilitative Training course, which is aimed at a simialr audience; Chiropractors, Osteopaths, Physiotherapists, Personal Trainers etc. as well as members of the medical profession. The education within these professions is adopting and encouraging a much greater biomechanical approach to pain and dysfcuntion. This is in an attempt to prevent acute and chronic pain from occuring, thus reducing the strain on the national health services. It is important however, that these professions work together, accepting that each has its limitations.

To add clarity to the text, the book contains a combination of maticulously put together illustrations and photographs. These, along with the text, have been crafted over the past three years to help the reader understand the content from a professional perspective.

My hope is that anyone who chooses to pick up this book will value the time dedicated to making it an interesting and informative read. As well as having a positive influence on their career and chosen profession in these incredible industries.

Ben J. Boulter

Acknowledgments

All books are written with help and support. So it no surprise, that there are a few people I wish to thank.

Firstly, I would like to thank my group of very close professional friends. Each of them has a different, but fantastic perspective on life and professional practice. Their diversity inspired me to embark on this journey: Matt, Phil, Ben, Joe, Neil, and Rob. I do and always will trust and respect each of your opinions.

To my illustrator, Victoria, thank you for putting up with my pedantic never-ending requests during our numerous Skype conversations, text messages and emails.

To Charlie and Chloe, thanks for making a daunting photo-shoot enjoyable and entertaining. They all look great.

Thanks to Elizabeth for your guidance and grammatical wisdom.

To Rachel, who has held the fort on the days that I have had to dedicate to writing the book and fully supported the idea, thank you.

I would like to extend my endless thanks to my parents, who each drive me to achieve something different. To my mum: thank you for believing in me to achieve anything. Dad: thank you for motivating me to complete everything. Martin: thank you for providing me with an unquestioned amount of support.

My family, friends and patients have been incredible, even inspirational. They are single handedly responsible for getting me to the finish line - I am, and will always be extremely grateful for your encouragement.

Finally, but by absolutely no means least, I would like to thank Holly. Your continued support and belief in me has always driven me to push myself. Thank you for adding something very special to my life.

Introduction

Pain relief is one of the most gratifying feelings one can empower within another. Not only is there a great sense of professional fulfilment, but also to watch a client/patient achieve something they were initially so wary of is an amazing sensation. Education and knowledge is a vital part of this course, because true pain or discomfort can be incredibly disabling, and more often than not a client/patient will just want to be 'fixed' without taking on any responsibility themselves. It is important that any professional working with clients/patients can pass on that responsibility through education of their functional/muscular imbalances or faulty movement patterns.

For many years, research has been produced stating how spinal manipulation has increased benefits to patients suffering with lower back, neck and shoulder pain compared to exercise treatment (UK BEAM Trial Team, 2004 and Twomey & Taylor, 1995). The results were generally weighted heavily in favour of manipulation as opposed to exercise intervention. However, there is one group whose response to pain relief is significantly better, and that is the group of combined spinal manipulation and exercise treatment (Erhard *et al*, 1994 and Meldrum, 2012).

Current research offers health and fitness professionals much support when justifying the validity and effectiveness of many interventions. Research is essentially a compilation of detailed experiences, a comparison of methods and the subsequent outcomes. Among its qualities, research can also be rather self-limiting, as research is quite often conducted to support a hypothesis. If that hypothesis is not proven to be correct or is insignificant then quite often the research will be dismissed and not published. This, along with the ever-increasing amount of informally published written material such as reports known as Grey Literature, can often make interpretation of possible methods and outcomes somewhat precarious.

A first person, hands-on experience can often be more advantageous to professional decision-making, acting as its own randomly controlled trial (RCT). Within the setting of a treatment room or an exercise facility, having the ability to think quickly and modify a method that is not working for one that might for another one that might work better is a skill. Like every skill it requires understanding, and then practice. Throughout a professional career no matter how long or short, there is still a wealth of experience to be gained and integrated within other methods of practice. The modern education of complementary medicines such as Chiropractic, Osteopathy and Physiotherapy teaches very detailed, invaluable knowledge and understanding of the neuromusculoskeletal system. However, these professions are not overtly encouraged nor taught how to physically train the neuromusculoskeletal system in the same manner as a fitness professional.

This course has been designed to open fitness professionals' perception as to the benefits they possess within themselves to be able to push, train and ultimately enhance client/patients' lifestyle through pain related functional training. It will also give complementary medical professions an insight into the physical capabilities that not only an athlete has, but also an average client/patient has. Thus, hopefully bridging the gap between evolving professions to form a well-rounded, more functional health-care system that doesn't just help people get better, but prevents people developing problems in the first place.

Function is defined as:

"An activity or purpose natural to or intended for a person or thing" or "to work or operate in a proper or particular way" (Oxford Dictionary, 2013).

The Institute of Functional Medicine proposes functional medicine "addresses the underlying causes of disease, using a systems-oriented approach and engaging both patient and practitioner in a therapeutic partnership" (2013). This means that, in a functional approach to musculoskeletal medicine, all of the body's systems are considered rather than the site of injury or pain, which can prove invaluable in the treatment or training of chronic musculoskeletal pain. This concept is shared by B2: Fitness Training Solutions, and is represented by the development of this course. Encouraging the progressive nature of complementary medicine to move into the 21st century of science-based medicine, means treating more than just the presenting symptoms of client/patients, but treating the person as an individual. It is important to expand on the aforementioned proposition by including not only the "cause of disease" but also addressing the cause of biomechanical dysfunction.

The Functional Rehabilitative Training course will take the skill and knowledge that healthcare and fitness professionals possess, and develop it towards working with sedentary and sporting dysfunctions. Teaching them the fundamentals in neuromusculoskeletal support and physical fitness (body composition, speed, flexibility, strength and endurance), and encouraging the use of motivation to train a client/patient to their individual physical limits (Mackenzie, 2000). A Functional Rehabilitative Trainer is safe but effective in aiding clients/patients achieve pain relief and maintain their normal function using specific exercises that focus on unique indiscretions rather than poor fitness. Anatomy will be used in a far more advanced way to build a catalogue of exercises and training methods to strengthen and support an individual's body, based on experience and integrated learning.

1. Muscular & Nervous System Anatomy

Learning Objectives

- To have a fundamental understanding, and ability to explain anatomical location using position and planes.
- To identify different muscle contractions, as well as practical application.
- To understand and appreciate various body compositions, as well as understanding how to measure somatotypes using skinfolds.
- To understand the importance and relevance of the nervous system on anatomical function.
- To understand the importance of the relationship between the spinal joints and the associated muscles.
- To be able to understand and recall significant muscles, including their origin, insertion, action and potential problems.

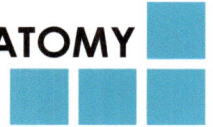

For any sports professional or athlete, having an appreciation about the body and how it performs is invaluable; it is not only interesting but also aids their perception of injury, performance and recovery. Accurate and relevant education of the body is becoming ever more fundamental, not only for people involved in sport, but also the general public. This is predominantly due to the increase in information on the Internet being misinterpreted and dramatized. For example, it may not be relevant for a 25-year-old male to know the thorough details of the pancreas if they are suffering with knee pain when running.

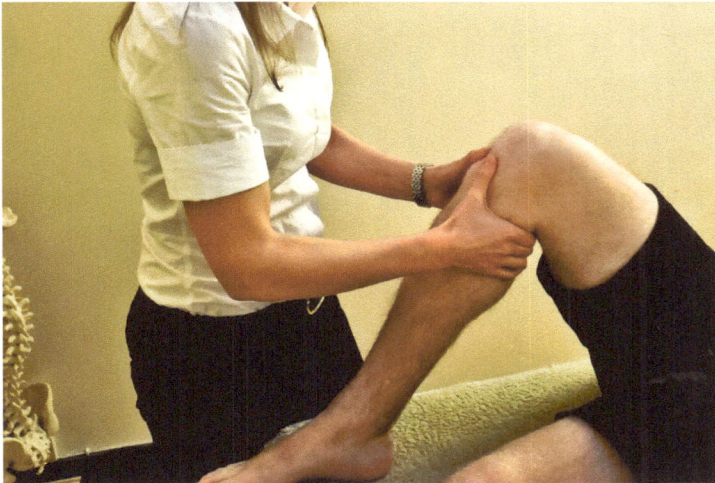

Physical assessment of the mobility of the knee

Understanding anatomy is the foundation to biomechanical and functional medicine, so a thorough appreciation is vital. Typically the term anatomy refers to either the gross anatomy (seen without the aid of magnification), or microscopic anatomy (seen with the aid of magnification) (Drake *et al*, 2005). A fundamental understanding will aid health and fitness professionals towards making an accurate interpretation of neuromusculoskeletal dysfunction, thus being able to correctly treat a client/patient safely and effectively. The process of learning anatomical structures and orientation is best done through the use of visualization and observation techniques, rather than lists and flow charts of muscles or arterial routes.

1.1 Anatomical Position & Planes

When describing the true anatomical location of certain structures there is a standard reference for the position, which is represented by the human body standing upright with the feet together. The hands are by the side of the body and the face looking forwards in a neutral position, neutral facial expression with a closed mouth also. The palms of the hands should be facing forwards and fingers extended. The feet should also be facing forwards (Drake *et al*, 2005).

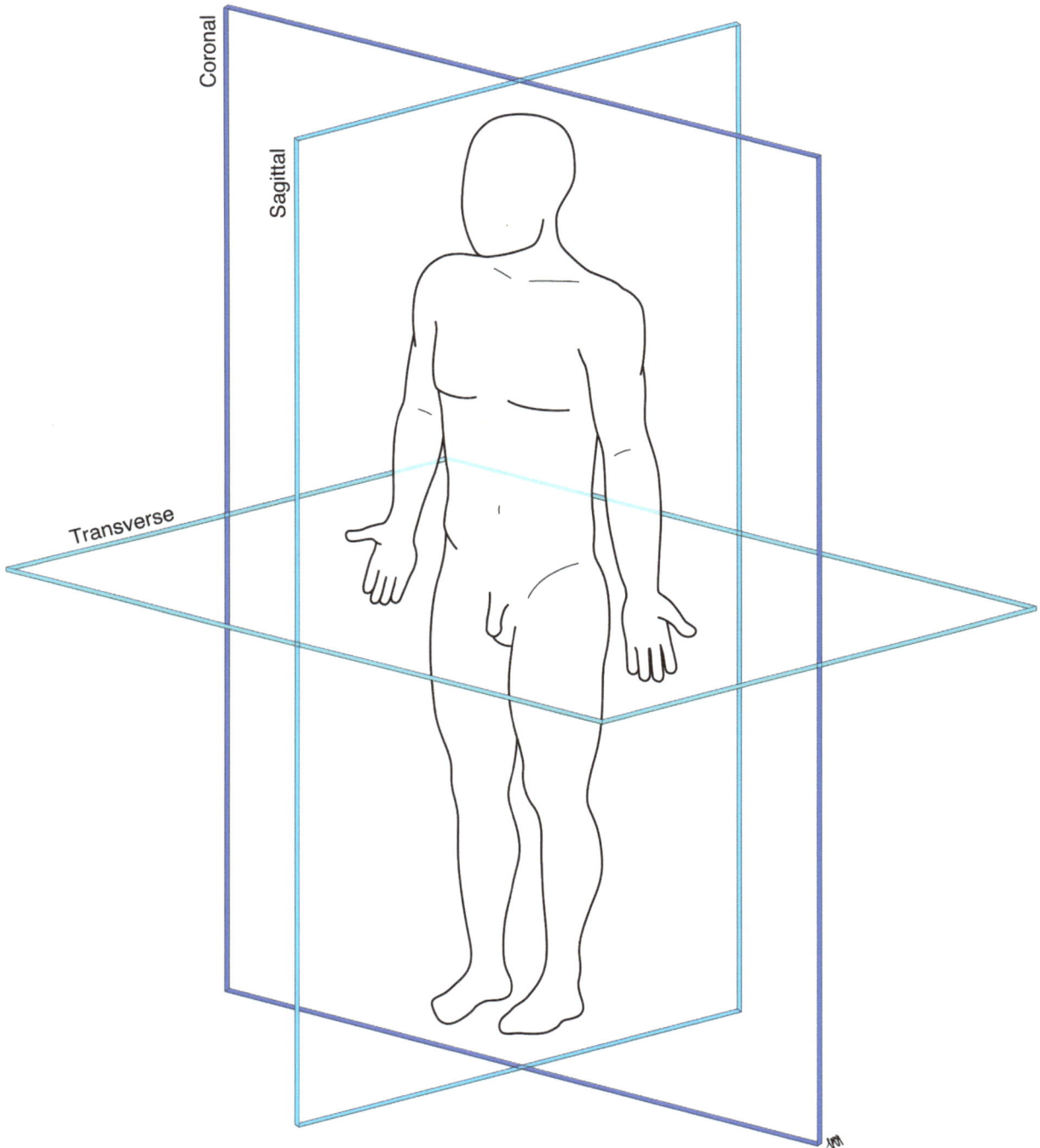

Figure 1: demonstrates the
three anatomical planes

MUSCULAR & NERVOUS SYSTEM ANATOMY

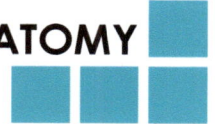

There are also three major groups of anatomical planes (Figure 1) to help explain and describe anatomical position:

- **Coronal Plane** – is orientated vertically through the body to divide it into anterior and posterior parts.
- **Sagittal Plane** – is also orientated vertically through the body, although it sits at a right angle to the coronal plane. It divides the body into right and left parts. The plane that passes through the body to divide equal right and left parts is known as the median sagittal plane.
- **Transverse or Horizontal Plane** – divides the body into superior and inferior parts.

As well as the planes, there are some pairs of terms to help accurately locate or describe certain structures as mentioned by Drake *et al* (2005):

- **Anterior and Posterior** – describe the position of the structures relative to the 'front' and 'back' of the body. For example, the nose is an anterior structure, whereas the spinal column is a posterior structure. The nose is also anterior to the ears, as the spinal column is posterior to the sternum.
- **Medial and Lateral** – are the terms used to describe the position of structures relative to the median sagittal plane and the sides of the body. For example, the thumb is lateral to the little finger. The nose is in the median sagittal plane and medial to the eyes, which are in turn medial to the ears.
- **Superior and Inferior** – describe the anatomical position of the structures in relation to the transverse plane. For example, the head is superior to the shoulder, whilst the knee joint is inferior to the hip joint.
- **Proximal and Distal** – describe being closer or farther away from the structure's origin, particularly the limbs. For example, the hand is distal to the elbow joint but the glenohumeral joint is proximal to the elbow joint.
- **Superficial and Deep** – describe the location of structures relative to the surface of the body. For example, the sternum is superficial to the heart and the stomach is deep to the Rectus Abdominus.

CHAPTER 1.

1.2 Muscle Contraction

Muscle contraction is coordinated by the nervous system to allow the body to perform certain movements and functions that the body requires to be able to survive. Skeletal muscles either work individually or within a group to manoeuvre the attached bones around a joint into position. They also work to prevent the joints being moved into a position past the physiological end point (Honeybourne *et al*, 2002). Sandoz (1976) explained this 'paraphysiological space' using Figure 2 to explain the total motion available at a joint, and consequently demonstrate at which point manipulation of a joint could occur. At the end of 'normal' joint motion, is what is described as an elastic barrier, which, when a joint loses a certain amount of flexibility, can be decreased. Various practices of joint manipulation have adopted different terms to describe this state. Chiropractors have used the terms "subluxation" or "fixation" (Gillet & Liekens, 1969); Osteopaths termed it "somatic dysfunction"; medical and physiotherapeutic specialists use terms such as "dysfunction", "barrier" and "loss of end-play". All of these terms contain the notion of "hypomobility" within a joint, and it appears the generically accepted term is "joint dysfunction" (Vernon & Mrozek, 2005).

There are four primary characteristics of muscle tissue:

- Excitability – they can respond to a stimulus from the nervous system
- Contractibility – they can shorten to apply a force to their connecting structures
- Extensibility – they can stretch past their normal length
- Elasticity – they can return to their original shape

The attachment points of the muscle to the bone are known as either the origin or insertion depending on the orientation. The origin of the muscle is the fixed stable end, proximal to the midline of the body. The insertion point of the muscle is usually attached to the bone that moves and is distal from the midline of the body. Movement around a joint should happen by the origin insertion being pulled closer to the origin of the muscle via muscle contraction. For example, when the Biceps Brachii contracts it

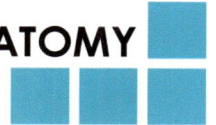

flexes the elbow joint, bringing the radius (insertion) closer to the scapula (origin).

Concentric or Isotonic Contraction

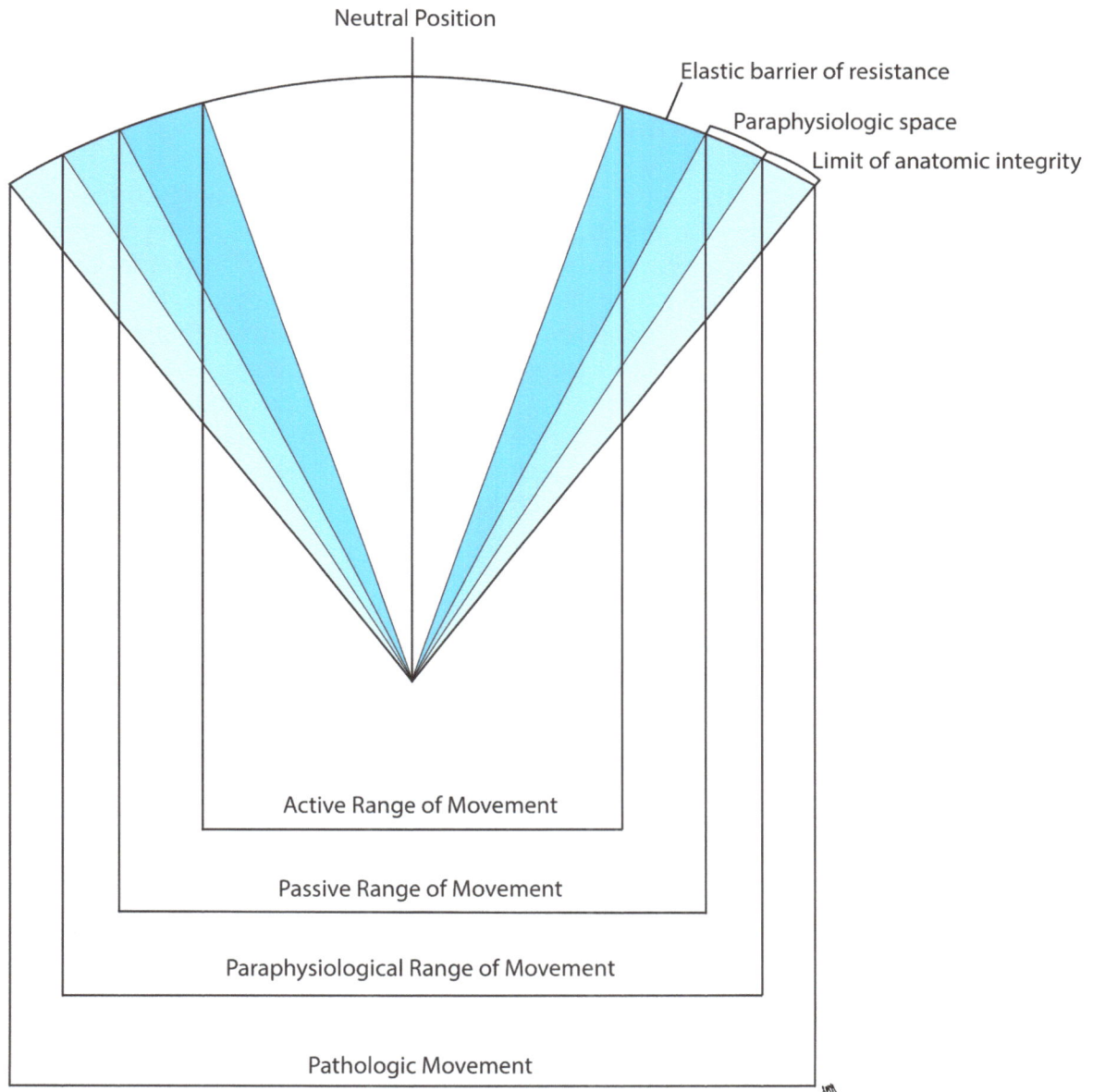

Neutral Position

Elastic barrier of resistance

Paraphysiologic space

Limit of anatomic integrity

Active Range of Movement

Passive Range of Movement

Paraphysiological Range of Movement

Pathologic Movement

Figure 2: identifies the total motion available at a joint, including its paraphysiological space

This is a form of muscular contraction that results in the muscle length shortening, producing a force to generate movement around a joint. The muscle is often a prime mover and is stimulated by the sliding filament theory (Faulkner, 2003). An example of concentric contraction would be the Biceps Brachii bringing the radius (insertion) closer to the scapula (origin), causing a flexed movement around the elbow joint.

Eccentric Contraction

This form of contraction is the opposing contraction to the concentric from. The muscle elongates under tension from the opposing muscle either decelerating movement or returning the muscle to its normal resting length. Muscles will suffer more damage during heavy eccentric loading compared to concentric loading. It is commonly suggested that muscles are approximately 40% stronger during eccentric contraction as opposed to concentric contraction (Roots, 2013; Raffle, 2012), although a reasonable theory, there appears to be a lack of empirical research to support it.

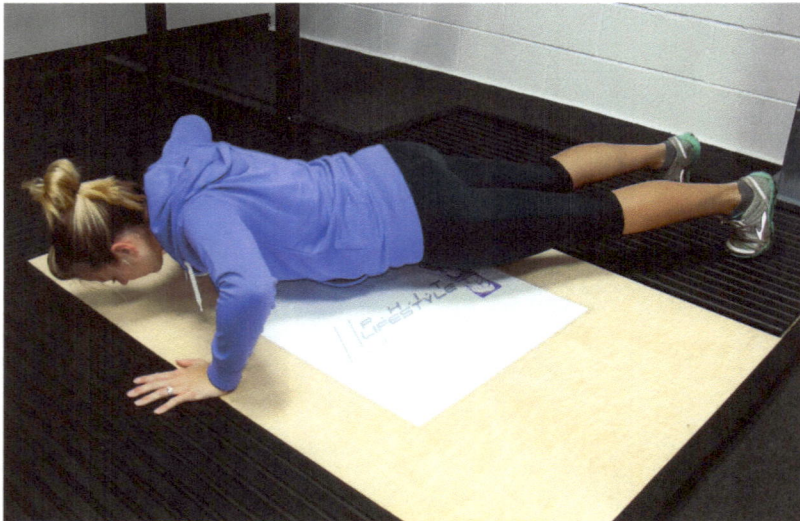

Eccentric contraction occurs in the Triceps during the lowering phase of a press-up

Performing a press up is a good example of eccentric contraction – during the downward (lowering) phase the Triceps Brachii contract eccentrically (lengthening under tension) to control the movement.

Eccentric contraction has been researched more recently with regards to its ability to rehabilitate weak or injured tendons. Injuries such as Achilles tendonitis have shown improvement through the use of highly weighted eccentrically loaded exercise (Satyenda & Byl, 2006; Alfredson *et al*, 1998).

Wall Squat is a good example of isometric contraction

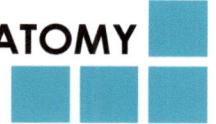

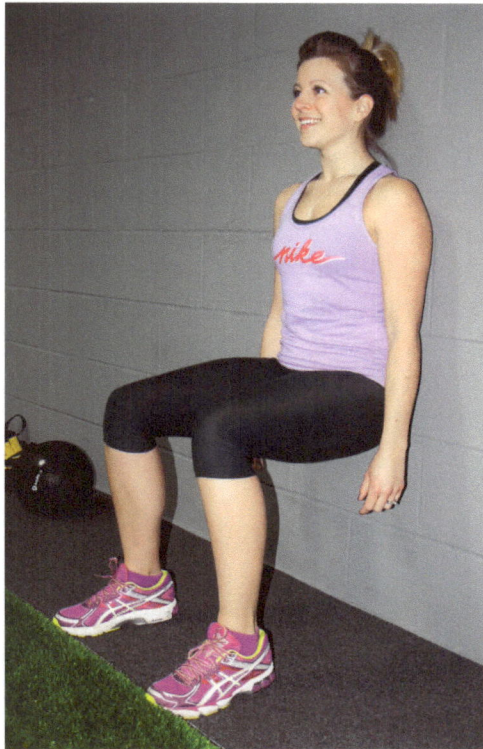

Isometric Contraction

The muscle will increase in tension but the length will stay the same, therefore there is no movement. This form of contraction happens when the muscle works against a resistance that it cannot overcome, an example of this would be when a rugby scrum engages with equal force, or during an even tug of war. It also occurs during a wall squat (Honeybourne *et al*, 2002).

1.3 Body Composition

Success of an athlete depends on several components such as skill, ability and body composition. Sheldon *et al* in 1940 suggested three extremes for expressing body composition: Endomorphy, Mesomorphy and Ectomorphy (Figure 3). This process then became known as somatotyping. Somatotypes are expressed using a numerical scoring system of 1-7 based on each individual extreme body type, which would have been interpreted as:

7 – Very High
6 – High
5 – Moderately High
4 – Average
3 – Moderately Low
2 – Low
1 – Very Low

Although absolute distinctions cannot be made, a person can be classified as being more of one type than another. This was done by visual analysis of three standardised photographs taken from front, side and rear views.

*For example, two, six, three (**263**) means: two (low endomorphy); six (high mesomorphy); three (low ectomorphy).*

Absolute distinctions are difficult to make with somatotypes because of the nature of subjective judgement. Inter-examiner reliability may deem one person's interpretation of an individual's physique as having a low mesomorph score, where another examiner may view them as having an average mesomorph score. Essentially, the judgement is based on the deposition of muscle and adipose tissue, which in itself is subject to change. A person's somatotype can, and is likely to, change over time due to exercise, diet, and hormones and inevitably age. However, the use of somatotypes is a useful tool to measure change within an individual. It can give a reasonable impression of before and after an intervention, such as a Functional Training programme to redistribute and reduce adipose tissue to lessen the risk of injury. As mentioned there are three characteristic somatotypes:

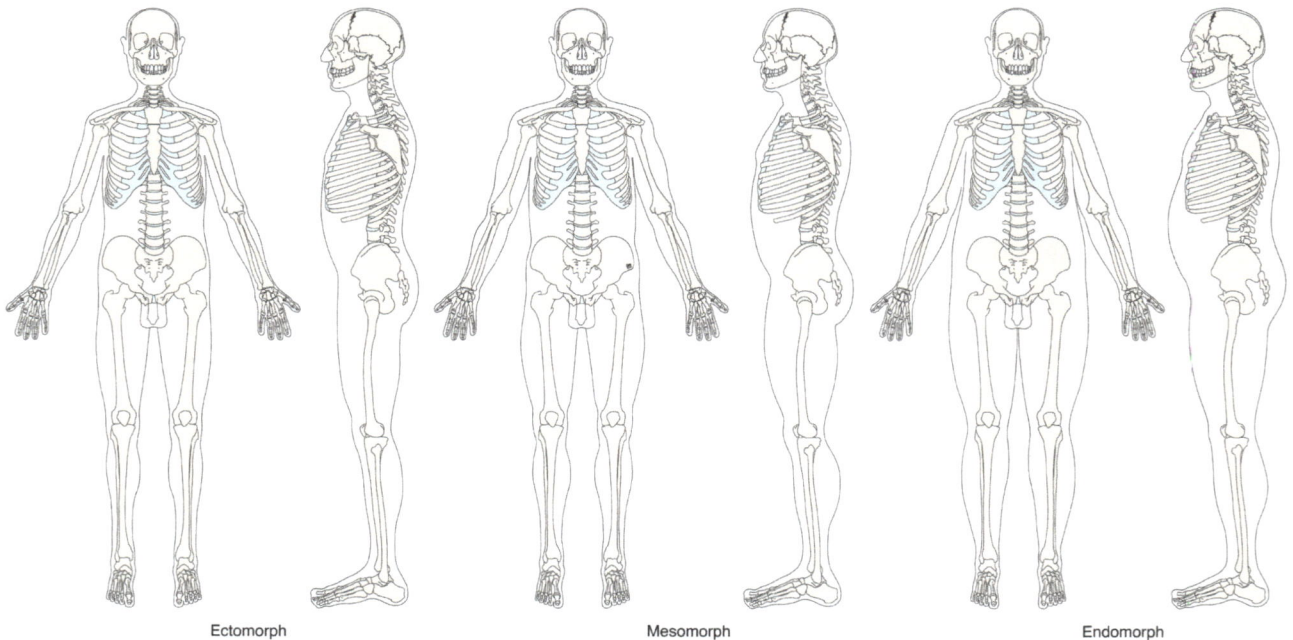

Ectomorph   Mesomorph   Endomorph

Figure 3: demonstrates the three different somatotypes; ectomorphs, mesomorphs, and endomorphs

Endomorphs

Usually have short arms and legs and a lot of mass around their frame. The mass often hinders their ability to perform well in sports that require a high level of speed and agility, and make endurance-based sports, such as running, difficult. Sports that

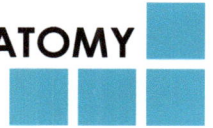

require strength and power, such as sumo wrestling and power lifting, are often best suited to endomorphs. They can gain weight and decondition quickly if training stops. In summary:

- Pear shaped body
- Rounded head
- Wide hips and shoulders
- Wider front to back rather than side to side
- Excess fat and mass around the body, upper arms and thighs

In sports, endomorphs are best suited to such sports as rugby as they can increase muscle mass more efficiently than an ectomorph. An endomorph will also have a large lung capacity, useful in sports like rowing – although training is often difficult as their muscle fibres are often Type IIb fast glycolytic fibres. This means their muscle contraction speed is fast and their strength high, however they fatigue quickly (Honeybourne *et al*, 2002).

Mesomorphs

In general will have a medium structure and height, they also have a tendency to gain muscle and strength easily. This, combined with their ability to sustain a low body fat and gain or lose weight quickly, makes them strong candidates to become top athletes. Mesomorphs often excel in speed, agility and strength. In summary:

- Wedged shaped body
- Cubical head
- Wide broad shoulders
- Arm and leg musculature
- Narrow hips
- Minimum amount of fat

Having a good response to cardiovascular and resistance training, makes the mesomorph the ideal somatotype to become an athlete. All muscle groups will adapt quickly to sporting requirements, as well as being able to gain or lose weight easily.

Ectomorphs

A long, thin and slender frame leaves the ectomorph susceptible to injuries in sports dominated by strength or power. Ectomorphs generally succeed at sports where endurance is important or sports such as gymnastics, due to their light frame. They can achieve low levels of body fat which can be detrimental to health, particularly women who participate in endurance sports can experience period cessation and iron deficiency. In summary:

- High forehead
- Receding chin
- Narrow shoulders and hips
- Narrow chest and abdomen
- Thin arms and legs
- Little muscle and fat

Ectomorphs have sporting benefits such as a previously mentioned light frame, which is suited to sports such as gymnastics. Efficient thermo regulation along with a smaller body surface area makes ectomorphs suitable for endurance activities.

Measuring Somatotypes

Using Sheldon's method, the interpretations can be placed onto a shield-like graph to demonstrate how varied body composition is (Figure 4).

Sheldon (1940) also developed the theory that a person's somatotype had a direct correlation to their temperament and personality (constitutional psychology). He claimed that endomorphs tended to be 'viscerotonic' (easy-going, sociable people who take pleasure in eating); mesomorphs tend to be 'somatotonic' (bold and competitive individuals who are risk-taking, adventure-seeking extroverts); and ectomorphs tend to be 'cerebrotonic' (solitary and hyperactive, with fast reaction times). In later chapters, schemas and learnt behaviours that mould an individual's personality are explored and discussed. However, to lightly touch upon it, Sheldon stated that a person's somatotype was not likely to change because these schemas and behaviours

Extreme Mesomorph
171

Weight Lifter ——————

—————— Gymnast

American Footballer ——————

—————— Sprinter

—————— Rugby League Player

Wrestler ——————

—————— Tennis Player

Sumo Wrestler ——————

Rubgy Union 2nd
Row Player

—————— High Jumper

711
Extreme Endomorph

117
Extreme Ectomorph

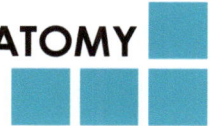

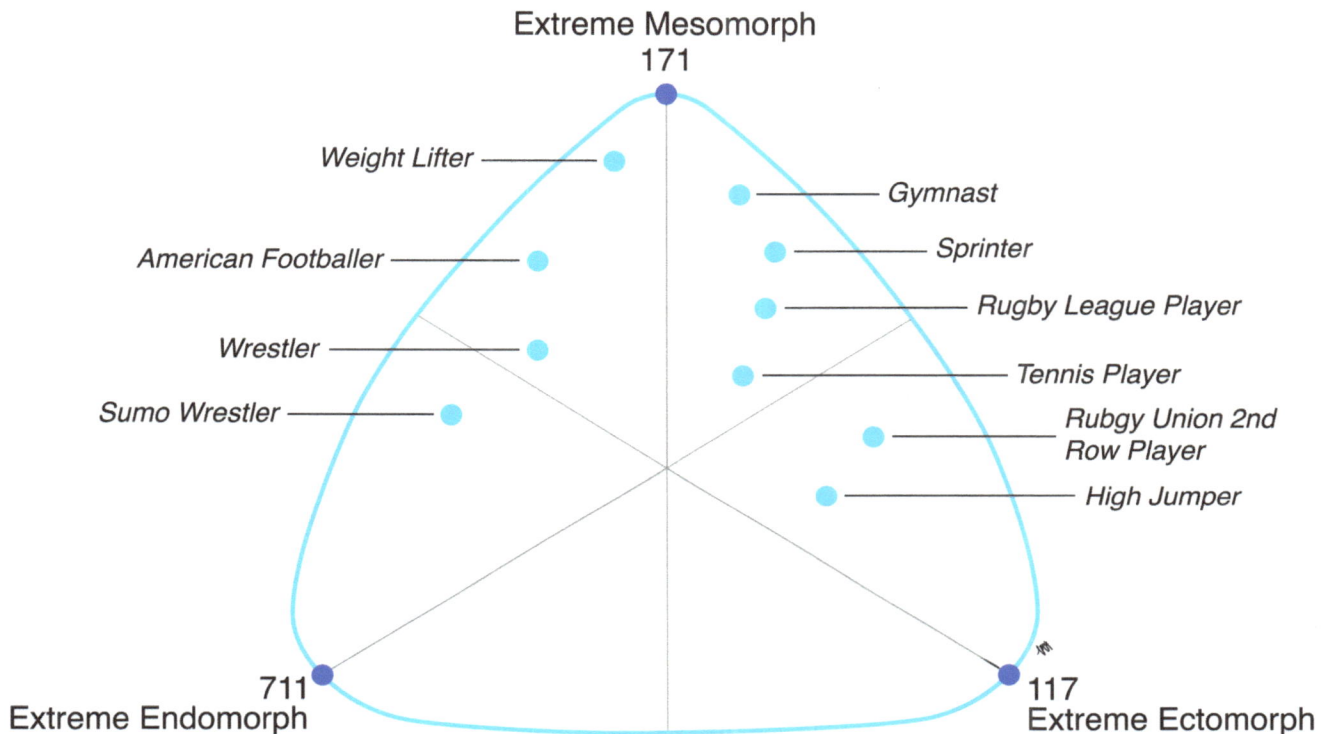

Figure 4: Sheldon's shield-like somatotype graph

were so ingrained within someone. This means that a person's somatotype, much like their personality, would remain constant throughout their life.

Sheldon's theory unfortunately is not generalisable. For example, a long-term smoker would be said to have an addictive personality (Lang, 1983), although if that person decided to stop smoking and succeeded, their 'addictive personality' may turn to exercise. If this happens, their personality, according to Sheldon's theory, will not have changed, but inevitably with the increased exercise, their body composition may have. Thus rendering Sheldon's theory unsuitable for this person.

Heath and Carter in 1967 took this a step further and suggested somatotypes can have a wide variation over time, whilst also encompassing Sheldon's characteristic descriptions and his suggested affiliation between personality traits. In doing this they developed the more commonly accepted Heath-Carter measurement system, which integrated the use of anthropometrical measurements as well as standardised photographs.

The system involves a more mathematical approach to somatotyping rather than just a visual adjudication of an individual's physique. It uses the chart in Table 1 to give a somatotype score that correlates to the already understood 1-7 values of each characteristic.

Measurement	Limit																	
Subtriceps / Subscapular / + Suprailiac / Total / - Calf / =	Upper Limit		10.9	14.9	18.9	22.9	26.9	31.2	35.8	40.7	46.2	52.2	58.7	65.7	73.2	81.2	89.7	98.9
	Lower Limit		7	11	15	19	23	27	31.3	35.9	40.8	46.3	52.3	58.8	65.8	73.3	81.3	89.8
Total Skin Folds																		
Endomorphic Component			0.5	1	1.5	2	2.5	3	3.5	4	4.5	5	5.5	6	6.5	7	7.5	8
Height (cm)		139.7	143.5	147.3	151.1	154.9	158.9	162.6	166.4	170.2	174.9	177.9	181.6	185.4	189.6	193.0	196.9	200.3
Humerus Bicondyle (cm)		5.19	5.34	5.49	5.64	5.78	5.93	6.07	6.22	6.37	6.51	6.65	6.80	6.95	7.09	7.24	7.38	7.53
Femur Bicondyle (cm)		7.41	7.62	7.83	8.04	8.24	8.45	8.66	8.87	9.08	9.28	9.49	9.70	9.91	10.12	10.33	10.53	10.74
Upper Arm Circumference (cm)		23.7	24.4	25.0	25.7	26.3	27.0	27.7	28.3	29.0	29.7	30.3	31.0	31.6	32.2	33.0	33.6	34.3
Max Calf Circumference (cm)		27.7	28.5	29.3	30.1	30.8	31.6	32.4	33.2	33.9	34.7	35.5	36.3	37.1	37.8	38.6	39.4	40.2
Mesomorphic Component			0.5	1.0	1.5	2.0	2.5	3.0	3.5	4.0	4.5	5.0	5.5	6.0	6.5	7.0		
Height (cm) = / Weight (kg) = / Height ÷ 3 √ Weight =	Upper Limit			39.65	40.74	41.43	42.13	42.82	43.48	44.18	44.84	45.53	46.23	46.92	47.58	48.25	48.94	49.63
	Lower Limit			less	39.66	40.75	41.44	42.14	42.83	43.49	44.19	44.85	45.54	46.24	46.93	47.59	48.26	48.95
Ectomorphic Component				0.5	1.0	1.5	2.0	2.5	3.0	3.5	4.0	4.5	5.0	5.5	6.0	6.5	7.0	7.5

Table 1: Heath-Carter somatotype measurement chart

Here is an example of how to work out a somatotype score:

Endomorphic Component

Multiply the skinfold measurement's from the Subtriceps, Subscapular and Suprailiac. Then deduct the Calf skinfolds from that total.

MUSCULAR & NERVOUS SYSTEM ANATOMY

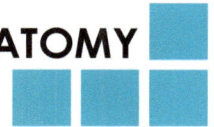

Subtriceps skinfold – with the client/patient's arm hanging loosely in the anatomical position, raise a skinfold at the back of the arm at halfway on a line connecting the acromion and the olecranon process and measure.

Subscapular skinfold – raise the subscapular skinfold on a line from the inferior angle of the scapula in a direction that is obliquely inferior and laterally at 45 degrees, and measure.

Suprailiac skinfold – Raise the fold 5-7cm above the anterior superior iliac spine (ASIS) on a line that is diagonally inferior and medially at 45 degrees, and measure.

Calf skinfold – Raise a vertical skinfold on the medial side of the leg, at the level of maximum girth, and measure.

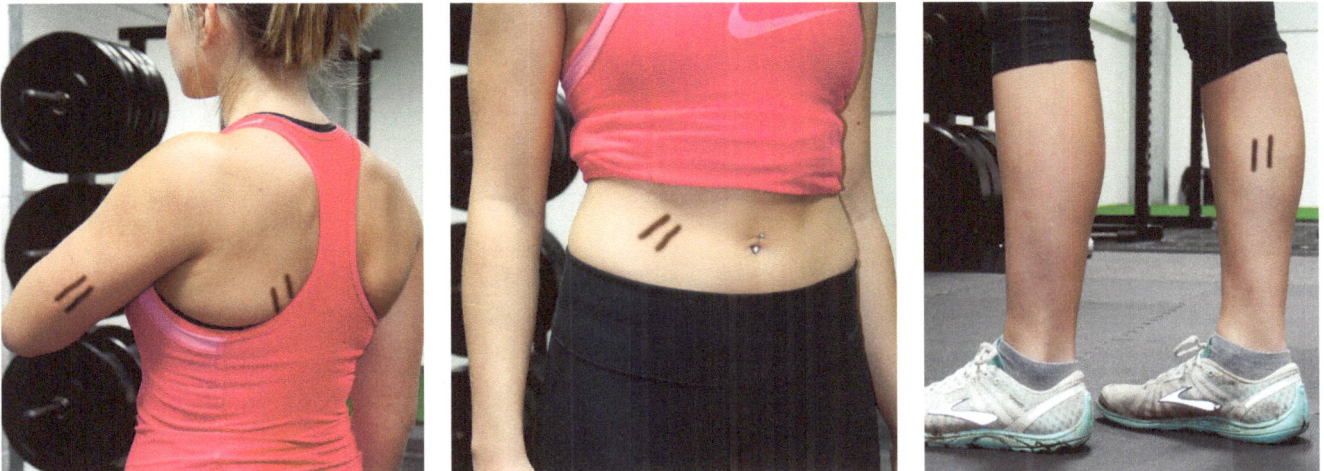

Markings for Subtriceps, Subscapular (left), Suprailiac (middle) & Calf (right) skinfold measurements

Subtriceps	6cm
Subscapular	4.5cm
Suprailiac	5cm
	15.5cm
Calf	- 0cm
Total	**15.5cm**

This score lies between 15 – 18.9cm on the chart, resulting in an Endomorphic Component value of **1.5**.

CHAPTER 1.

Mesomorphic Component

Typically the most complicated aspect, as it involves various sums. Firstly measure Height, Humerus Bicondyle, Femur Bicondyle, Upper Arm Circumference and Calf Circumference.

Humerus Bicondyle – is the width between the medial and lateral epicondyle of the humerus with the shoulder and elbow flexed 90 degrees.

Femur Bicondyle – is the greatest width between the medial and lateral epicondyles of the femur with the client/patient seated and their knee bent at a right angle.

Upper Arm Circumference – the client/patient flexes the shoulder to 90 degrees and the elbow to 45 degrees, clenches the hand and maximally contracts the arm. The measurement should be taken at the greatest girth of the arm.

Calf Circumference – the client/patient stands with feet slightly apart, and the measurement of maximum girth should be taken.

- Circle the values numerically closest to the client/patients results on the Heath-Carter chart (if however the measurement falls directly between the two values, circle the lower value. This is approached conservatively because the largest girths are recorded).

- From this point, the chart should only be viewed in terms of columns, rather than numerical values:

  » Column deviations to the right of the height column are +ve deviations. Deviations to the left are –ve deviations and values in the same column as the height value have deviations of zero or are ignored.

  » Calculate the sum of the ± deviations (D). Use the formula $(D \div 8) + 4.0$. Round the obtained value to the nearest 0.5 unit along the Mesomorphic Component scale.

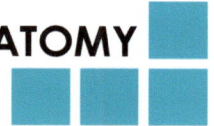

Continuing with the example:

Height   172cm
Humerus Bicondyle 6.5cm
Femur Bicondyle   9.1cm
Arm Circumference 30cm
Calf Circumference 36.8cm

After the column deviations the sum is:

(+1) + (+1) + (+3) = +5

Then, using the formula (D ÷ 8) + 4.0, the Mesomorphic value can be calculated:

(5 ÷ 8 = 0.625) + 4.0 = 4.625

Rounded to the nearest 0.5 makes the Mesomorphic Component **4.5**.

Ectomorphic Component

This value uses two mathematical equations. The first is to calculate the cube root of the client/patients weight, for example:

$\sqrt[3]{58.5kg}$ = **3.88**

The height (172cm) should then be divided by that number (3.88):

172 ÷ 3.88 = **44.32**

That number can then be transferred to the chart, where it lies between 44.19 – 44.84. Giving an Ectomorphic Component value of **4**.

The final somatotype value is scored as:
Endomorphic: 1.5
Mesomorphic: 4.5
Ectomorphic: 4

The values are rounded up, making the somatotype number for this example **254**. This value can be recorded along with standardised photographs to monitor and demonstrate change in an individual as time progresses.

Somatotypes can, and are used by health and fitness professionals to advise on nutrition, exercise and supplementation if they and the client/patients feel it is something that can be used to improve their health or function. This makes it a valuable consideration when trying to identify and highlight why certain lifestyle modifications are necessary to an individual.

1.4 Nervous System

The nervous system can be divided into parts depending on structure and function (Drake *et al*, 2005):

- Structurally, it comprises the central nervous system (CNS), which is made up of the brain and the spinal cord, and the peripheral nervous system (PNS). This is composed of all the nervous structures outside of the CNS.

- Functionally, it can be divided into somatic and visceral parts. The somatic part innervates the skin and most of the skeletal muscle, and is involved with responding to information from the external environment. Whereas the visceral part innervates the organs, smooth muscle and glands. It responds to information from the internal environment.

Dermatomes

Each spinal nerve (PNS) carries somatic sensory information from a very specific area of the skin on the surface of the body. A dermatome is that area of skin supplied by a single spinal cord level, or on one side, by a single spinal nerve. There is often an overlap in the distribution of dermatomes.

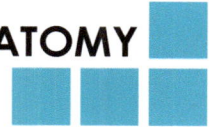

Myotomes

Each spinal nerve also carries somatic motor fibres that correlate to a single spinal cord level. A myotome is the portion of skeletal muscle innervated by the single spinal nerve (Drake *et al*, 2005).

Myotomes are often much more difficult to identify than dermatomes as skeletal muscles may have more than one spinal level of innervation.

Neuromuscular Control

Human movement is under the control of the electrical stimuli, conducted from the brain to the muscles via the nerves. Neural feedback is what creates this neuromuscular response. The feedback is supplied from various structures such as the muscles, joints, eyes and ears, before being interpreted by the brain.

One individual motor neurone branches off and can stimulate between 15 and 2000 muscle fibres – this necessitates fewer motor neurones. The motor neurone and its respective muscle fibres are known as a motor unit, and are subject to the 'all or none' law; once the motor unit is stimulated, all the connected muscle fibres will contract (Honeybourne *et al*, 2002).

Proprioception

The term proprioception has appeared in scientific literature since 1906. Sherrington first proposed its existence as a 'secret' sense, along with the partnering terms interoceptors (sensations from organs and pain) and exteroceptors (sight, hearing, smell, taste and touch). Current literature still fails to agree on an accepted definition. Sherrington's suggestions and more recent proposals from Day (1969) and Mergener *et al* (1993) support the theory that proprioception is an interaction between kinesthesis and vestibular afferents.

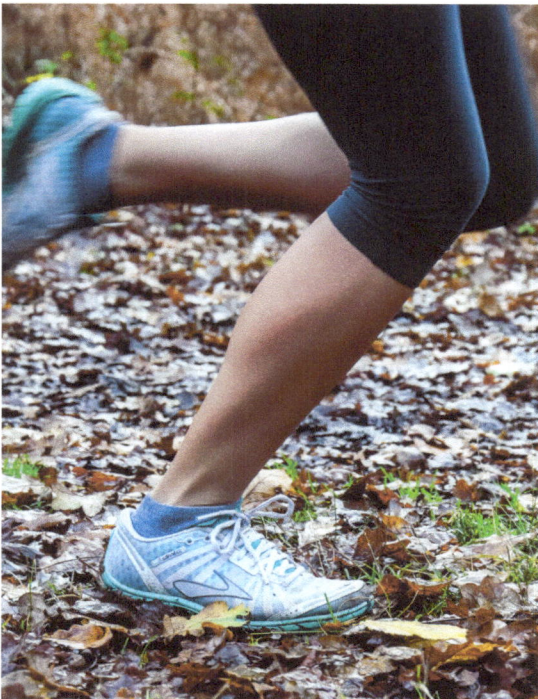

The muscles and joints respond to uneven ground through proprioception when running

18

CHAPTER 1.

Proprioception consists of two key components:

- **Kinesthesia** – is the awareness of the position and movements of body parts using the sensory receptors in joints and muscles. Often kinesthesia and proprioception are used interchangeably, although they have very different implications (Konradsen, 2002). For example, an inner ear infection will disturb the sense of balance required for proprioception, although it will not affect the kinesthetic sense.
- **Joint Position Sense** – is the ability to recognise and respond to an externally passive movement, understanding the position of a joint without visually being aware of it. An example of this is the response of the ankle joint to cross country running – the ankle adapts to the terrain to support itself depending on its joint position.

Although it appears as though there are only two key components of proprioception, without visual or vestibular input the ability to recognise equilibrium or surroundings would be detrimental to the contraction of muscles and consequently stabilisation of the joints. For example, for a trampolinist on a descent, without the sense of rotation and acceleration from the vestibular system, or visual input from the environment, certain muscles and joints required for a soft impact would not be stabilised.

The vestibular system acts in response to rotational and linear acceleration by sand-like crystals (known as otolith crystals) moving around the semi-circular canals of the inner ear and displacing tiny hair cells. Then the information is sent to the brain (Lindsay & Bone, 1998).

The body will use visual sensory information to perceive the movements of objects in the environment, in conjunction with the vestibular system, joint position sense and kinesthesia to modify its movements adequately. Boucher (2013) suggests peripheral vision plays a key role in space perception, locomotion, postural control and kinesthesia. Individuals with impaired peripheral vision will ultimately be prone to losing balance while standing and walking.

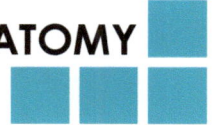

Considering the various mechanisms that enable proprioception (kinesthesia, joint position sense, vestibular and visual systems), suggests proprioception is less of a 'secret sense' as suggested by Sherrington, and more of an integration of senses. This integration enables us to observe our environment and skilfully manoeuvre through it. Expanding on this further, we define proprioception as:

> *"The ability to sense the position, location, orientation and movement of the body and its parts in relation to space."*

Although it is now understood that proprioception is an integration of senses, there is also a consensus that one aspect contributes to proprioception more than any other; cutaneous receptor feedback – more specifically, feedback from the muscle spindles (Kandel *et al*, 2000; Smetacek & Mechsner, 2004).

Cutaneous Receptors

These receptors are known as sensory receptors and relay information regarding pain, temperature, vibration, touch and pressure. They are technically located in the dermis or epidermis of the skin, although there are two sensory receptors that are located along the muscles and tendons – these are known as proprioceptive sensory receptors (or mechanoreceptors), which provide information on muscle length and tension (Table 2).

The variations in proprioceptive sensory receptors include:

*   **Muscle Spindles** – These are located in the belly of the muscle and relay information about the length of the muscle, which is then processed by the brain to interpret the position of certain body parts. The muscle spindles are orientated parallel to the extrafusal muscle fibres and have both sensory and motor functions. They have a vital role in the stretch reflex, by responding to the sudden change in length and velocity.

*   **Golgi Tendon Organs** – They sense the change in muscle tension. Located within the tendons of musculature at both the origin and insertion. Unlike the muscle spindles, the golgi

tendon organs are arranged in series rather than parallel to the muscle fibres.

Following an investigation by Collins *et al* (2005), it is now understood that inputs from cutaneous and proprioceptive receptors combined are likely to contribute to kinesthesia at the joints of the body.

With regards to training and an individual's function, Lephart *et*

Sensation	Cutaneous Receptors
Pain	**Free Nerve Endings** – They respond to multiple modalities (polymodality) that can cause pain such as temperature, stretch, pressure and touch.
Pressure	**Pacinian Corpuscles** – They may be used in the detection of surfaces (rough and smooth) through vibration as well as gross changes in pressure. They are rapidly adapting receptors, which decrease any overload in information from excessive pressure on the skin, such as clothes. **Ruffini Corpuscles** – Slowly adapting receptors that respond to sustained pressure. They demonstrate very little adaptation qualities. They are sensitive to skin stretching and joint deformity, as well as displaying thermoreceptor properties towards warmth. **Merkel Cells** – Another slowly adapting receptor, although possibly the most sensitive of the pressure receptors. They relay information mostly on texture based on two-point discrimination from pressure on the skin.
Temperature	**Krause Corpuscles** – Known as thermoreceptors, they detect cold temperatures. They are mostly found in the lips, tongue, penis, clitoris and certain synovial joints such as the metacarpophalangeal joints. **Ruffini Corpuscles** – Detects warmth
Touch	**Meissner's Corpuscles** – Rapidly adapting receptor, highly sensitive to light touch. They are very superficial and found predominantly in the lips and fingers. They do not detect pain or deep pressure, which is achieved by the Free Nerve Endings and Pacinian Corpuscles, respectively. **Pacinian Corpuscles** **Hair Follicle Receptors** – Respond to the positioning of the hair mostly affected by the wind or clothes.
Vibration	**Meissner's Corpuscles** **Pacinian Corpuscles**

Table 2: description of various cutaneous receptors and their associated sensation

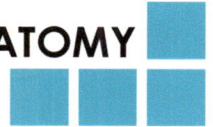

al (1997) suggest that neuromuscular feedback is impaired with injury or abnormality, and that to ensure restoration of this any rehabilitation should include a proprioceptive component. They propose that it focuses on spinal reflexes, brainstem activity and cognitive programming. To achieve this, exercises such as single arm cable work or dumbbell work, or wobble board exercises can aid the progression and recovery of proprioception with shoulder and ankle injuries, respectfully.

1.5 Spinal Anatomy & Joints

The bones of the spine are known as the vertebrae (Figure 5), which are separated into specific regions identified as the Cervical, Thoracic, Lumbar, Sacrum and Coccyx. These collectively are known more commonly as the spinal column, and together, along with the skull, scapulae, ribs and bones of the pelvis provide the framework of the back and sites for various muscle attachments (Drake *et al*, 2005).

The approximate 33 vertebrae of the spine individually have various jobs depending upon location and anatomical orientation:

Key Point: It can never be factually stated that the spine consists of 33 vertebrae, as there are cases where an individual has 6 Lumbar vertebrae or even 8 Cervical vertebrae. This may be completely asymptomatic and just a finding upon x-ray.

The *Cervical* region is made up of seven vertebrae, although it consists of 8 sets of nerves. The vertebrae are relatively small in size in comparison to the rest of the spine and they also have a small hole known as a foramen that travels inferiorly through each of the transverse processes, which houses the artery supplying blood to the head and brain (Drake *et al*, 2005). There are also other defining characteristics such as:

* A short and bifid spinous process, which is often not easily palpable in the majority of the cervical spine due to the lordotic curve of the cervical spine.
* The first and second cervical vertebrae, known as the Atlas and Axis, are unique to the cervical spine as they accommodate the movement of the head, approximately 60% of cervical rotation occurs between C0-C2 (Pettman, 2006).
* The joints of the cervical spine are typically sloped from anterior to posterior, which aids the flexion and extension movement available at the neck.

The *Thoracic* spine consists of twelve vertebrae with distinctive articulating surfaces for the ribs. The vertebrae are larger in size than the cervical vertebrae, and also have a circular vertebral foramen to accommodate the narrowing of the spinal cord through the thoracic region (Drake *et al*, 2005). Other characteristics include:

- A long, elongated and inferiorly placed spinous process that should be easily palpable due to the thoracic kyphotic curve.
- The facet joints of the thoracic spine are orientated vertically in order to limit the amount of flexion and extension, but also to enable rotational movement.

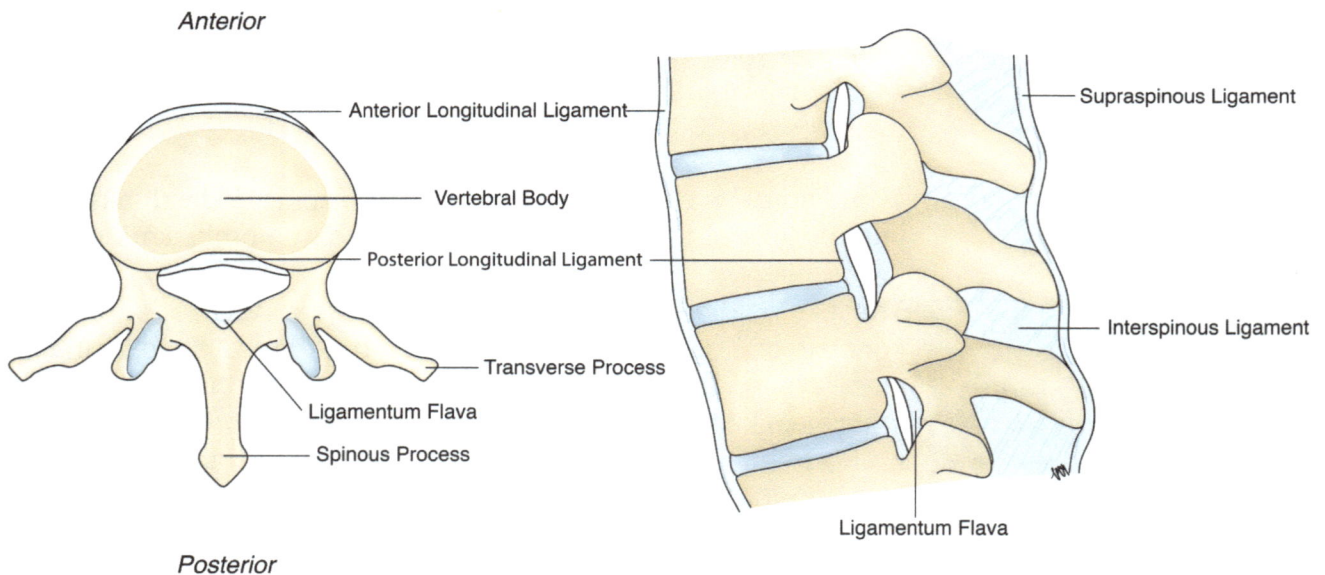

Figure 5: Spinal unit anatomy

There are five *Lumbar* vertebrae, which are recognisably larger in size compared to the other regions of the spine. As they do not articulate with the ribs, they have long and thin transverse processes, as well as a larger vertebral foramen than the thoracic region to accommodate the Cauda Equina. Other lumbar characteristics include:

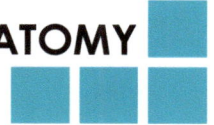

- The spinous processes of the lumbar spine are thick and shorter than the thoracic spine, and similarly to the thoracic spine should be palpable.
- The joints of the lumbar spine are curved and interlock to limit excess movement that may place an increased load upon the intervertebral disc.

The *Sacrum* consists of five single vertebrae that are fused to form one single bone. It has two articulating surfaces on the posterior surface that articulate with the last lumbar vertebrae, and then two larger laterally placed articulating surfaces that create a joint between the sacrum and the pelvic bones.

The *Coccyx*, the final part of the spine is usually made up of three to four fused bones that make a small triangular shaped bone that articulates to the base of the sacrum.

Zygapophysial (Facet) Joints

There are two types of joints between the vertebrae (Drake *et al*, 2005):

- Symphysis joints occur between the vertebral bodies (intervertebral discs)
- Synovial joints are found between the articular surfaces of the vertebrae.

An individual vertebra will commonly have a total of six joints with the adjacent vertebrae (four synovial and two symphyses). However the thoracic vertebrae have between eight and ten, as they have additional articulating surfaces for the attachment of the ribs.

The main type of joint found within the spine is the zygapophysial joint, or facet joint, which is a type of synovial joint. It has all the characteristics of a typical synovial joint:

- A thin layer of hyaline cartilage that covers the articulating surface of the bone.
- A synovial membrane then encloses the articular cavity. The

membrane itself receives a good vascular supply in order to produce synovial fluid, which maintains the joints lubricated ability to move. It also is a semi-permeable membrane, which means that it can prevent the passage of some substances but allow the passage of others.

- A final fibrous layer is found superficially to the synovial membrane that surrounds the synovial capsule to add stability and support to the joint.

The facet joints of the spine are unique as they allow different regions of the spine to undergo more than one direction of movement at one time, for example in the Cervical and upper Thoracic spine, lateral flexion occurs with axial rotation in the same direction. This combined movement is called *Coupled Motion*. The spine is able to produce gross ranges of motion because of this attribute. The limitations and restraints placed on the individual joints by the orientation of the facet joints along with the structures such as the vertebral discs and ligaments of the spine mean that a single segment alone cannot achieve a wide range of motion (Banton, 2012).

In the Lumbar spine, the motion of lateral flexion is coupled with axial rotation in the opposite direction. However, movement of the middle and lower thoracic appears inconsistent and apparently dependent upon which movement is initiated first (Banton, 2012).

Intra-articular Pressure

The pressure within the enclosed synovial capsule is known as the intra-articular pressure. This pressure is usually below atmospheric pressure and around -4mmHg in a resting human knee joint, and it decreases further with the contraction of the Quadriceps. The slightly negative pressure aids the stability of the joint by holding it together by adding resistance to distraction of the joint.

Exercise or an excess in a certain or particular movement will cause an increase in the intra-articular pressure (Gaffney *et al*, 1995). This increase in intra-articular pressure will often result in

> **Key Point**: Coupled motion is an important consideration in the rehabilitation of diseases such as scoliosis.

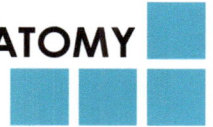

the joint becoming restricted, which may even cause pain. Once the intra-articular pressure has lost equilibrium and the joint has become restricted, the stability of the joint can be challenged with the application of traction. This traction will often result in a cavitation of the joint, causing a cracking sensation, which is the release of built-up gas in the synovial capsule (Matsen *et al*, 2009).

1.6 Muscle Anatomy

For the purposes of understanding Functional Rehabilitation, only certain muscles have been selected and described in this chapter. Inevitably, every muscle supporting and responsible for movement of the skeleton is essential to function. However the muscles that have been selected pose some direct functional relevance and are often the most commonly imbalanced or impaired during function for various reasons.

This section can be used in conjunction with a good quality gross anatomy textbook, for reference to other muscles that may not be discussed. Each of the muscles included in this chapter will include descriptions of its origin, insertion, action, nerve root supply and commonly seen dysfunctions associated to that muscle.

The ***origin*** is a bony point to which the muscle attaches. It is usually proximal, and it is the most stable of surfaces that the muscle attaches to (Honeybourne *et al*, 2002). An example of this is the Biceps Brachii, which originates from the scapula – the most proximal and stable of the two attachment points of the Biceps Brachii.

The ***insertion*** of a muscle is usually the structure that is to be moved, it will often be a distal bony landmark that has greater motion during contraction. Using the Biceps Brachii an the example once again, the insertion point is the radius – distal in comparison to the radius and more mobile.

Splenius Capitus

Origin: Spinous Processes of C3-T4 and Nuchal Ligament

Insertion: Mastoid Process of Temporal Bone and Occiput

Action: Ipsilateral Rotation and Lateral Flexion of the Head and Neck, as well as Extension of the Head

Nerve Supply: C2-C6

Problems: The *Splenius Capitus* (Figure 6) muscle is a broad muscle and is an important muscle in relation to stabilisation of the head. The average head weighs between 4.5 and 5kg, which then balances on the neck, a considerably narrower structure in comparison. This means that the muscles of the neck have to be remarkably strong in order to maintain control of the head.

The Splenius Capitus muscle, due to its close relationship with the cervical spine, can often have a significant role in cervicogenic headaches – a headache associated with dysfunction of the cervical spine and cervical musculature.

In today's society of increasing sedentary postures, the muscle is being contracted for longer periods of time due to the rise in *Upper Crossed Postures* (see Chapter 3.2). This overuse can result in the muscle becoming tighter and placing a greater strain on the attachment points, causing an anterior head carriage, as well as the muscle referring pain across the posterior and superior aspects of the head due to the development of trigger points.

It can prove rather difficult to effectively train the Splenius Capitus. The most effective and beneficial way of reducing strain to the muscle is to teach the client/patient how to utilise and correct their posture.

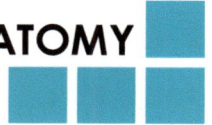

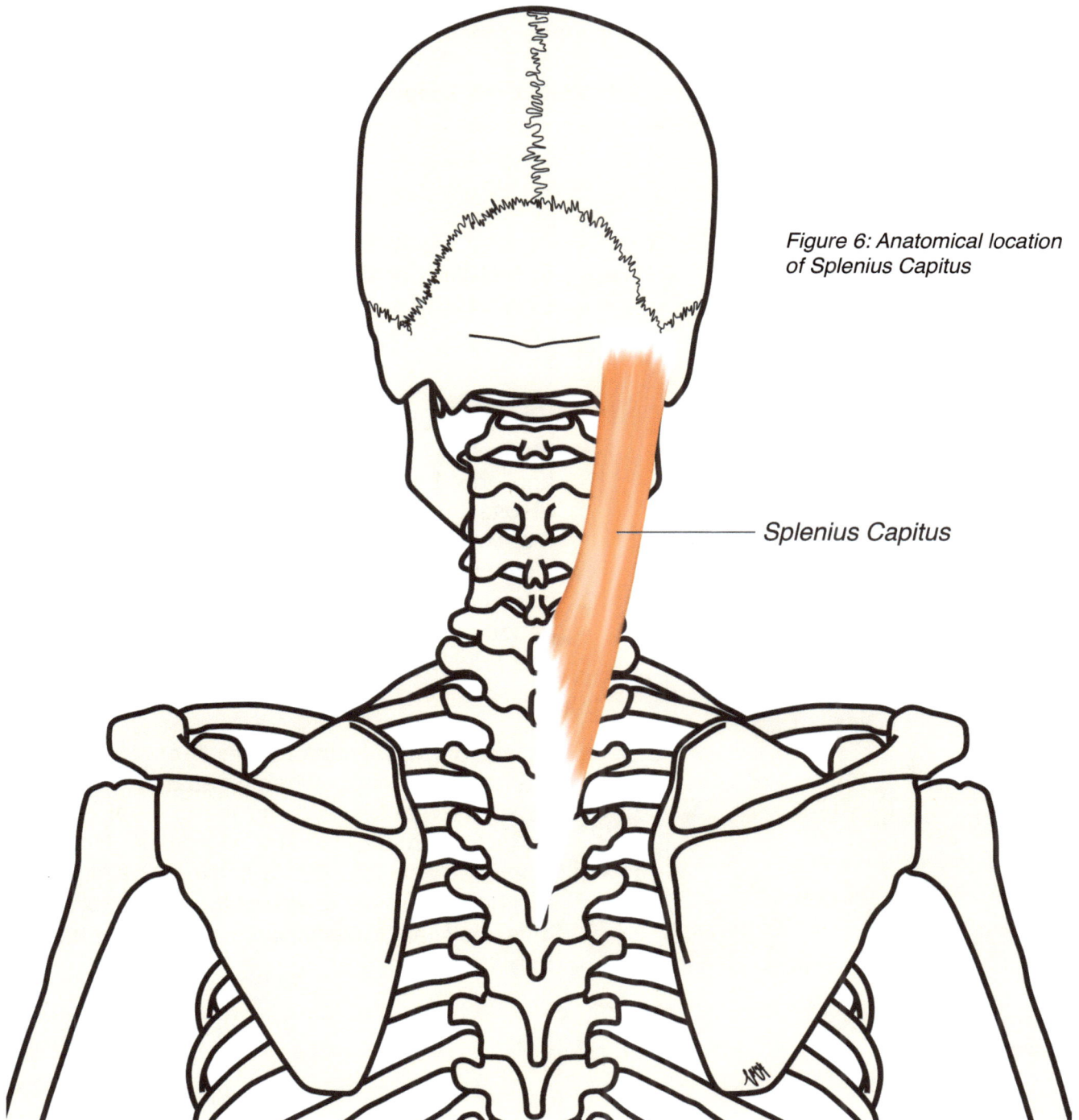

Figure 6: Anatomical location of Splenius Capitus

Splenius Capitus

Levator Scapulae

Origin: Transverse Processes of C1-C4

Insertion: Superior-medial angle of the Scapula

Action: Elevation of the Scapula and Extension & Lateral Flexion of Neck

Nerve Supply: C3-C5

Problems: Due to its orientation, the *Levator Scapulae* (Figure 7) has very similar implications to the Splenius Capitus. It is a slightly longer and stronger muscle, and is primarily involved with shrugging the shoulders up towards the ears.

It is very much a muscle associated with posture, particularly seating posture (see Chapter 3.1) and the body's affinity to slouch. Slouching results in many biomechanical stresses, none more so than an exaggerated *Upper Crossed Posture* (see Chapter 3.2), causing an increased demand on the Levator Scapulae, as well as various other muscles. As it becomes tight, pain can refer up into the base of the skull or across the shoulder, due to its anatomical orientation.

Education and reinforcement of the correct posture, especially when seated, is the most beneficial tool for reducing the amount of strain placed upon the Levator Scapulae. However, *Shoulder Shrugs* offer a form of training that can help improve the strength and control of this muscle. It can prove difficult to isolate this muscle from the Trapezius.

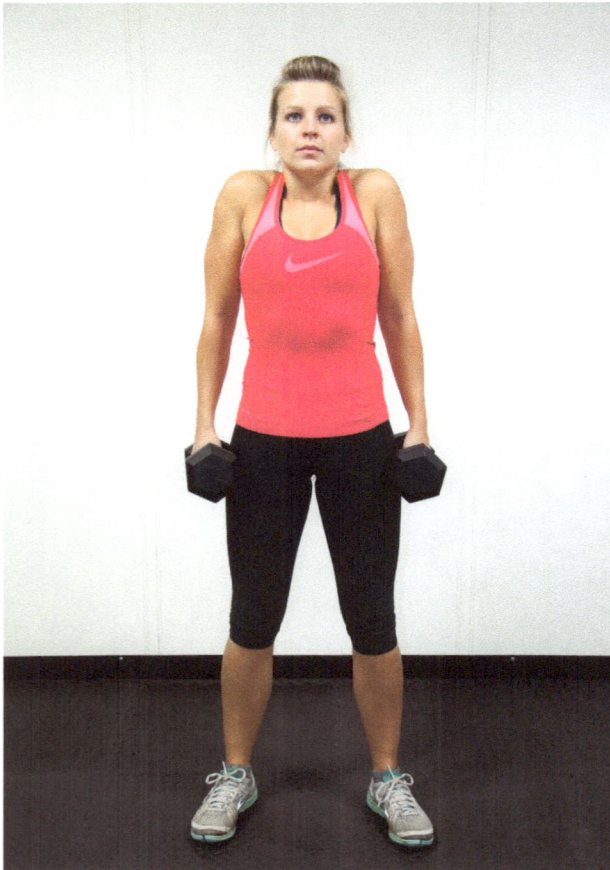

Shoulder Shrugs are an effective exercise to train the Levator Scapulae

Levator Scapulae

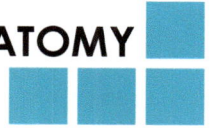

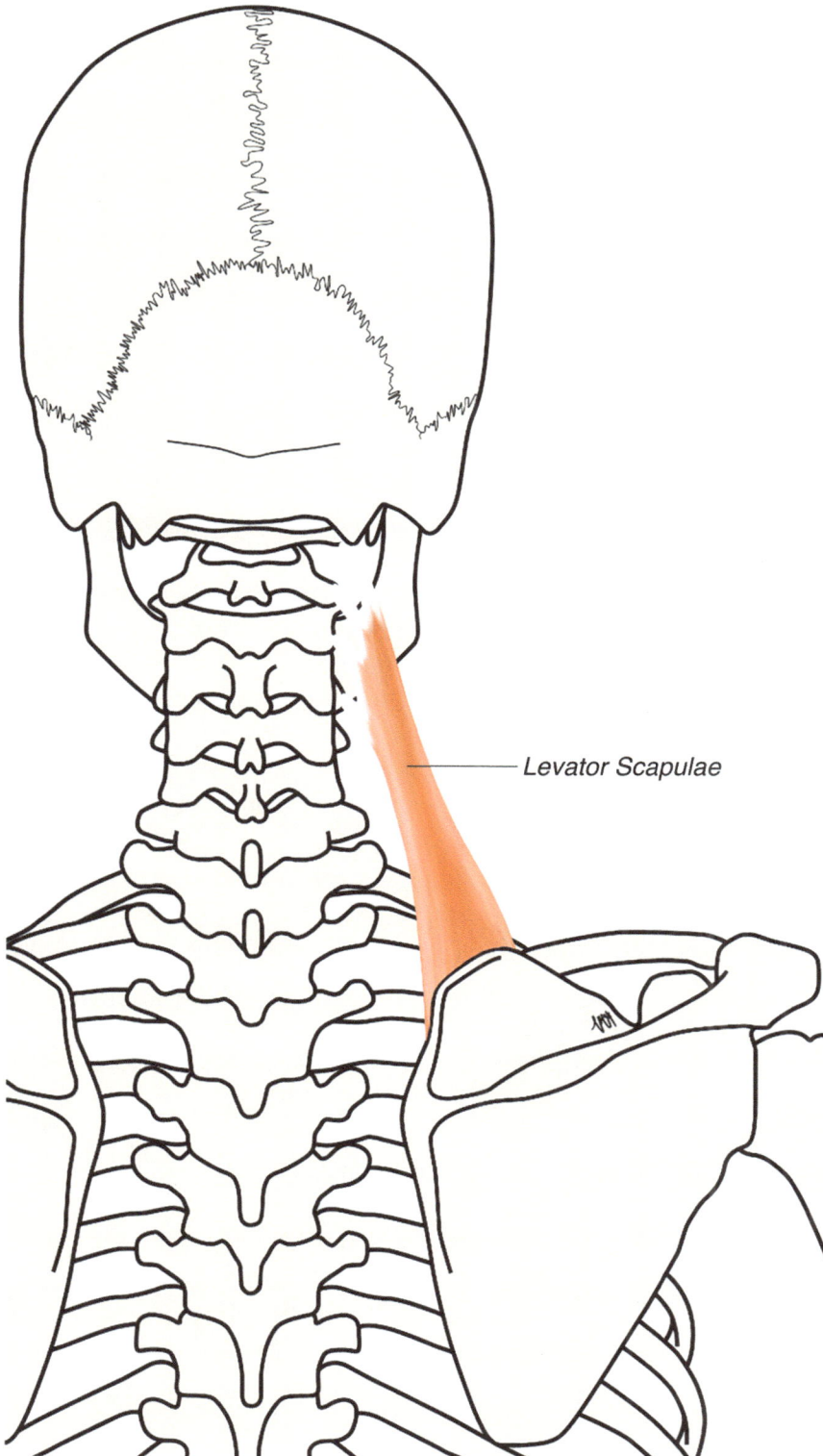

Figure 7: Anatomical location of
Levator Scapulae

Trapezius

Origin: EOP, Medial Side of the Superior Nuchal Line, Spinous Processes C7-T12

Insertion: Lateral 1/3 of Clavicle, Acromion, and Spine of Scapula

Action: Elevation & Retraction of the Scapula, Lateral Flexion and Extension of the Head

Nerve Supply: CN XI and C2-C4

Problems: Understandably problems are plentiful with this muscle. As the main shoulder stabilizer, the *Trapezius* (Figure 8) is often very tight and commonly refers pain down the arm and into the neck and head. It is also commonly linked to stress, tension and anxiety, which may be more of a circumstantial primitive reaction rather than a biomechanical strain.

As this muscle spans such a vast area, and crosses many spinal joints it will often create or react to spinal dysfunctions at the cervical and thoracic regions, and especially at the cervico-thoracic junction. It may also become hypotonic (reduced muscle tone), particularly in the *Lower Trapezius* – this is often as a result of an *Upper Crossed Posture* (see Chapter 3.2), which protracts the scapula and causes the internal rotation of the glenohumeral joint, rendering the Lower Trapezius inactive.

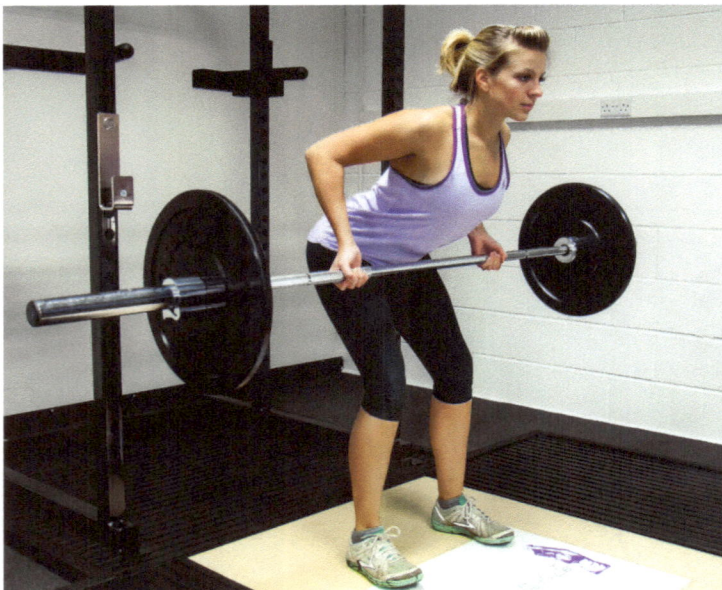

Barbell Bent-over Row is an effective exercise for the Trapezius

Fortunately there are many ways to activate and train the Trapezius muscle, with adequate modifications for isolating the Upper, Middle and Lower Trapezius, including exercises such as a *High Row, Bent-over Row and Incline Row* respectively.

Trapezius

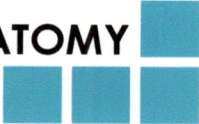

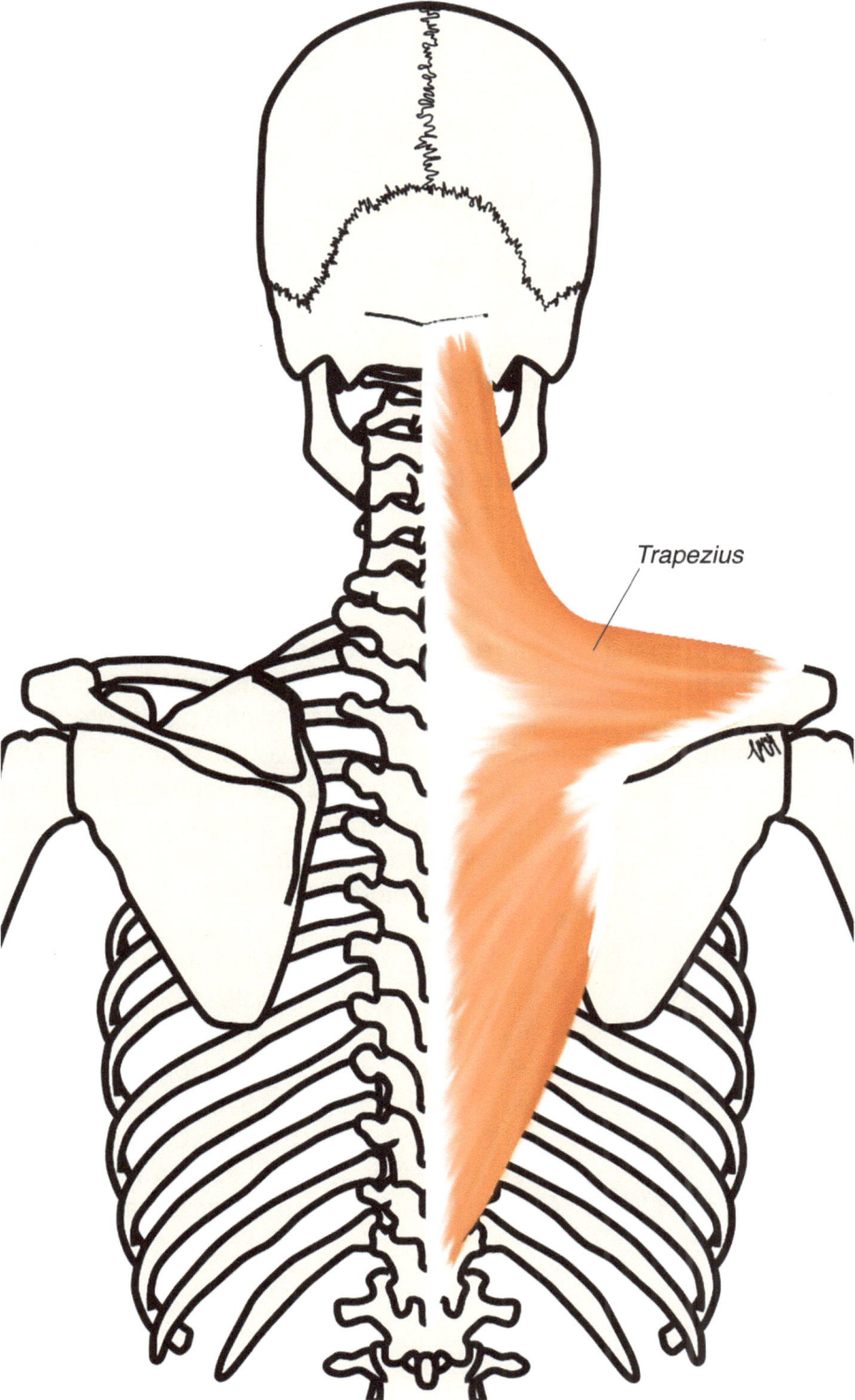

Figure 8: Anatomical location of the Trapezius

Rhomboids

Origin: Spinous Processes of C7-T1 and T2-T5

Insertion: Medial Border of the Scapula

Action: Retraction of the Scapula

Nerve Supply: C4-C5

Problems: The increasing prevalence of sedentary postures is having a dramatic effect on the strength and tone of the *Rhomboid* (Figure 9). This is due in large part to the tightness created at the pectoral muscles. The consequent 'rounding' of the glenohumeral joints, causes the scapulae to become protracted, which holds the rhomboids in a constant stretched state. Once a muscle is stretched, it requires a greater force to contract the muscle due to the cross-bridges between muscle fibres being further apart.

This over-dominant posture often causes a secondary problem at the Rhomboids, in the form of excessive contraction and the development of trigger points. Trigger points can often refer pain up towards the shoulder and laterally out towards the ribs. The mal-positioned shoulder blade may also result in other secondary conditions, such as impingement syndrome or faulty shoulder biomechanics.

Fortunately the Rhomboids are a relatively easy muscle to isolate with regards to training. Exercises such as *Reverse Flyes, Seated Row and Single Arm Rows* are effective at working the Rhomboids, but can also be modified to isolate left from right in order to train a specific side for muscular imbalance.

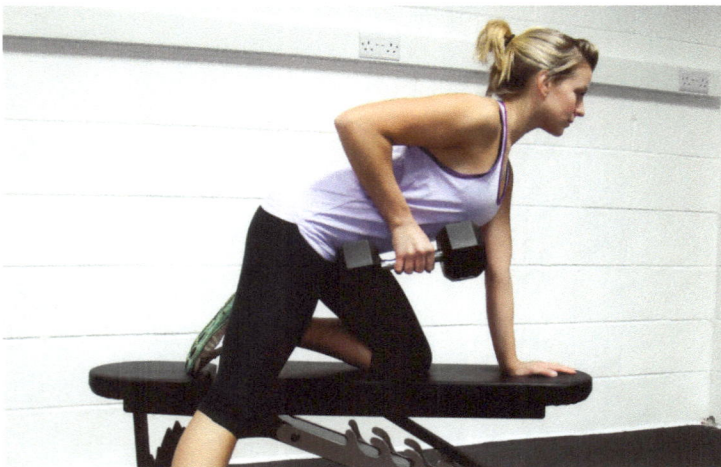

Dumbbell Single-Arm Row is an effective exercise for the Rhomboids

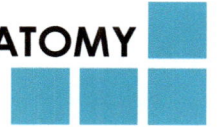

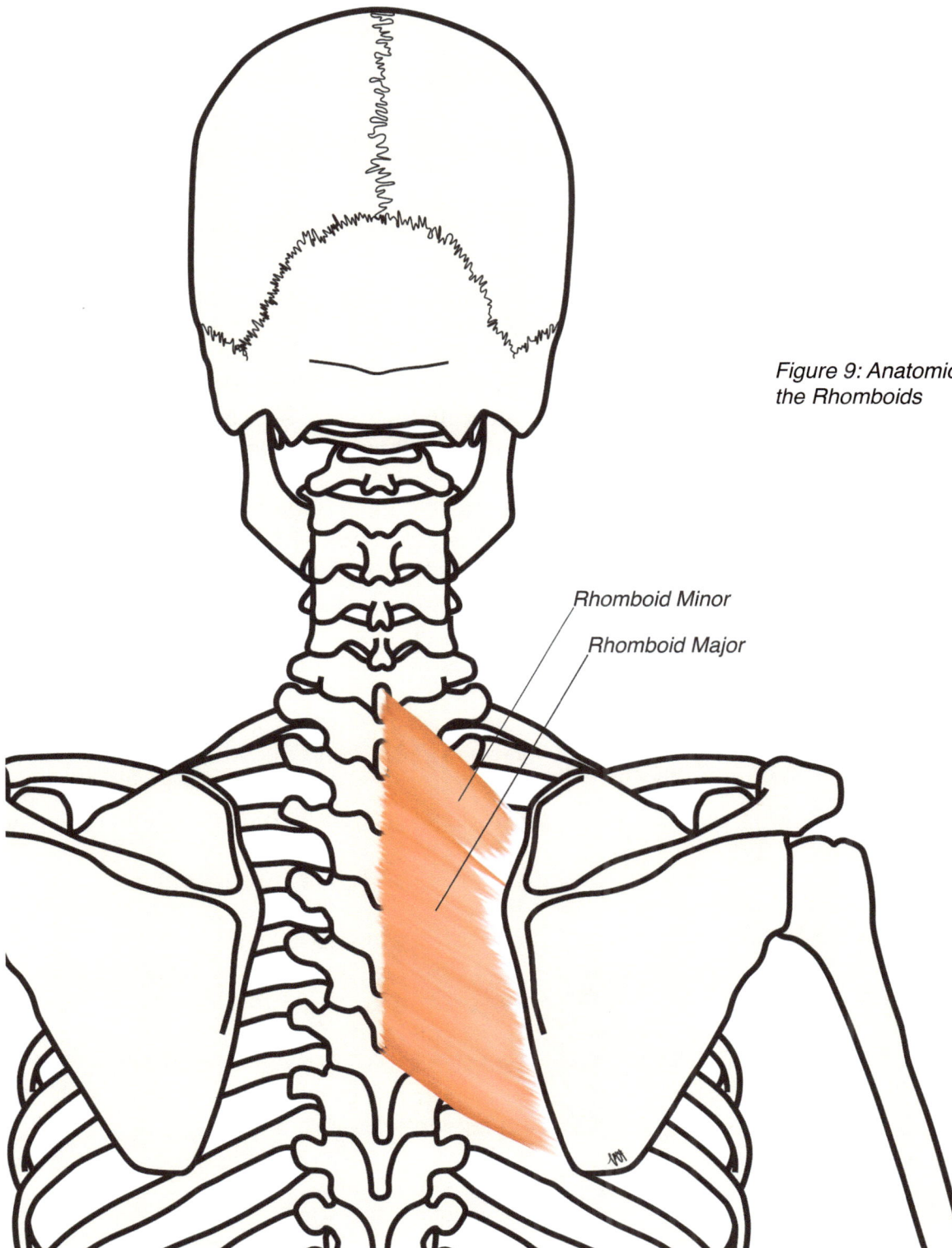

Figure 9: Anatomical location of the Rhomboids

Rhomboid Minor

Rhomboid Major

Supraspinatus

Origin: Supraspinous Fossa

Insertion: Greater Tubercle of Humerus

Action: Abduction of Shoulder

Nerve Supply: C5-C6

Problems: Not unlike the other muscles in the upper quarter, the *Supraspinatus* (Figure 10) is quite often a victim of posture-related injuries. Its orientation, particularly with the shoulder blade means that it is very susceptible to even very small biomechanical changes in the shoulder.

The muscle itself originates from the superior fossa of the shoulder blade, and then passes underneath the joint created between the clavicle and acromian (AC joint) before attaching to the humerus. The space in which the tendon passes under the AC joint can become significantly narrow as the scapula protracts, causing compression and an increase in fiction on the tendon as it contracts and relaxes. The added friction may cause micro tears or trauma to the tendon, resulting in the development of injuries to the tendon (tendinitis, tendinosis, tendinopathy).

The Supraspinatus is difficult to isolate from the Trapezius and Deltoid muscle due to their combined action to create abduction of the shoulder. An effective exercise is to use a slightly modified *Front Lateral Raise* – raising the arm in the plane of the scapula with the shoulder internally rotated.

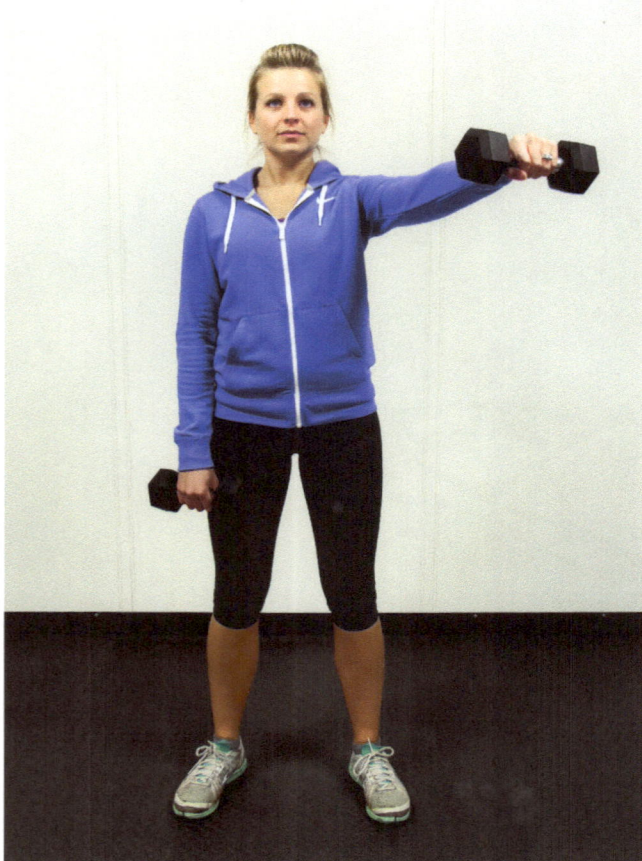

Dumbbell Lateral Raise in the neutral plane of the scapula is an effective exercise for the Supraspinatus

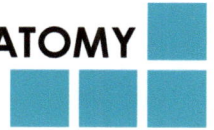

Figure 10: Anatomical location
of the Supraspinatus

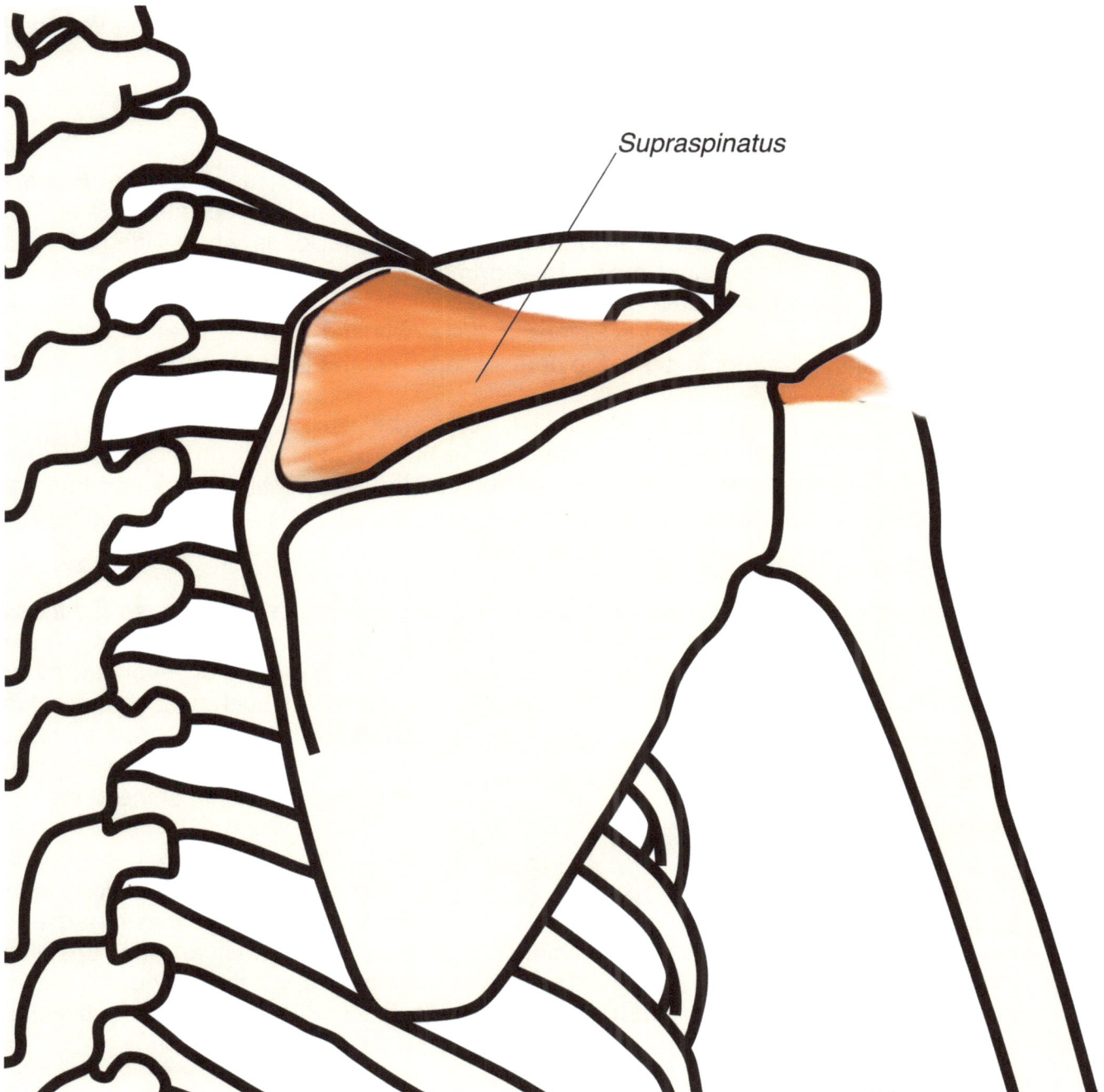

Supraspinatus

Erector Spinae

Origin: Iliac Crest, Posterior Sacrum and Lumbar Spines

Insertion: Rib Angles, Cervical TVP's and Mastoid Process

Action: Stabilisation of the Trunk and Extension of the Vertebral Column and Head

Nerve Supply: Dorsal Rami of Spinal Nerves

Problems: The group of muscles that make up the *Erectus Spinae* (Figure 11) can easily become injured due to repetitive extension movements or excessive loads whilst lifting. This is because the muscles primary purpose is to stabilise the spine and maintain posture. Unlike the Quadriceps or Biceps for example, the Erectus Spinae is not a 'working' muscle, meaning that it is not designed to perform large contractions to induce movement.

The Erectus Spinae group can be placed in the category of a trunk muscle, which means it will have a close working relationship with other trunk muscles such as the Rectus Abdominis and Internal and External Obliques. This identifies its role in supporting the spine during movement.

Activities such as rowing and lifting can often cause tightness within sections of the group, which may cause pain. If the Erectus Spinae is overworked, other local muscles such as the Quadratus Lumborum will activate to compensate and support the demand placed on performing extension of the spine.

The key to preventing the Erectus Spinae group from overworking is to maintain good form with regards to lifting and to maintain a neutral, strong posture with repetitive activities. The group can be successfully trained by using a gym ball to perform a *Dorsal Raise*, which will help develop its strength.

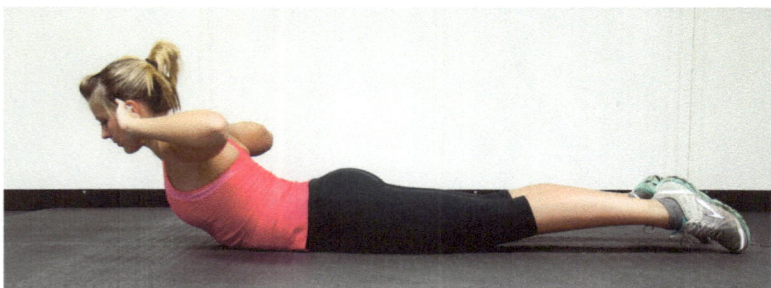

Dorsal Raises are an effective exercise to train the Erector Spinae muscles

Longissimus Capitus

Spinalis Cervicis

Spinalis Capitis

Iliocostalis Cervicis

Longissimus Cervicis

Iliocostalis Thoracis

Spinalis Thoracis

Longissimus Thoracis

Iliocostalis Lumborum

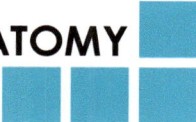

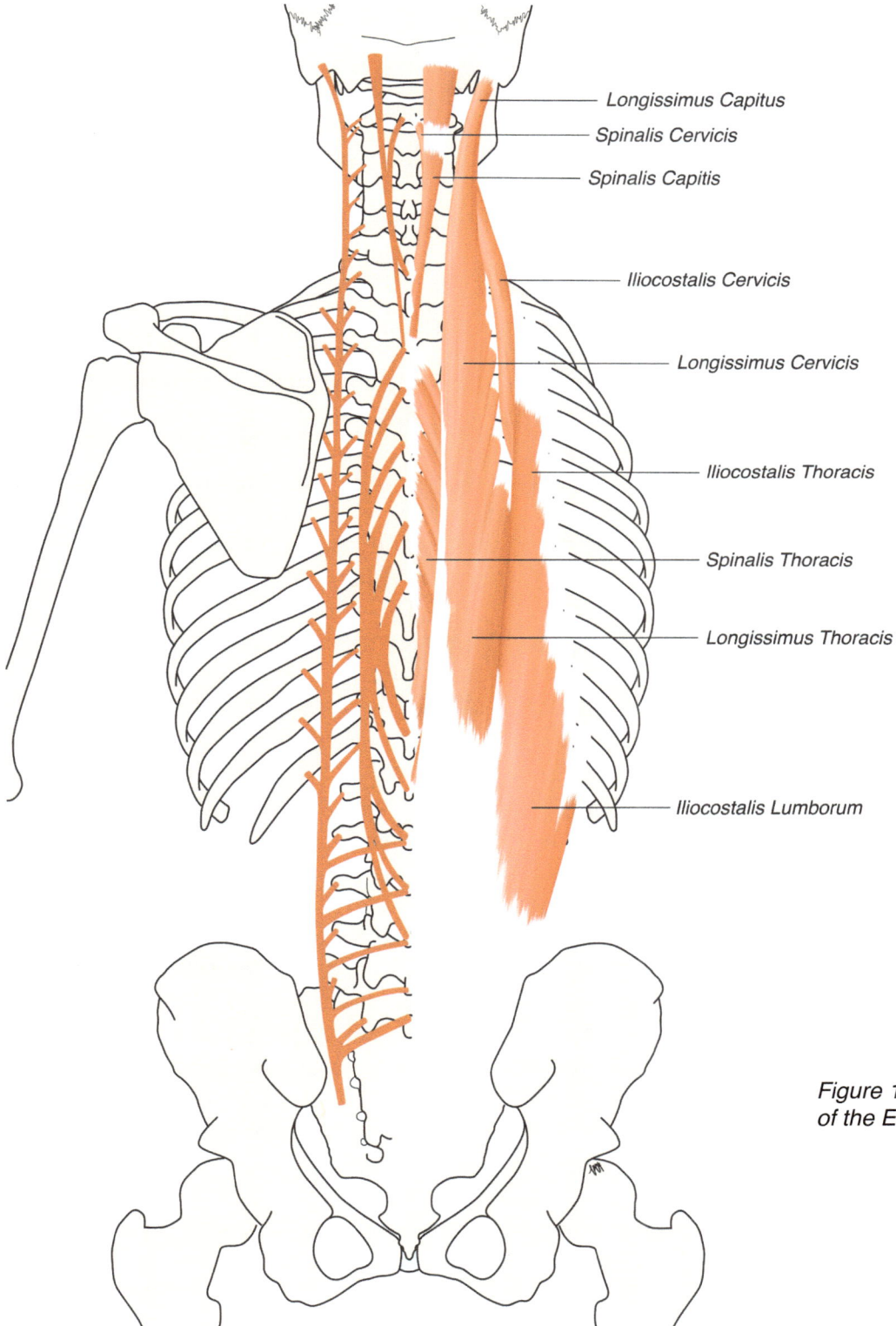

Figure 11: Anatomical location of the Erectus Spinae

Quadratus Lumborum

Origin: 12th Rib and TVP of L1-L4

Insertion: Iliac Crest & Iliolumbar Ligament

Action: Extension and Lateral Flexion of the Lumbar Spine

Nerve Supply: T12-L3

Problems: The *Quadratus Lumborum* (Figure 12) is one of the most important muscles with regards to dysfunction and imbalance within the body. Its anatomical orientation means that it has several roles, including pelvic stability, postural control and support of the trunk. The combined action of the Quadratus Lumborum will support the trunk when extending from a flexed position. However, individually they are involved in assisting the other trunk muscles to perform various movements.

Firstly, the Quadratus Lumborum will often spasm or become hypertonic, in response to trauma to the lower back. Its close attachment to the lumbar spine means that if a disc becomes herniated/prolapsed or the facet joint becomes sprained, the immediate response of the Quadratus Lumborum is to contract in order to protect the already damaged structures. It also has the ability to become overworked as well as contracting to support the trunk.

The natural, neutral position of the Quadratus Lumborum is to maintain the lordosis of the lumbar spine, where the muscle is balanced between relaxed and contracted. If however a client/patient slumps for a sustained period of time, the Quadratus Lumborum will constantly be trying to contract to activate regain the lumbar lordosis. This sustained, repetitive contraction will cause the muscle to fatigue along with the development of trigger points within the belly of the muscle.

As with the majority of problematic muscles, correct postural control will reduce the amount of stress the muscle is placed under. Encouraging the use of good form when sitting and lifting

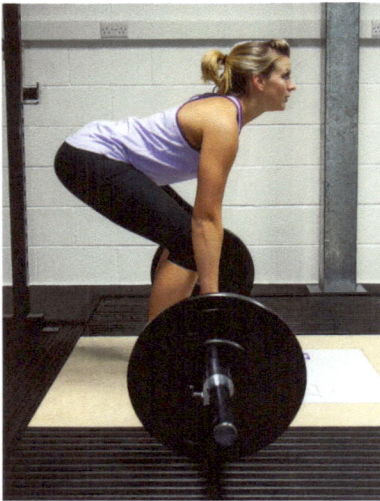

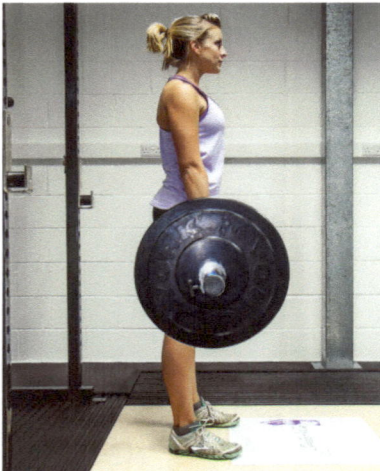

Deadlifts are an effective exercise for training the Quadratus Lumborum & Erector Spinae muscles

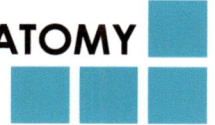

is paramount. An effective training exercise for improving the strength and control of the Quadratus Lumborum is with use of *Deadlifts* and its various modifications, such as performing it with a Single Arm or a Kettlebell.

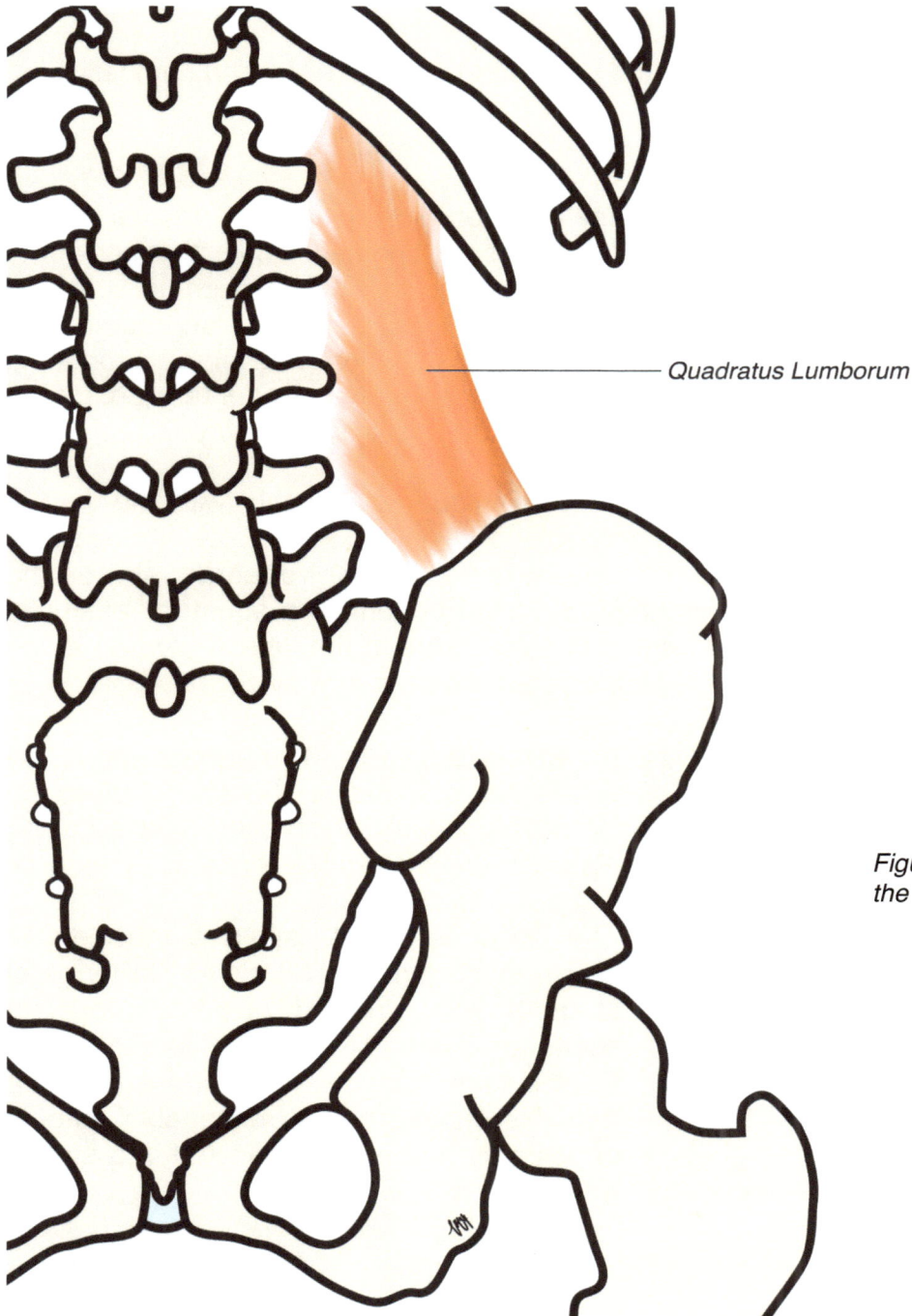

Quadratus Lumborum

Figure 12: Anatomical location of the Quadratus Lumborum

Iliopsoas

Origin: TVP's L1-L5, Vertebral Bodies of T12-L5 & Iliac Fossa

Insertion: Lesser Trochanter of Femur

Action: Flexion and Lateral Flexion of the Hip and Lumbar Spine

Nerve Supply: L1-L3

Problems: Due to the deep positioning of the *Iliopsoas* (Figure 13), it can be difficult to assess its tightness and activity. Its ability to flex the hip joint often means that it can become tight and overused particularly in long distance runners, and sports that involve a kicking action. It is also common to observe a shortening of this muscle in client/patients who have a sedentary job, mainly due to the sustained hip flexion and lack of activity.

The Iliopsoas also has a unique relationship with the way in which the pelvis anteriorly and posteriorly rotates. It originates from the anterior surface of the lumbar vertebrae, and as the pelvis anteriorly rotates at the bottom of a squat for example, the Iliopsoas begins to tighten due to the flexion created at the lumbar spine, which can restrict the range available.

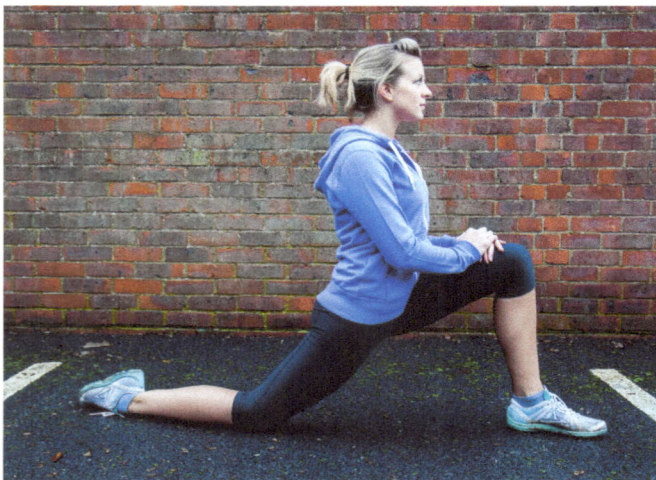

Another example of the relationships it has with other muscles is the role it plays on Hamstring length, which can be tested using *Passive Straight Leg Raise* (see Chapter 8.7).

The Iliopsoas is not usually a muscle that needs much functional 'training', in terms of strength work. However due to its constant sedentary overuse it is subject to shortening. For this reason, it is more important to ensure that this muscle has a reasonable amount of flexibility and is not neglected in a stretch routine.

Stretching the Iliopsoas can greatly improve the its flexibility

41

Psoas Major

Iliacus

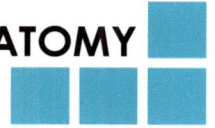

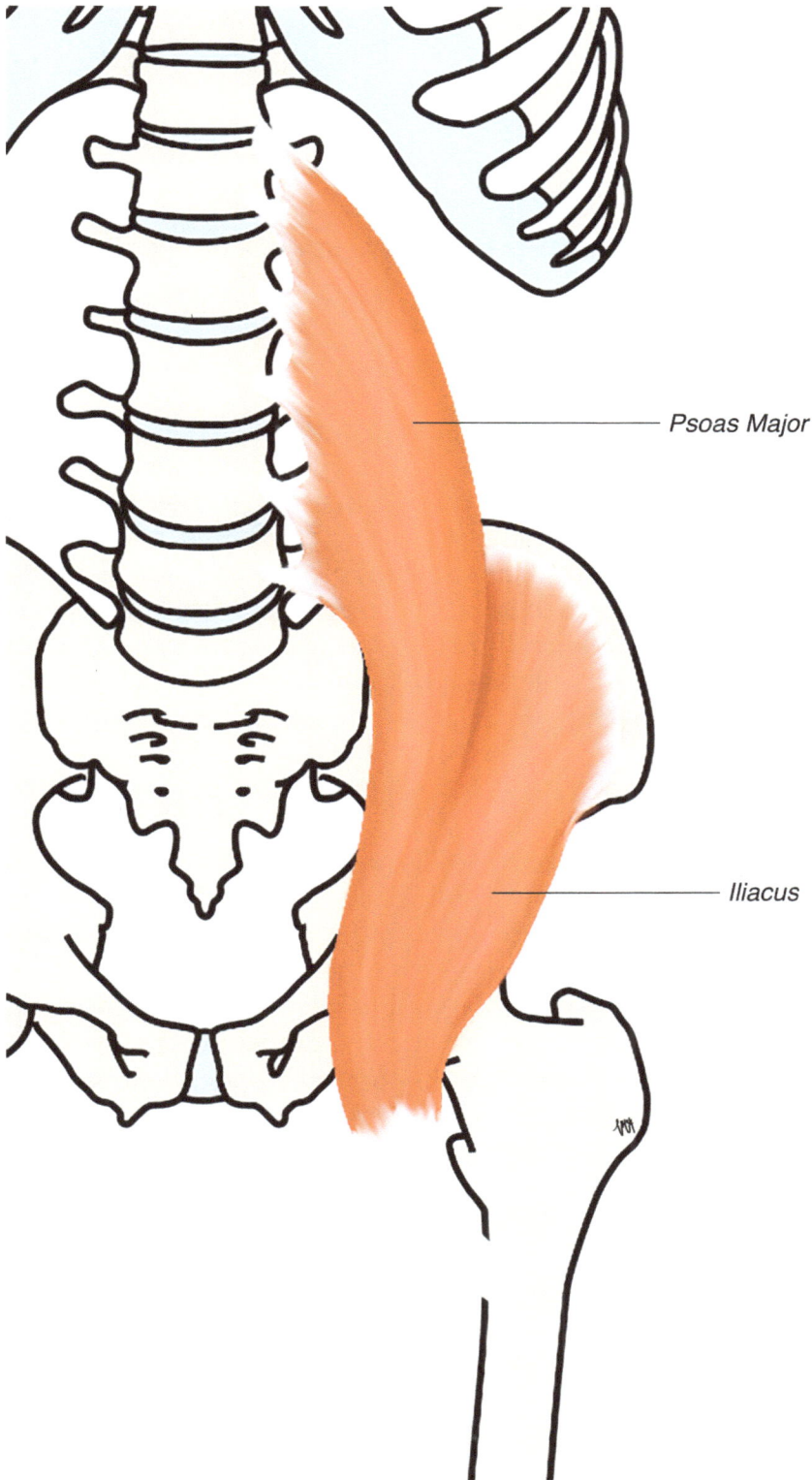

Figure 13: Anatomical location of the Iliopsoas

Gluteus Medius

Origin: Outer Ilium

Insertion: Greater Trochanter

Action: Abduction of the Hip and Stabilisation of the Pelvis during Gait

Nerve Supply: L4-S1

Problems: It is often either weak or detrimentally strong. This muscle, not unlike others, has a very close relationship to the Quadratus Lumborum. This is due in large part to their paralleled actions, which firstly include stabilising the pelvis and lumbar structures, and also initiating and controlling *Hip Extension* (see Chapter 8.8). Although most of the movement itself should be performed by the Gluteus Maximus, the *Gluteus Medius* (Figure 14) will also activate to stabilise the hip and pelvis through various stages of the gait cycle.

There is an obvious relationship that can be observed when assessing the Gluteus Medius & Quadratus Lumborum muscles. This association will also have input from various other muscles depending on the action. An example of this is during gait as the hip extends. The four muscles can be thought of as having an equal role during this pattern, with each muscle working in conjunction with the muscle diagonally across from it (right Quadratus Lumborum working with the left Gluteus Medius). Quite often one muscle in particular or group of muscles can become more dominant than the others, which is usually the Quadratus Lumborum. This is mostly due to a lack of Gluteus Medius activation, which can result in the other muscles being overused to compensate.

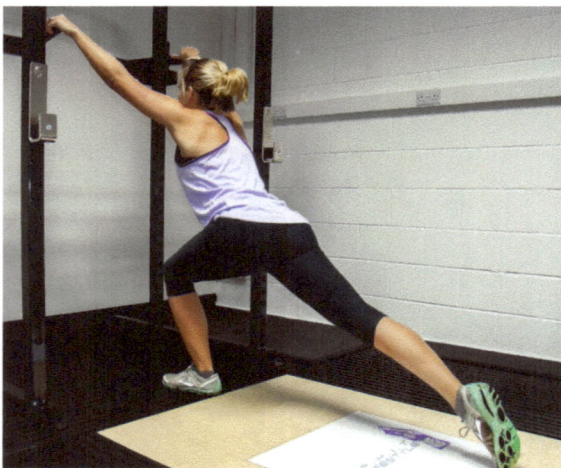

A Functional Squat is an effective exercise to activate both the Gluteus Medius & Maximus muscles when performed correctly

The development of trigger points within this muscle as a result of overuse can cause referred pain to travel laterally towards the hip or inferiorly to the posterior aspect of the thigh.

The Gluteus Medius can be effectively trained using exercises that encourage stabilising the pelvis one leg at a time, such as a *Functional Squat* or a *Side-lying Leg Raise*. The majority of training that this muscle often requires will revolve around teaching the client/patient to consciously activate the muscle during certain movements and activities.

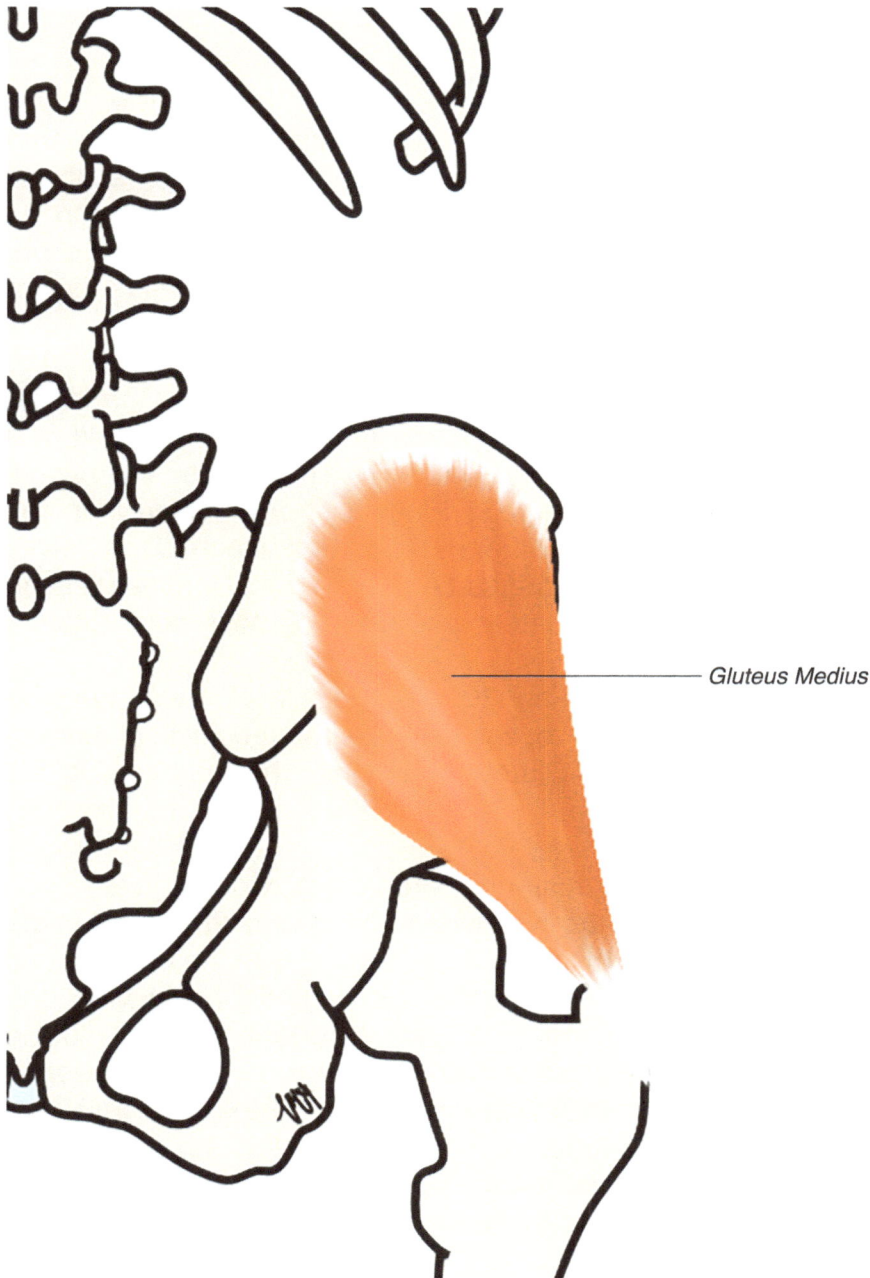

Gluteus Medius

Figure 14: Anatomical location of the Gluteus Medius

Hamstrings

Origin: Ischial Tuberosity

Insertion: Medial Condyle of the Tibia & Head of the Fibula

Action: Flexion of the Knee and Extension of the Hip

Nerve Supply: L5-S2

Problems: The *Hamstrings* (Figure 15) are a well-documented problematic muscle, particularly in sporting settings such as football and cycling. Its anatomical position in relation to its pelvic attachments, as well as its primary decelerating action, can put it under high loads and stress, thus increasing its risk of spontaneous injury such as tears and strains.

The common sedentary seated posture does not aid the length of the Hamstrings, in which typically the Hamstring is held in a shortened (partially contracted) state. This may cause the muscle to become tight and inflexible. Placing stress not only on the muscle itself, but also the other muscles that attach to the pelvis. Muscles such as the Quadratus Lumborum and Iliopsoas rely on the pelvis' ability to adequately anteriorly and posteriorly rotate.

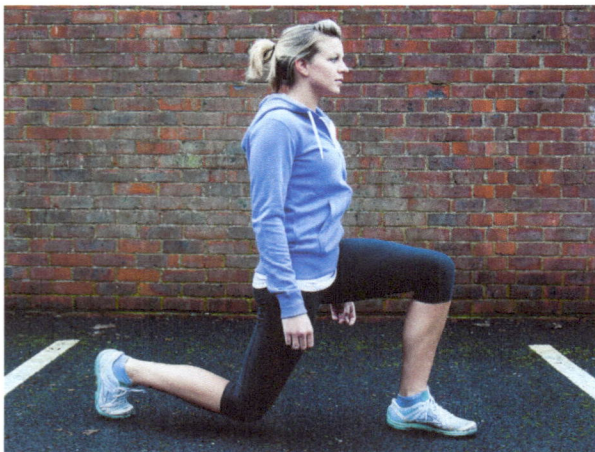

It may also typically overwork and develop tightness to compensate for the lack of activity from the Gluteus Maximus when performing hip extension.

The Hamstrings are often worked very well during the downward phase of a *Squat* or *Lunge*, however they can be isolated with the use of a *Leg Curl*. Due to the prevalence of tightness within the Hamstrings, it is also important that the muscle is stretched regularly for the majority of people, particularly with an increase in exercise and age. When teaching Hamstring stretches, ensure that the Hamstring itself, and not the sciatic nerve is being stretched at the posterior aspect of the knee.

The downward phase of a Lunge will be controlled by the Hamstrings

45

Semitendinosus

Biceps Femoris, Long Head

Biceps Femoris, Short Head

Semimembranosus

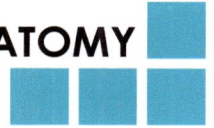

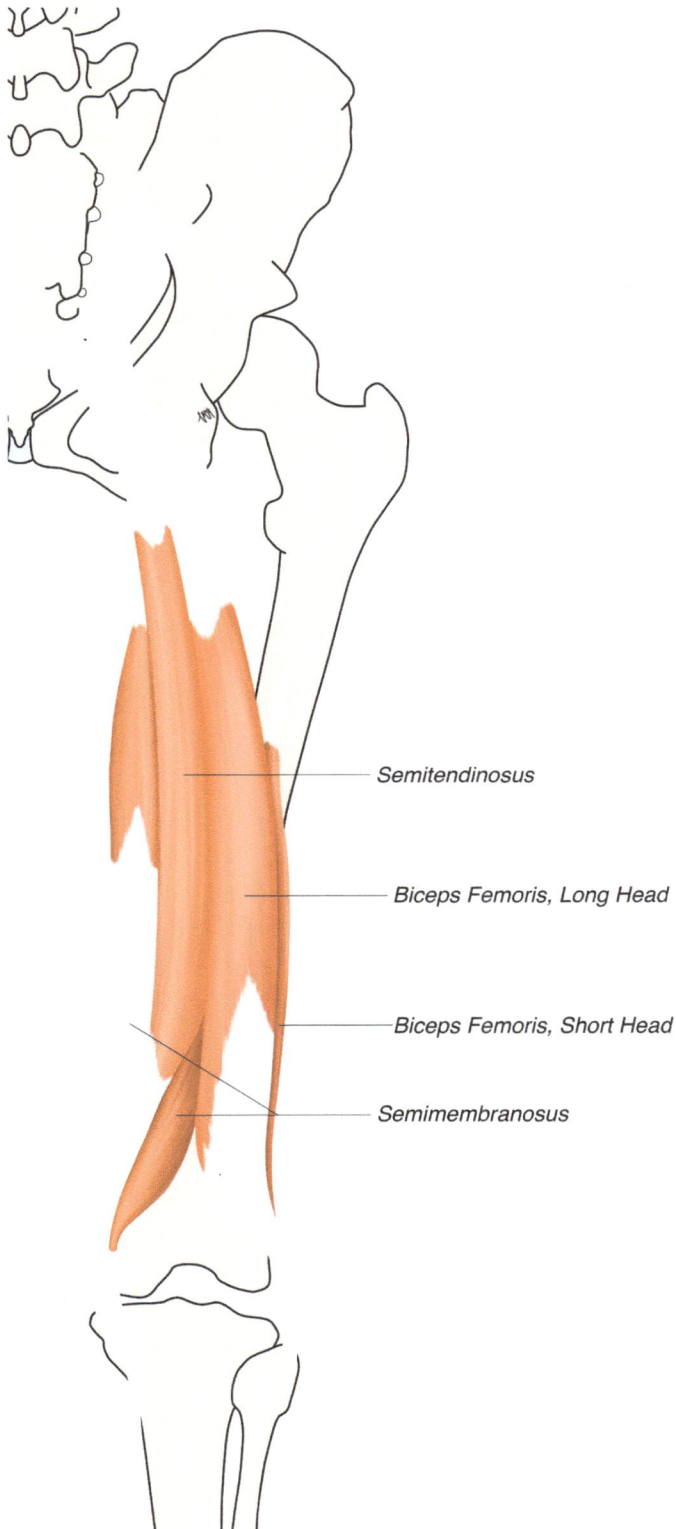

Figure 15: Anatomical location of the Hamstrings

Vastus Medialis Oblique

Origin: Intertrochanteric Line

Insertion: Medial Aspect of the Patella & Patella Tendon

Action: Extension of the Knee

Nerve Supply: L2-L4

Problems: This muscle has an important relationship with the Vastus Lateralis – the most lateral of the Quadricep muscles. The activity and control of both of these muscles should always be balanced and equal due to their insertion points. The *Vastus Medialis Oblique* (Figure 16) inserts into the medial aspect of the patellar tendon, whilst the Vastus Lateralis inserts into the lateral aspect of the patellar tendon. The two muscles therefore are primarily responsible for the tracking of the patella through the patellar groove at the knee joint.

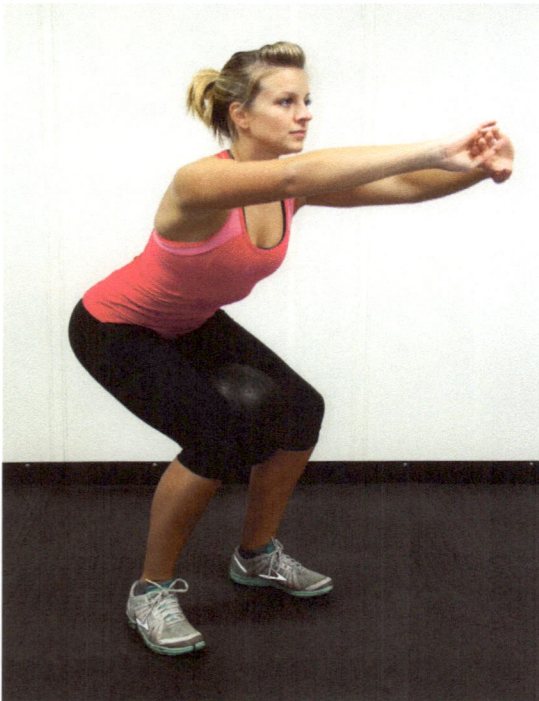

Due to this relationship, it is often associated with Patellofemoral Pain Syndrome or otherwise commonly known as Runner's Knee. This may be caused by tightness in the Vastus Lateralis or by a weakness in the Vastus Medialis Oblique, which results in the patellar tracking more laterally, creating friction and pain at the knee joint.

The Vastus Medialis Oblique can be trained using a slight variation to a Squat, known as a *VMO Squat*, which utilises a partly inflated ball, or medicine ball between the knees to ensure the Vastus Medialis Oblique remains active throughout the exercise. It is also important to ensure the Vastus Lateralis is stretched regularly to ensure it does not become tight and shortened, thus placing more tension upon patella.

Neurologically isolating the contraction of VMO is impossible. However, functionally, it can be isolated using a VMO Squat, which utilises a partly inflated ball or medicine ball

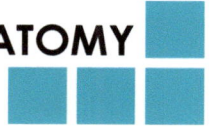

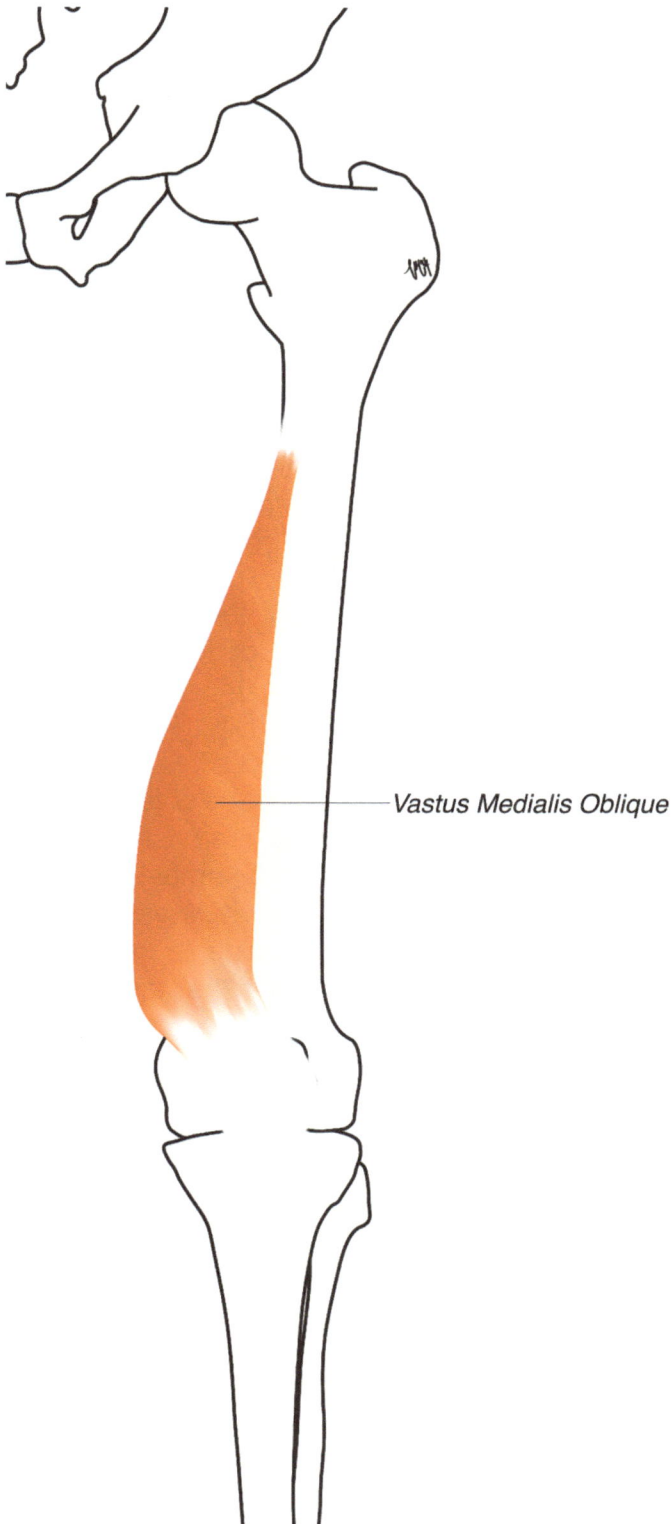

Vastus Medialis Oblique

Figure 16: Anatomical location of the Vastus Medialis Oblique

Peroneus Longus

Origin: Head of Fibula & Proximal 2/3 Fibula

Insertion: Base of 1st Metatarsal and Cuneiforms

Action: Eversion and Plantarflexion

Nerve Supply: L4-S1

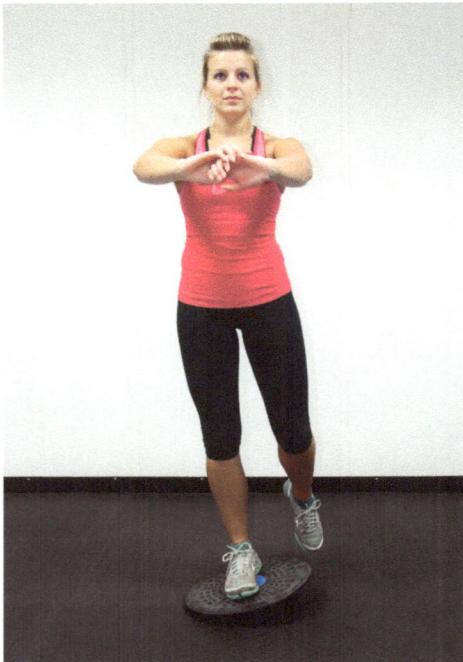

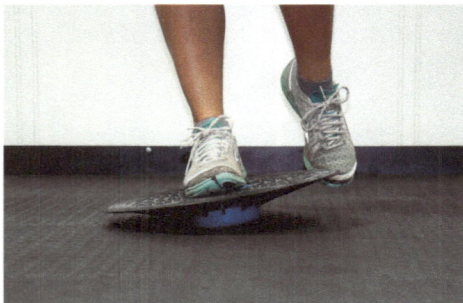

Wobble Board exercises are effective at training the stabilising muscles of the ankle, such as the Peroneus Longus

Problems: The *Peroneus Longus* (Figure 17) is a particularly long muscle that can often become damaged during an inversion sprain of the ankle due to it overstretching. A balanced relationship between the Peroneus Longus and the Tibialis Posterior will aid in the preservation and support of the longitudinal arch of the foot. This is due to their anatomical orientation, and their long tendon that travels across the posterior aspect of the foot to their insertion point.

A weakness of the Peroneus Longus has been linked with the development of excess pronation of the foot, or more commonly flat feet during gait cycle (see Chapter 7). A general cause for excess pronation still remains unknown, with theories in existence for muscular weakness, structural deformity, conditional behaviour and laziness, there is room for argument. However, it is understood that the Peroneus Longus has a significant role in ankle stabilisation during standing, walking and running. This, along with the paralleled antagonist action of the Tibialis Posterior, provides essential strength and proprioception to support the ankle joint.

Due to the muscle's length and action it can prove difficult to exercise effectively, however the proprioceptive function of the Peroneus Longus can be trained using *Wobble Board* exercises for the ankle joint. The more unstable the terrain, the more active the Peroneus Longus will be. A *High Calf/Heel Raise* will also challenge the muscle at an extreme range of motion.

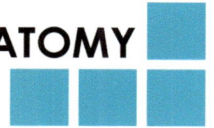

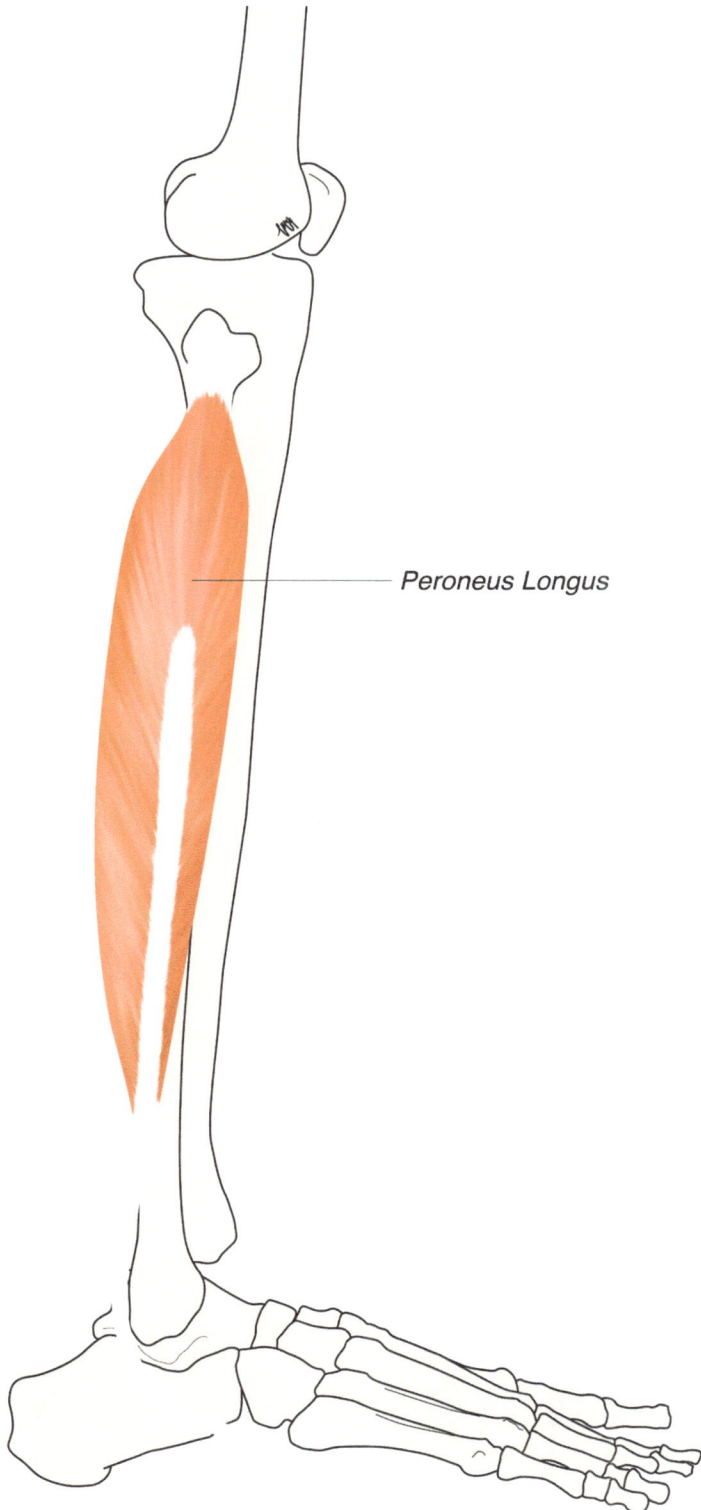

Figure 17: Anatomical location of the Peroneus Longus

Peroneus Longus

Soleus

Origin: Soleal Line of Tibia & Proximal Fibula

Insertion: Calcaneus

Action: Plantar Flexion of the Foot

Nerve Supply: S1-S2

Problems: The general public, including clients/patients, do not often know too much about the *Soleus* (Figure 18). However, it is a muscle the majority of exercisers, particularly those that run, should be aware of due to its function and anatomical position in relation to the Gastrocnemius.

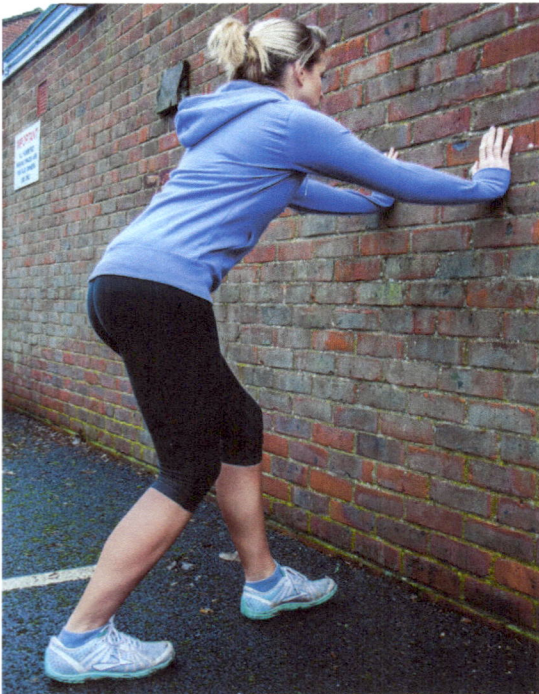

Stretching the Soleus will reduce the stress being placed upon the Achilles Tendon

The Soleus is a longer muscle than is often realised, as it originates deep to the Gastrocnemius and travels inferiorly until it reaches the Achilles. Due to its position, the sheath that surrounds the muscle naturally has less elastic properties than that of the Gastrocnemius. This means that the sheath will not readily expand with increase work and blood flow. This may cause some pain and discomfort particularly if the muscle is not adequately stretched after and between exercising.

So much depends upon the proper use of the 'calf' muscles, rather than the strength of them. Proper use will coincide with the correct running style (see Chapter 7.2) for the distance and speed being run. *Calf Raises* are the preferred exercise to train the Soleus and Gastrocnemius complex. However it is also important that the client/patient understands how to stretch both adequately in order to reduce the load and stress being placed upon the Achilles tendon.

Soleus

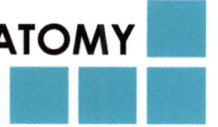

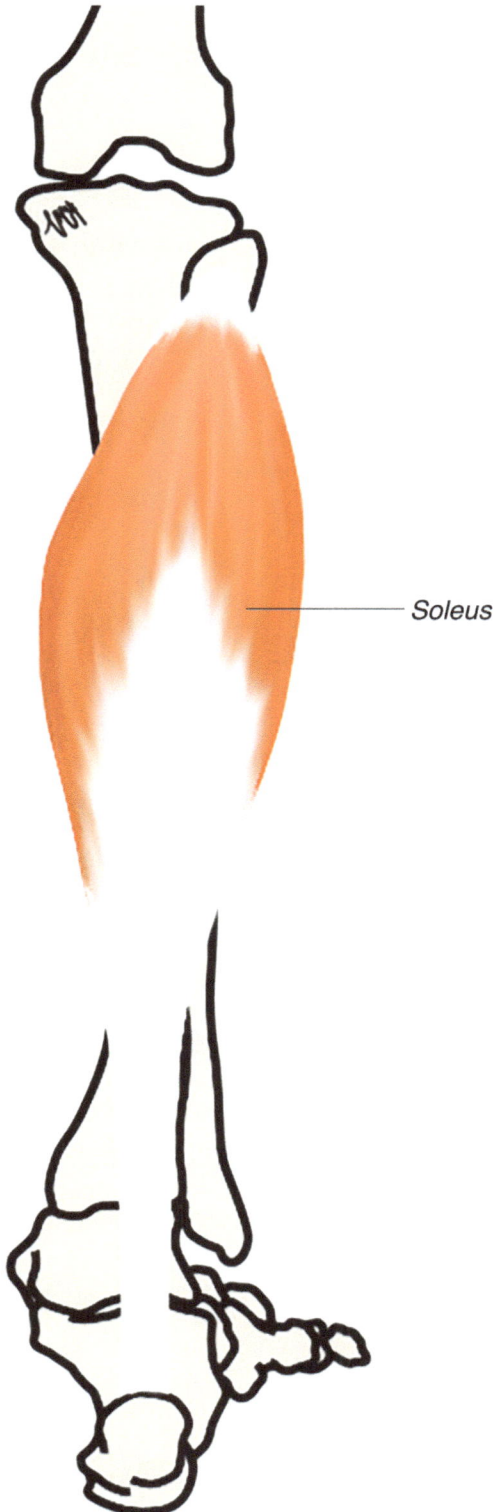

Figure 18: Anatomical location of the Soleus

CHAPTER 1.

At the end of each chapter, each case study and questions will be relevant to the knowledge acquired in the previous chapter(s).

Case Study 1

A 27-year-old female tennis player presented to a Chiropractor 2 weeks ago with 1-month history of pain in the anterior aspect of her upper right arm, at the proximal end of the humerus. The pain is generally worse with tennis, especially as the game goes on. It then continues to throb for a few hours post-exercise.

Following an examination of the shoulder joint, the associated musculature, and the thoracic and cervical spine. The Chiropractor diagnosed the client/patient with:

Subacute moderate mechanical biceps tendonitis (R)

They explain to the client/patient their options for treatment, such as acupuncture, massage, eccentric loading etc. Between them they decide, based upon the client/patients desire to continue training that the best option would be to combine rehabilitative exercise with massage. It is the first time the client/patient has been trained specifically for sport and rehabilitation.

They are referred to you...

1. Using all of your knowledge, list all the muscles associated with the shoulder girdle?

2. Can you explain how eccentric loading may benefit this client/patient, and suggest an exercise that would be relevant?

3. What would be an ideal somatotype for this client/patient? Please explain your answer, along with a hypothetical somatotype score.

Notes

2. Psychological Behaviour & Pain

Learning Objectives

- To understand and appreciate the value of schemas in a professional environment.
- To understand the different ways of learning behaviour.
- To understand motivation and how it is influenced by goal setting and feedback.
- To understand how social learning theory can influence learnt behaviour
- To appreciate how pain can affect a person's behaviour, and how this can lead to feeling helpless.

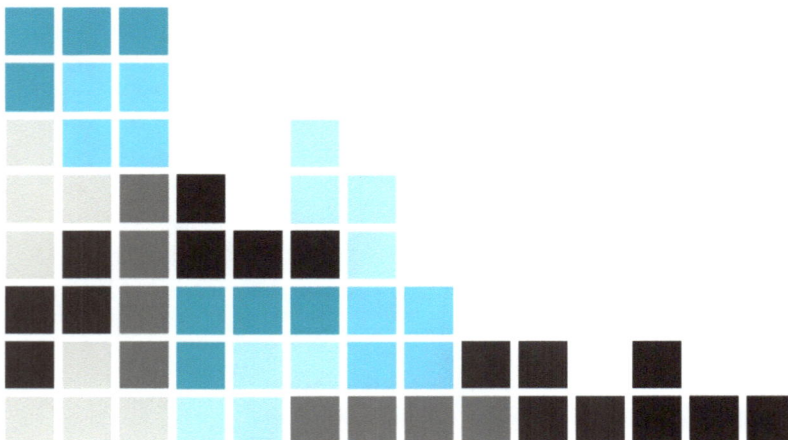

PSYCHOLOGICAL BEHAVIOUR & PAIN

Behaviour and response to pain are two aspects of human psychology that prove very difficult to generalise, due to an individual's unique personal experiences throughout life. This is known as 'subjective well-being', suggested by Diener (1984). It refers to how people experience the quality of their lives based on emotional reactions and cognitive judgements about specific areas of their lives. We have developed traits that are common among the population, although they are also influenced by social and environmental factors. Thus, making behaviour rather difficult to predict. Although, Fishbein and Ajzen (1975) proposed the theory of reasoned action, which suggests a person's behavioural intention depends on the person's attitude about the behaviour and subjective norms (for example, peoples beliefs). This highlights that it still remains a much-debated area in psychology. Regardless, a greater appreciation for why people behave in a particular way can enable a health and fitness professional to get the best out of them, as much as their ability will allow.

Pain, inevitably, is incredibly difficult to gauge, as it is such a subjective sensation of nervous input that can be quite easily increased or decreased depending not only mental state, but mood and time of the day. Clients/patients may present with no pain one day and in severe distress the next. It is important to be able to understand the basic psychological implications this can have on their lifestyle and their ability to exercise. Furthermore, being able to recognise how pain avoidance behaviour can be accommodated for and conditioned to make certain, usually painful, activities comfortable is the foundation of being a Functional Rehabilitative Trainer.

2.1 Schemas

When faced with a decision or proposition, we consciously and unconsciously think and process all the variables surrounding that situation. Psychologists explain this complex integration of personal experience, expectations and images as a schema. Bartlett suggested the concept of schemas in 1932 during research into memory, although the concept originates from Piaget, as early as 1926. Woolfolk (2013) describes schemas as the knowledge structures that organise vast amounts of information. This information is organised mentally into a recognisable framework to the individual that will help guide their perception of what could and might happen in a situation, based on past experience. (Sternberg & Sternberg, 2012).

Schemas start to form with every new experience we encounter from birth, helping us individually make the world more predictable. Inevitably making the learnt experiences and behaviours we witness from our parents some of the most significant (Bandura, 1977). Schemas work like a manuscript, which has been written and modified throughout life. Details can be added and deleted to keep up with an individual's conception of the world, continually reconstructing how situations, and the world is viewed and perceived, and ultimately our response to it (Gross & McIlveen, 2004). Schemas can be either 'dynamic', whereby they change based on experience, or 'fixed', such as the response of a suckling baby. It is possible though for a perception to lead to significant dynamic distortions in comparison to social norm. This will obviously depend on the experiences a person will have had, creating human error, cultural diversity etc., meaning that a person's schema may twist unfamiliar or unconsciously unacceptable information 'to fit' in with their existing knowledge.

An example of this is demonstrated in research conducted by Allport & Postman (1947), where white participants were shown a picture of two men involved in a dispute (Figure 19).

The participants were asked to briefly look at the picture and then describe the scene to someone who hadn't seen it. Then that person was asked to describe it to another based on the information they had been told. As the information was being passed, some of the key components of the picture changed, most notably the knife was reported to be in the black man's hand. This demonstrates that the memory is an active process and can be changed to 'fit in' with what is expected to happen based on knowledge and understanding of society.

Schemas should play an important role when trying to highlight and exemplify when new learnt behaviours should be applied, as a previously understood dynamic schema may contradict

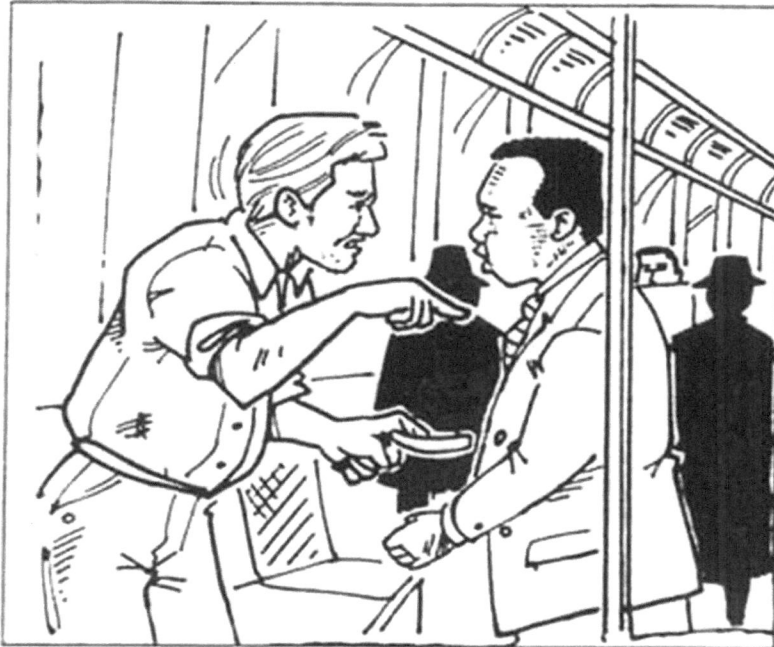

Figure 19: The picture from Allport & Postman's (1947) study of a white man holding a knife to a black man

what is being taught. For instance, asking a new mother who displays signs of an introverted personality (quiet, reserved, thoughtful and introspective), to perform a fully functioning squat in the supermarket to pick up her child, may prove initially too much of a challenge to her perception of social etiquette, based on her experiences or desire to not 'stand out'. Thus, challenging her schema of how to perform or act in public. By encouraging her to start implementing change to the way in which she performs tasks around the home would reduce the risk of her fear and anxiety towards doing something that maybe the general public does not subscribe to. This may be due to the vast majority of the public being either unaware of the proper way to squat, or fearing judgement from others. Also by continued practice of the corrective movement within the home, the movement itself then becomes the 'norm' over a period of time, meaning that it will not have to be thought about quite so consciously when out in public. Consequently, all health and fitness professionals should employ a duty of care towards their clients/patients, to reduce fear-avoidance behaviour. This will aid their receptiveness towards changing their behaviour, and consequently their schema, thus hopefully reducing the risk of their pain reoccurring.

2.2 Learning and Conditional Behaviour

The majority of clients/patients that are referred for functional rehabilitative training will have most commonly suffered from a spontaneous or mechanical injury. This stress may be something everyday and mundane such as picking up a child or putting on a sock, but it can still have very painful consequences. These situations however do not just happen. Pain is often the last symptom of a mechanical dysfunction, and over a period of time other muscles, joints and ligaments may have been compensating for the imbalance of dysfunction. So even when a client/patient is pain free, that activity or movement may still put those vulnerable structures under stress. This is why learning and behaviour, particularly operant conditioning behaviour, is a very useful tool. The benefit of using operant conditioning is highlighted in the flowing scenario because in order to produce a successful response to a problem, the mother must find a solution. If the solution works and the problem is resolved, they will be rewarded and are then more likely to repeat the behaviour.

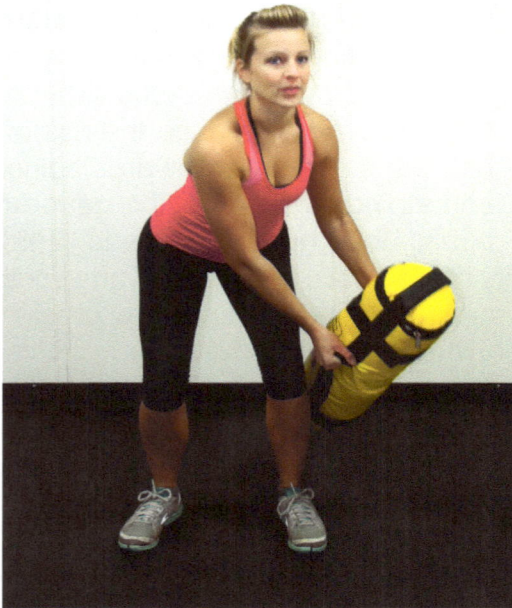

For example, a new mother consistently throughout the day picks up her new born with minimal effort, but equally poor form, and inadequate engagement of the trunk stabilisers when doing so. Spontaneously three months after birth, her lower back "goes" whilst picking something up off the floor. Once she is pain free, it is also important to educate her to engage her trunk and strengthen it for function. It isn't just a case of physically training that client/patient. They also have to learn that certain movements and activities can put the mechanical structures at risk of injury, and that certain situations require the engagement of specific muscles in order to protect those structures.

This demonstrates how important the role of aiding conditional behaviour can be, especially with pain and function. Learning is often described as a hypothetical construct, as it cannot be directly observed, but it can be inferred as a construct based on observable behaviour.

Repetitive movement patterns need reinforcing and strengthening

Classical Conditioning

This is often referred to as 'associative learning' or 'Pavlovian' conditioning. Pavlov (1927), a physiologist, noticed during an experiment into dogs' digestion, that dogs would start salivating before any food was given to them. This suggested the dog learned or acquired a response to a stimulus, such as looking at the dog bowl or hearing the footsteps of the laboratory assistant,

that didn't stimulate a response before. This classical response is likely to be involuntary, such as an emotion or physiological response.

A good example of this physiological response is the 'Little Albert Experiment' conducted by Watson & Rayner (1920), whereby a 9-month-old infant was shown a white rat, a rabbit, a monkey and various masks. He initially showed no fear to any of these, he did however demonstrate fear towards a steel bar being struck with a hammer behind his head. The sudden noise caused 'Little Albert' to burst into tears.

When 'Little Albert' was 11 months old he was presented with the white rat and seconds later the bar was struck with the hammer. This was done 7 times over the next 7 weeks and each time he burst into tears. After the 7 weeks 'Little Albert' would only need to see the rat and he would display signs of fear. Watson & Rayner demonstrated in this experiment that classical conditioning could be used to create an irrational response that was out of proportion to the presented danger – they had created a phobia.

This type of conditioning (classical) is not relevant to a functional training setting, as eliciting an emotional or physiological reaction will not be helpful to the client/patient or appropriate to the purpose of training. The reason is that the client/patient needs to learn a voluntary response to a stimulus rather than an involuntary response. Although a valid point that can be appreciated is that a stimulus will become more or less liked when it is consistently paired with a stimulus that is respectively positive or negative (De Houwer, Thomas & Baeyns, 2001). Much like clicker training with a dog, behaviour that is positively reinforced is more likely to repeated, as opposed to behaviour that has negative consequences. This concept can be applied using praise and positive reinforcement of good technique during training.

Operant Conditioning

Although the suggestion of classical conditioning chronologically appeared first, Skinner (1938) argued that most behaviour was a voluntary response associated to a specific stimulus. He saw learning as an active process, whereby small actions produced a consequence to the surrounding environment. This resulted in not only humans behaving in a certain way, but also non-humans, depending on their immediate environment.

	Stimulus Added	**Stimulus Removed**
Behaviour Increases	**Positive Reinforcement** Giving praise to a footballer for turning his marker and getting a shot at goal on target makes this behaviour more likely to occur again.	**Negative Reinforcement** A coach who continually shouts criticism at his players becomes quiet, which portrays his satisfaction, making it more likely to happen again.
Behaviour Decreases	**Positive Punishment** A coach, who generally praises players, criticises some sloppy defending. The players become aware that the coach is unhappy and will strive to avoid a repeat.	**Negative Punishment** A coach who usually gives a lot of praise and encouragement withdraws this type of feedback. Players perceive that the coach is not happy and this acts as a type of punishment.

Table 3: This demonstrates examples of how rewards and punicshments can be used to motivate an increase or decrease in behaviour

Skinner demonstrated just this with his rat experiment in 1948. It was initially a variation of the puzzle-box first designed in 1898 by Thorndike to study law of effect (an early theory that progressed into what we now know as operant conditioning). Cats were held inside the puzzle-box until they learnt to operate the catch that would release the escape door, at which point they were rewarded with food. Each time they were returned straight back to the box and each time it took them less time to escape. Skinner's rat experiment took this one step further as it was completely automated, meaning the rat was responsible for immediate repetition of the positive reinforcement it received rather than the cat having to be placed back into the box. The rat was placed in a box, and within the box a lever that when pressed delivered food to a tray also inside the box.

This explains how either rewarding or reinforcing behaviour can make it more likely to reoccur, with punishment making it more likely to reduce the chances of that behaviour occurring again in the future (Table 3). Both rewards and punishments can be used as motivators.

Any one of these approaches can be tailored to an individual's coaching or teaching style, so long as good performance/ behaviour is rewarded and poor performance/behaviour is punished. It is important that whichever approach is used, it is consistent with individual client/patients.

2.3 Motivation

The ability to learn or acquire new motor skills is driven by a motivation to do so, a reason to achieve. In 1974, it was proclaimed by Sage that motivation is 'the internal mechanisms and external stimuli which arouse and direct our behaviour'. This suggests that we have an inner drive towards achieving a goal that is dependent upon our perceived external (environmental) pressures and rewards. This directs the intensity of our behaviour to learn.

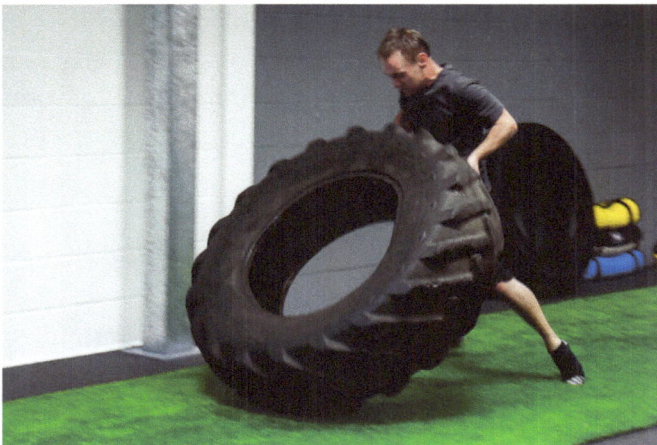

There is a clear distinction between intrinsic and extrinsic motivation

A clear distinction can be made between different forms of motivation, most commonly whether motivation is intrinsic or extrinsic. Intrinsic motivation can be described as the natural tendency to explore and conquer challenges through our personal interests. When we are intrinsically motivated, there is no need for rewards or punishment, because the activity itself can be enjoyable, fun or satisfying. Personal accomplishment and gaining a sense of pride can also be intrinsic motivators (Honeybourne *et al*, 2000; Woolfolk, 2013). This form of motivation can be used with a client/patient when explaining how certain exercises or movements can reduce the risk of reoccurrence of their injury.

In contrast, extrinsic motivation is demonstrated by incentives such as earning a good grade, to please parents, or even to avoid punishment. This form of motivation is mostly associated with negative emotions, poor academic achievement and maladaptive learning strategies (Corpus *et al*, 2009), suggesting that extrinsic motivation is driven by what can be gained from a task rather than the task itself.

Whether a person is intrinsically or extrinsically motivated is difficult to detect, as it depends solely on the students' reason for undertaking the task; their locus of causality. This identifies whether the motivation is coming from either inside the person (for example, a person that reads or exercises based on their personal interests), or outside the person (someone or something else is influencing them). A health and fitness professional looking to optimise the effects of motivation, be it intrinsic or extrinsic, should consider involving the client/patient in the decision-making. This will help incentivise a sense of personal achievement, which the client/patient will take a direct interest in.

2.4 Feedback

Feedback is a vital part of any activity or performance. It involves using the information available either during or after an activity to modify it. This can be done during the activity or when next it is performed – essentially adding to the schema that has developed around the activity itself. Honeybourne (2000) suggests there are several forms of feedback:

- **Continuous** – musculoskeletal feedback, such as proprioception or kinesthesis during an activity.
- **Terminal** – feedback that is in response to the activity being completed.
- **Knowledge of Results** – a type of terminal feedback, whereby the client/patient receives information about the end result of the activity (e.g. a lap time at the end of a race).
- **Knowledge of Performance** – this provides the client/patient with information about their movement during the activity, rather than the end result (e.g. a football manager explaining to a player his marking positioning from the side-line).

- **Internal/intrinsic** – a type of continuous feedback, specifically from the proprioceptors.
- **External/extrinsic** – feedback from external sources, such as sound and vision (e.g. a crowd's reaction).
- **Positive** – reinforces skill learning and will give the client/patient information about a successful activity.
- **Negative** – provides information of an unsuccessful activity, from which, information can be used to create a more successful strategy.

Most of the time, clients/patients' objectives are not only to be pain-free, but also to be able to maintain that state themselves. Initially knowledge of performance and positive feedback will be the most beneficial forms of feedback from the professional. However, it is important to instil a sense of self-awareness so that the client/patient is receiving continuous feedback.

Knowledge of performance is particularly important early on, as it is normally associated with external feedback about the movement that has taken, or is taking place. As the client/patient becomes more astute about their own performance, they will then be able to distinguish between good and poor movement. During the stage whereby external feedback is being given, it is with care that it should be delivered. The client/patient should develop an internal feedback system, because if they rely too heavily upon the external feedback, this may not develop. Consideration for the ability of the client/patient, the task being undertaken, and the client/patient's personality should be taken as different people will respond differently to different types of feedback.

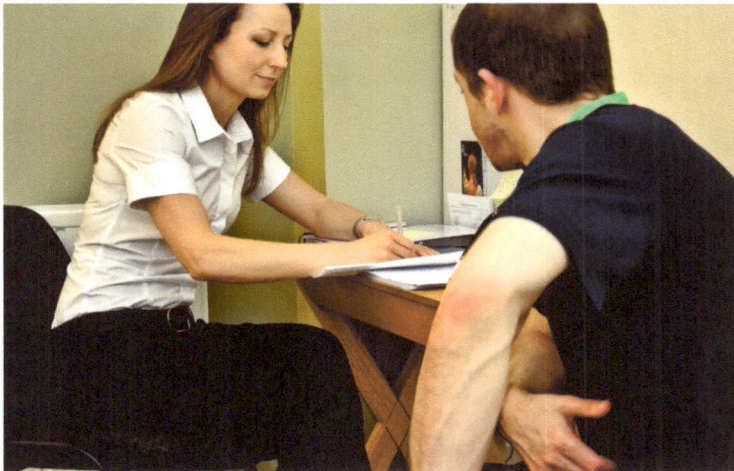

Discussing goals and giving feedback on progress with clients/patients can be a very useful tool

A study by Magill & Schoenfelder-Zohdi (1996) adds an interesting point to the way in which movement can be taught. They found that gymnasts who were shown an expert model demonstration of a motor skill needed less knowledge of performance than gymnasts that weren't shown the demonstration. This suggests the use of visual aids adds a significant advantage towards the learning of motor skills.

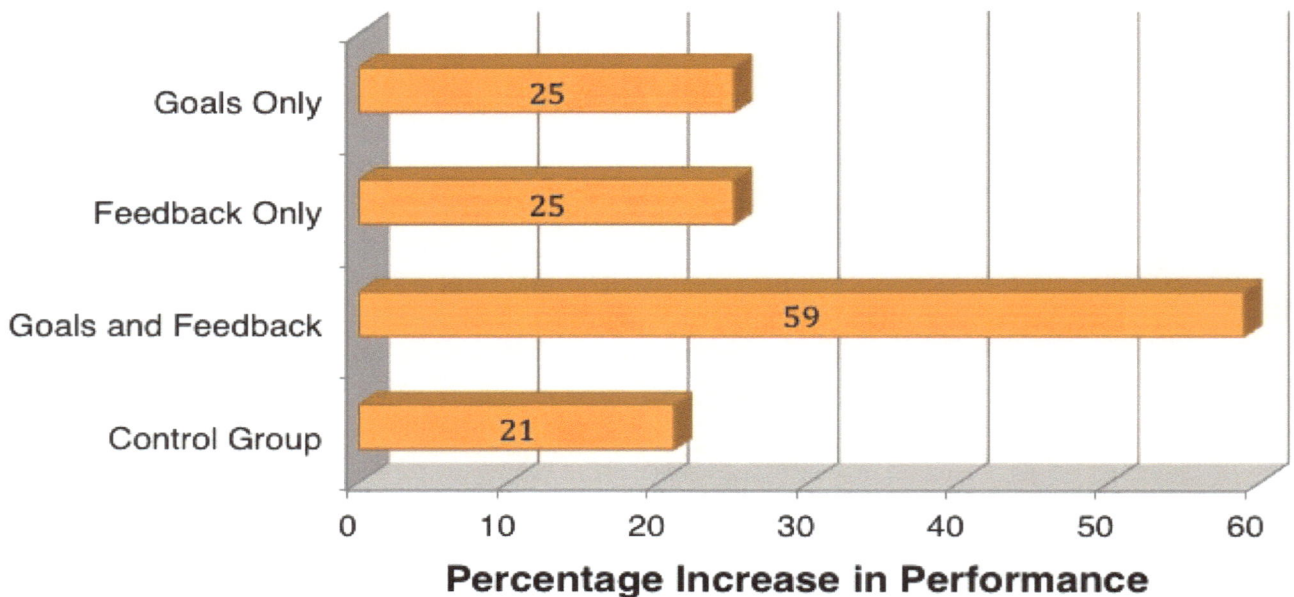

Graph 1: A representation of how goals and feedback can affect performance in cyclists, according to Bandura & Cervone (1983)

Feedback and Goal Setting

A goal is an achievable outcome or end result that is set either internally or externally, by a teacher or parent etc. Goals can be a helpful and useful tool when identifying "where a person is" and what can be done to help them achieve "where they want to be". Locke and Latham (2002) suggested four reasons why goal setting can improve performance:

1. To direct attention to a specific task and away from distractions

2. It can energise effort. Often the more challenging the goal, the greater the effort will be to achieve it.

3. It can increase an individual's level of persistence. A clear goal will result in the individual being less likely to give up.

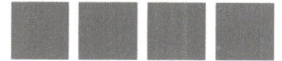

4. To promote the development of new skills and knowledge, to encourage the formation of new strategies when previous ones fail.

Bandura and Cervone (1983) concluded that performance in cyclists following feedback and goal setting was enhanced when compared to a feedback only, goals only and a control group, demonstrated in Graph 1.

Understandably, an improvement in the way a client/patient performs a certain movement or behaves with their posture is what is being attempted, to reduce their risk of injury and improve their muscular control. Using realistic goals and feedback, specific to that individual, will aid the process of both learning and application of what has been learnt into everyday tasks that involve movements such as lifting and twisting.

2.5 Social Learning Theory

Human beings naturally have a desire to be accepted by others and form groups or communities. Most of human behaviour is

copied and learnt from others as we grow. People we hold in high-regard, respect and trust will often influence our behaviour more positively, rather than unimportant people we may fear.

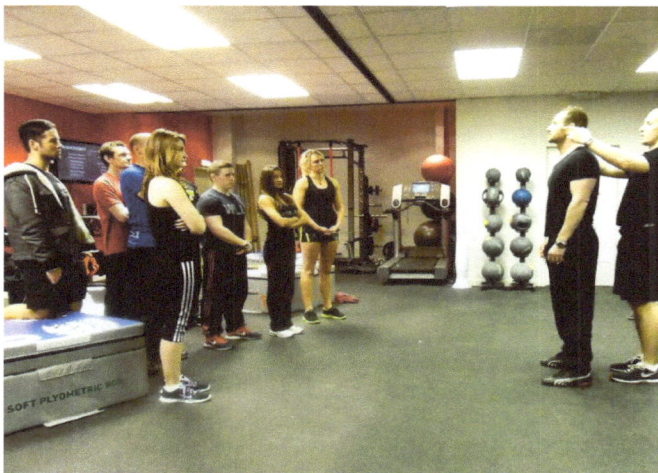

Social learning theory (SLT) is the process that helps us integrate into a group or community by copying learnt behaviour, making us more acceptable. Bandura first suggested SLT in 1977, when he explained how we learn through the observation of our environment. Stating that we learn from significant individuals, known as models,

The majority of behavioural accommadation occurs unconsciously, however it is always important to consider the audience when teaching

individuals such as parents, TV characters and friends from within a peer group.

Using the example of a child, according to Bandura people are more likely to imitate models they perceive similar to themselves, meaning they are more likely to imitate people of the same sex. In addition to this, the response of the people around them, whether it be either reinforcement or punishment will affect whether the child performs that particular behaviour again or not.

When teaching any individual functionally, a consideration for their personality, schemas, and their relationship to pain, their goals and many other attributes should be accommodated. Most accommodation will happen unconsciously, some aspects however may not be quite so natural. The ability to recognise and improve on those skills will separate a great health and fitness professional from the good ones.

2.6 Pain and Behaviour

Often associated with the sensation of pain is a physical, organic origin of where the pain is being stimulated. Pain that is either very acute or has turned chronic and has been lingering for a considerable period of time (more than 3-6 months), can start to affect the mental state of a person. Their mood may become affected as the pain disrupts their lifestyle, interfering with sleep and adding unnecessary stress to daily activities. Any form of pain can easily result in low self-esteem due to work, legal or financial issues, depending on the mentality of the person in pain (Hall-Flavin, 2013).

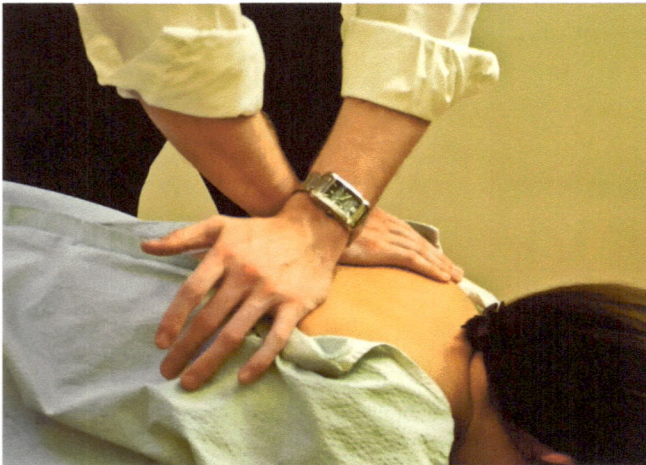

The majority of clients/patients coming through functional strength training will have been suffering with pain for a considerable time, and the use of strength exercises may have been overlooked initially. When a client/patient plateaus in their recovery from pain, much like when they plateau during weight loss, it can become frustrating for both the client/patient and the professional. At that point other options may be considered.

Clients/patients may initially try other interventions such as Chiropractic, Osteopathy or Physiotherapy

When those clients/patients visit you for the first time, it may be helpful to the therapeutic alliance to empathise initially towards

how this 'pain' is disrupting the clients/patient's life, especially before throwing them into a tough functional routine. Appreciate the individual's tolerance to pain. An appreciation for this starts at the initial assessment and will continue to develop as more time is spent with them. The bond that will develop between the health and fitness professional and the client/patient is known as the therapeutic alliance, Ardito and Rabellino (2011) state that the quality of the therapeutic alliance is a reliable predictor of a positive clinical outcome. This suggests that a strong relationship between the two will result in a more positive outcome, in this case towards pain relief and strength of functional movement.

Experience will guide an understanding towards pain behaviour, whether or not, and how much pain a client/patient is experiencing. This is often due to the individual's subjective perception of what pain is, based on their exposure to it and their dynamic schemas surrounding the situation (Sullivan, 2004). Importantly, pain is not the same as pain behaviour. There could be a presence of pain without pain behaviour, and the opposite is also true, most obviously in modern football, whereby players are 'diving' and rolling around in apparent agony without the presence of pain. This is demonstrated once the free kick is given, as the player miraculously springs to his feet. However, pain behaviour may include involuntary physiological responses (sweating etc.), as well as more complex behaviours such as medicating or taking time off of work, or even rolling around in agony etc.

In order to gauge an individual's pain, it may prove helpful to use a scale to monitor not only improvement but also how far a client/patient can be pushed. A typical example of such a scale would be 0-10 Individual Pain Scale (IPS) (Figure 20). On the initial assessment it is always worth explaining that throughout the functional strength programme, aspects of training may be painful or uncomfortable due to the physiological activation and remodelling of muscle fibres, and the stretching of joints and ligamentous tissue. This pain is a 'good' pain, although to ensure that the structures are not pushed too far it is important to set limits. The client/patient should be asked to place their current pain at 0 on that scale, from that point on they should work up towards a 5 on that pain scale but not above, this ensures they have an accurate baseline measurement of their subjective pain. They need to be very honest with themselves about what constitutes a level 5, some individuals will feel they have to push themselves too much, and some will feel they are at a 5 when in fact they are closer to a 3. A constant vigilance towards the client/patient's body language and pain behaviour will prove a useful tool when identifying whether they are working sufficiently hard. The use of such a scale can help maintain a positive approach towards training by providing a measurable representation of improvement. It will also aid the therapeutic alliance by enabling the client/patient to feel that the professional cares about their progress, at the same time of restricting the pain reoccurring and causing damage. This improves the relationship the client/patient has with pain and the behaviour associated with pain.

Individual Pain Scale (IPS)

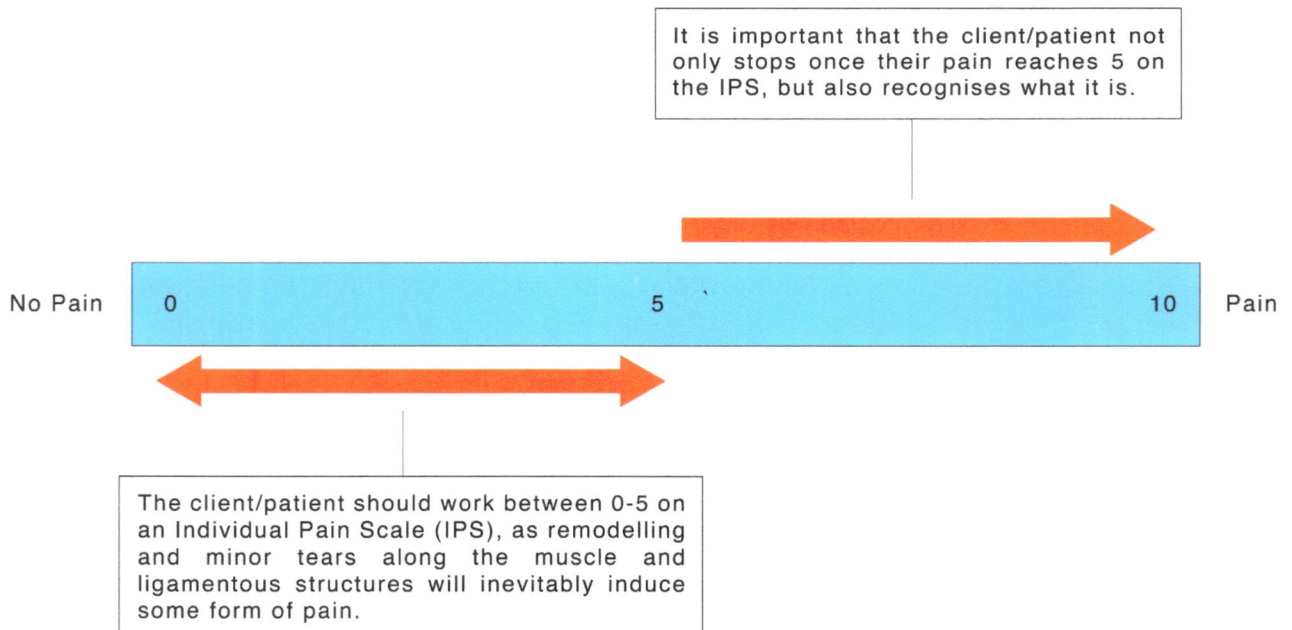

It is important that the client/patient not only stops once their pain reaches 5 on the IPS, but also recognises what it is.

| No Pain | 0 | | 5 | | 10 | Pain |

The client/patient should work between 0-5 on an Individual Pain Scale (IPS), as remodelling and minor tears along the muscle and ligamentous structures will inevitably induce some form of pain.

Figure 20: A representation of how the Individual Pain Scale should be utilised

Consequently, if the experience of being in pain can be approached positively and with the intention of handing the responsibility of recovery back to the client/patient, through the

use of goal setting, motivation and feedback, then they will be less likely to develop a depressive state by suffering with chronic pain. The physiological link between chronic pain and depression is still relatively unknown. However, chronic pain is thought to worsen depression symptoms and is also a risk factor for suicide (National Institute of Health, 2005).

2.7 Learned Helplessness

When a person feels that they have little or no control over the outcome of their lives, they are said to have developed "learned helplessness" (Seligman, 1975). Clients/patients that feel hopeless because their pain has existed for too long, and believe they have tried every form of intervention, will have developed an expectancy to fail. This will inevitably have an affect on their motivation, as they will feel that whatever they do is pointless. Their pessimism towards change will often result in them not practicing or utilising new learnt skills at home or in general life. Where they may view this as the functional intervention not working, it will actually be due to the fact that they are not aiding the process. This falls in line with responsibility for pain, and whose it is. Ultimately the emotional and physical responsibility has to lie with the client/patient, who can be encouraged by the health and fitness professional.

Woolfolk (2013) states that once the effects of learned helplessness (depression, anxiety, lethargic etc.) have developed, they are very difficult to reverse. People who display learned helplessness are often inclined to dispute this, as they are unwilling to accept they have an irrational or maladaptive mentality. They may suggest using techniques such as motivation, goal setting and feedback to reverse the effects. This is because they are effective tools in cognitive reconstruction (Martin & Dahlen, 2005).

Although these client/patients only account for a small proportion of the total number of client/patients that a health and fitness professional may have, they may require a more considered plan of action than the average client/patient, due to their emotional and physical demands. If they do not respond positively to functional training, consider being more deliberate in how

CHAPTER 2.

praise or encouragement is delivered. Initially the Functional Rehabilitative Trainer's mind-set may be driven more towards assessing and correcting the appropriate function, where in fact with clients/patients in a learned helplessness mentality, the emphasis should be on motivation, goal setting and feedback.

At the end of each chapter, each case study and questions will be relevant to the knowledge acquired in the previous chapter(s).

Case Study 2

Another practitioner refers a client/patient to you.

A 49-year old male, initially presented with lower back pain after "over-doing it". The client/patient is a baggage handler at a local airport, where over the past few years he has had numerous lengthy spells off of work due to injuries and pain. He is currently liaising with a union official regarding an injury last year when a bag fell on his foot – it appears non-problematic at present.

The client/patient is clinically obese, which he knows is to do with his diet and lack of activity. Following several treatments, the range of pain free motion improves, however he still complains of pain that he describes as 5-7 on the IPS. He is occasionally chirpy, but the majority of the time he is negative about work, life and his injuries.

On his 4th treatment he mentioned he enjoys coming, as he feels better after, but he has "money problems" and asked if there was anything that can be done. The practitioner suggested a payment plan. During the following treatment he explains that his mother-in-law passed away recently, so he and his wife are selling their house and moving in to her house, as "it's bigger".

He admits he doesn't do any of the stretches or exercises that were recommended, as he's lazy.

The practitioner feels the patient should be more active and that they have done everything they can with manual care, so they refer the client/patient to you.

1. Based on your understanding of schemas, is there anything regarding this client/patient that concerns you and your approach to their care? If so, why?

2. How do you intend to encourage this client/patient to take an active role in their prescribed care?

3. Does this patient's negative attitude and subjective response to pain concern you with respect to on-going care? Please explain your answer.

CHAPTER 2.

Notes

3. Posture & Function

Learning Objectives

- To understand what posture is and what an ideal posture looks like.
- To understand the importance of correct standing posture, as well as being able to correctly and efficiently assess standing posture.
- To understand the proper seated position along with possible implications of poor seated position.
- To understand what neutral spine is and how to teach a person to achieve it.
- To understand upper and lower-crossed postures along with associated muscle involvement.

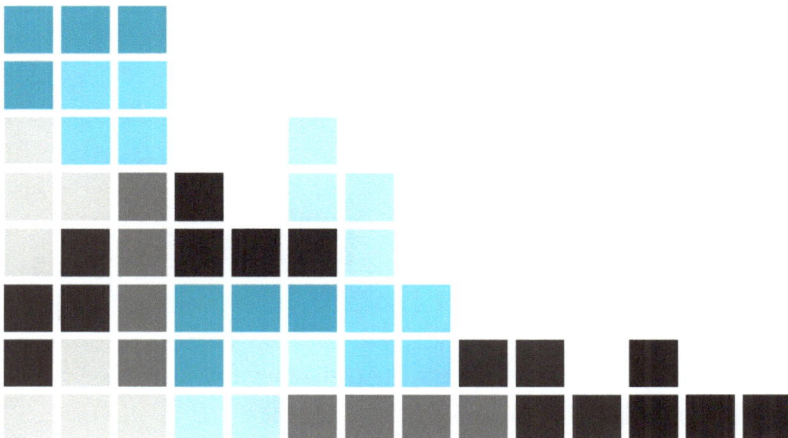

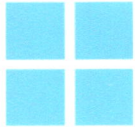

CHAPTER 3.

3.1 Posture

Posture is the position in which your body is held in relation to gravity, whether it be sitting, standing or even lying. A good posture will allow the least amount of strain to be placed upon the supporting musculature and ligaments during weight bearing movements.

An ideal posture will:

• Keep bones and joints correctly aligned
• Decrease the stress placed upon ligaments in the spine
• Reduce the risk of spinal unit restriction
• Decrease the stress on other joints (shoulder, hips, knees etc.)
• Reduce muscle fatigue in postural muscles (QL, Erectus Spinae etc.)
• Promote a good, confident appearance

According to Picard (2012), sitting is the new smoking when it comes to negative affects on health and lifestyle. He makes this suggestion based on work by Wilmot *et al* (2012), who identified that an increased sedentary (sitting) lifestyle time is significantly associated with the risk of diabetes and cardiovascular disease, and consequently premature mortality. This information doesn't conclude anymore than is currently understood through numerous anecdotes, in particular that exercise reduces these risks. However, as the rate of sedentary jobs within the world soars, rising by 83% since 1950 (American Heart Association, 2013), posture and back pain have become significant aspects of working life. Although its importance increases, it is quickly becoming a go-to reason for many healthcare and fitness professionals when diagnosing or surmising a client/patients complaint. The population are demanding more than ever, specific causality and reason as to why they are having complaints. This is due to the ease and accessibility of information from websites and books. If the true reason for a client/patient's complaint is posture, a health and fitness professional should commit to that reason decisively, and then advice can be given based on first-hand knowledge.

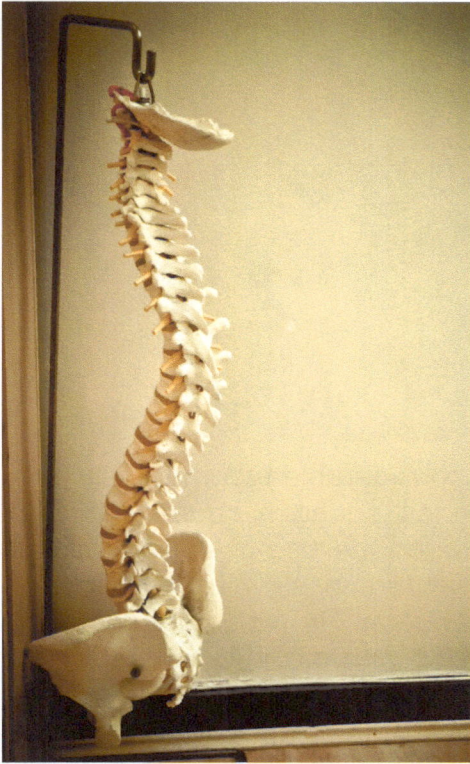

The curves of the spine should be maintained as often as possible

The spine is made up of 33 vertebrae, and all have a vital role in posture, whether it is sitting, standing or lying. Correct posture identifies when the three natural curves of the spine are present, two lordosis' at the cervical (C1-C7) and lumbar spine (L1-L5), and a kyphosis at the thoracic spine (T1-T12). The sacrum (S1-S5) and coccyx (4 fused bones) rest between the pelvic bones (Kendal *et al*, 2005). The spine is designed in such a way to allow a wide variety of movement, but also to act as a spring-like structure, able to absorb shock, provide strength and offer stability against other forces acting upon it from other aspects of the skeleton. Also when correct, the joints of the spine (known as the facet joints) are held in their correct positions, allowing the nerves to freely supply and receive the correct information to and from the body and brain.

When the curves of the spine are lost for a long period of time, the spine becomes more susceptible to degeneration or "wear and tear" due to excess stress being placed upon compensating structures, such as peripheral joints and muscles. Any excessive stress or injury can lead to pain and discomfort around the spine and other associated areas. This may be due to the facet joints becoming restricted, but also because of the subtle weaknesses that develop in various muscle groups offering support to joints, such as the knees and ankles. Steindler in 1955 applied an early concept of mechanical structure (Reuleaux, 1876) to the way in which the human body moves via overlapping segments of joints and soft tissue, which he termed the kinetic chain. An injury or excessive stress on a joint or soft tissue structure would constitute a 'break' within the kinetic chain. Thus potentially reducing the human body's complex performance.

Reuleaux originally used the term kinematic chain to describe a structure rather than a movement. Steindler later changed this to kinetic chain, but also with the additional prefix of open or closed, to categorise exercises. An open kinetic chain (OKC) exercise involves the distal joint of the limb being freely mobile; an example would be a dumbbell bench press. Whereas a closed kinetic chain (CKC) exercise is defined as a condition or environment

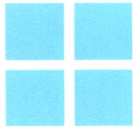

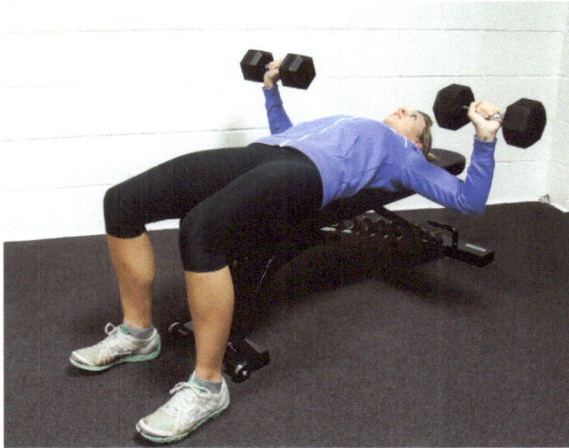

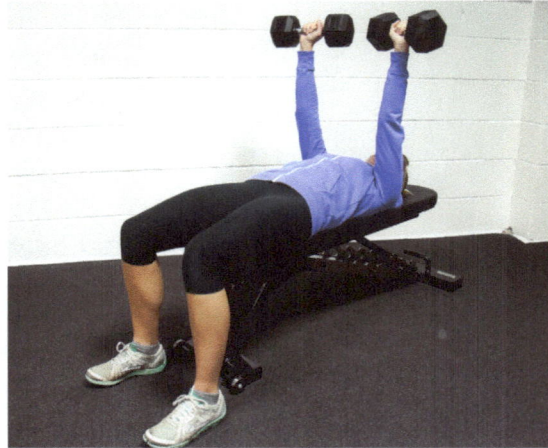

A Dumbbell Bench Press is an example of an open kinetic chain exercise

A Squat is a good example of a closed kinetic chain exercise due to the feet

in which the distal joint meets considerable external resistance and restrains movement, such as during a squat (Steindler, 1955). Di Fabio (1992) discouraged the use of open or closed kinetic chain terms, as he felt it undermines clinical research, as they are not descriptive enough. He uses the example of the isolated knee extension and a squat, whereby both could be viewed as CKC exercises because the lower leg meets considerable external resistance. However one exercise requires the feet to be restrained to the floor and in the other the feet are freely moveable. Although there is ambiguity, realistically in practice it is unnecessary to expand on the definitively correct terminology.

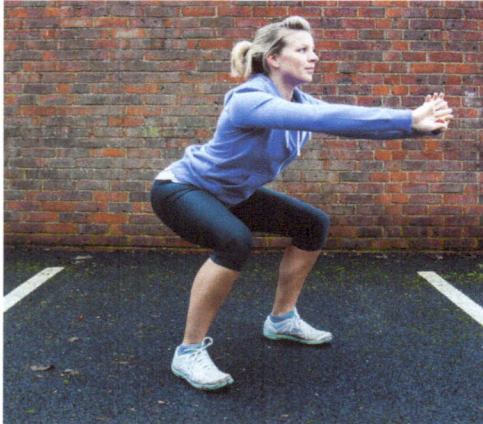

This kinetic chain (Figure 21) is an important aspect when considering postural implications of prolonged sitting, standing and in the performance of routine or sporting movements.

Research indicates that the risk of back pain and injury increases with static work postures that exacerbate poor posture and an increased period of time for which it is held (Andersson, 1997). As a response to this, governing bodies such as the NHS and British Chiropractic Council, plus many others, now advocate some form of physical activity along with stress on ergonomic assessments, and moving frequently if a certain position has been held for a sustained period of time. Throughout this chapter, variations in posture and the implications towards the kinetic chain will be discussed.

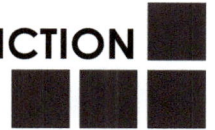

Standing Posture

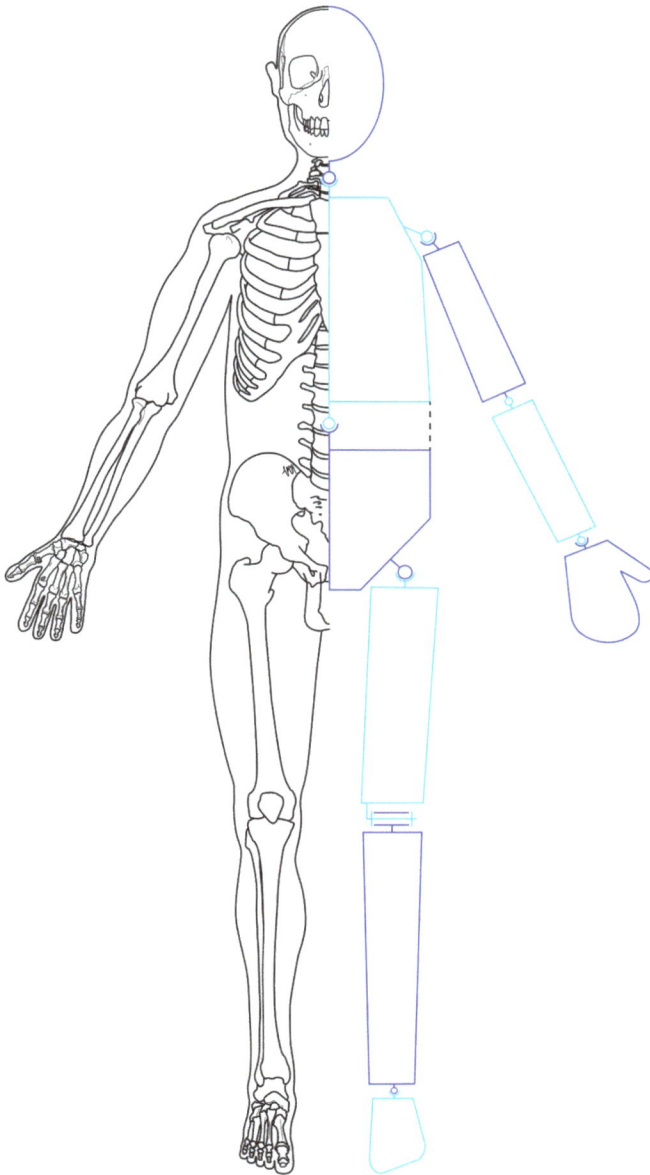

The vast majority of the population understand what it is to have poor posture and will very easily be able to actively demonstrate the general perception of what poor posture is – a slouched, hunched position, which exaggerates the thoracic kyphosis and encourages an anteriorly positioned head. Additionally, a good proportion of the population will also understand the term good posture, and will often demonstrate it by accommodating an upright body position with their chins held up, shoulders depressed and the curves of the spine being well maintained.

Postures that people assume, particularly when standing, are not only a useful tool to aid a health and fitness professional in identifying the condition of the body, with respect to injury or trauma, but also how a person feels about themself – confident, anxious, their enthusiasm etc. People who feel confident, motivated and optimistic will often display a tall posture with their chest out, chin up and a wide stance. In contrast, a person feeling anxious, demotivated and pessimistic may appear to have shifted their weight towards one leg (making them less stable), be looking at the floor with rounded shoulders, and possibly with their arms crossed in front of them (Johnson, 2012).

Figure 21: Demonstrates the human body's kinetic chain

This highlights how posture identifies alignment discrepancies, and also the emotional state of a person.

For example, a patient/client that has a decreasing motivation for a job that they no longer enjoy may demonstrate a less than enthused posture to coincide with their feelings. This may later result in an increasing stress being placed on certain joints,

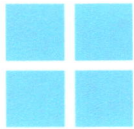

ligaments or muscles, resulting in pain. Consequently, even though they may have been referred for Functional Rehabilitative Training to improve their postural performance, the underlying fact is that they accommodate that particular posture due to something that is out of the health and fitness professionals' control – their demotivating job.

This example highlights the importance of listening to subtle clues when talking to a client/patient. They may not be forthcoming about their feeling towards work, although they may appear unenthusiastic when discussing it during training sessions. If there is suspicion of unrest towards something such as work, home or another aspect of life, then as a professional, approach it sensitively. If the client/patient is not comfortable discussing it, then that decision should be respected. However the importance of asking from a professional perspective to understand a client/ patients lifestyle, can often prove incredibly insightful in better helping the client/patients recovery.

Observation and assessment of posture during a Functional examination should eventually account for a very small proportion of the actual assessment, and should be able to be performed within five minutes. Although quick, the postural aspect of the examination offers vital information towards understanding body position, muscle tone, and even body language. For this reason, and also because of its simplicity, it should be the first part of the Functional Assessment, as it will give the health and fitness professional a brief, but broad overview of the client/patient.

Posture Assessment

The postural assessment is a lot easier to perform if the patient is shirtless, so it is important that the patient feels comfortable and this is done professionally. It may be helpful to have access to a private room in order to perform this. With all client/patients, but females particularly, it is important to explain that it is necessary to gain an understanding of their true posture and if they are uncomfortable in just a bra, advise wearing a sports bra or crop top. If this is dealt with professionally and respectfully there is no reason why it should be uncomfortable for either party. Where possible shorts or tight fitting trousers would also be appropriate to allow anatomical evaluation of the knees and ankles.

Side View
- EAP (external auditory meatus)
- Anterior body of C3 (visualise)
- Shoulder Joint
- Body of L4 (visualise)
- Hip Joint
- Lateral Knee
- Lateral Malleolus

Posterior View
- Mastoid Processes
- Acromion Processes
- Keyholes
- Superior Ridge of Iliac Crest
- Gluteal Folds
- Knee Creases
- Malleolus

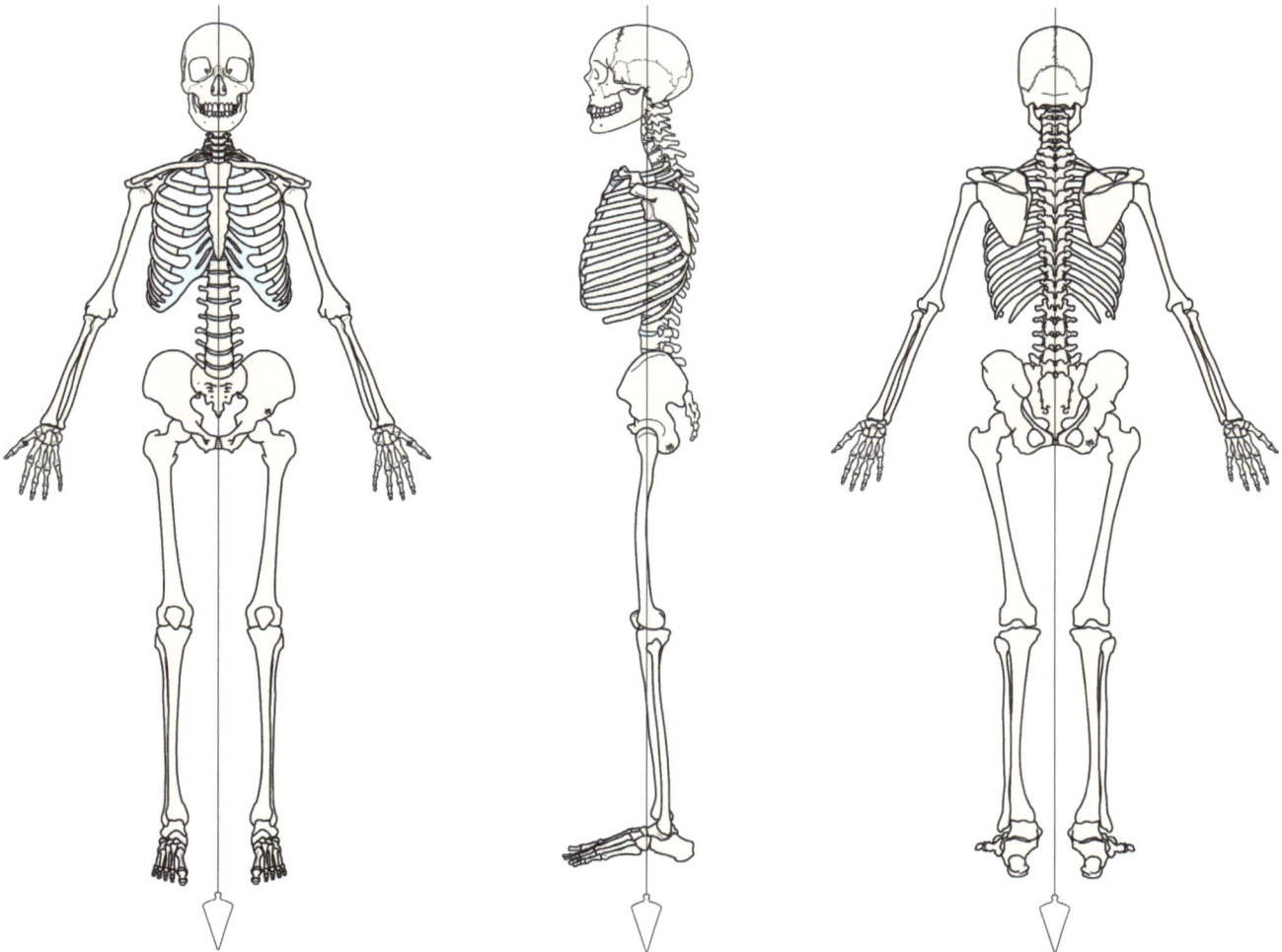

Figure 22: True anatomical position of anterior, side view and posterior skeleton with plumb line

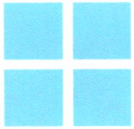

CHAPTER 3.

Posture traditionally is assessed using a plumb line, which technically is a weighted line hanging vertically that lies in front/superimposed on the client/patient through the body via certain points. These points are known as reference points, which on a side and posterior view can be seen in Figure 22.

The more observation on posture is performed, the less reliant the health and fitness professional may become on the plumb line. When practicing, it may prove helpful to use a plumb line and possibly a china body marker to identify key landmarks such as the borders of the scapula or crease of the knee. It is also helpful to have a checklist to refer to and mark against when assessing posture. Knowledge of muscle anatomy and actions is fundamental. Below is a guide to what landmarks should be considered:

Posterior View

1. **Head & Neck**: the head/neck or both may appear laterally deviated to either side, which may indicate a possible tightness in muscles such as the Upper Trapezius, Levator Scapulae and Sternocleidomastoid. This may be evident by the unlevelled appearance of the mastoid processes. A severe deviation with associated pain may be known as torticollis.

2. **Head Rotation**: a rotation of the head to either side may suggest a tightness of the Sternocleidomastoid or Scalene muscles.

3. **Shoulder Level**: by observing the level of the acromion processes it will be apparent as to whether one shoulder is either depressed or elevated. The Levator Scapulae muscles are the prime elevators of the shoulders, although it is usually the more dominant shoulder that is depressed.

4. **Shoulder Bulk**: an increase or decrease in shoulder bulk can provide an indication of overuse or injury. Client/patients involved in jobs that require carrying or lifting heavy objects may display a greater bulk in the Upper Trapezius and Rhomboids. Whereas a client/patient who has suffered with a

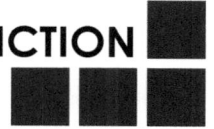

frozen shoulder or had the shoulder immobilised for a period of time may have some wasting of the Supraspinatus and Infraspinatus muscles, due to their reduced activity to stabilise the shoulder.

5. **Scapula Position**: the medial border of the scapula should appear to the same equal distance from the spine as each other. Protraction of the scapula during a static posture may indicate a weakness of the Rhomboids. Quite often it is misinterpreted as the Serratus Anterior being weak, however this is demonstrated by "winging" of the scapula, where the medial inferior angle of the scapula appears to lift away from the rib cage.

6. **Spinal Alignment**: the spine should appear neutral, relaxed and straight. Most people may display a mild functional scoliosis due to muscular tightness. However, a structural scoliosis according to the National Scoliosis Foundation (2013) is only present in 2-3% of the population.

7. **Keyholes**: the space between the client/patients arm and their body is known as the keyhole, and should appear equal bilaterally. An exaggerated or increased keyhole space may indicate tightness within the abductors of the arm, the Upper Trapezius, Supraspinatus or Deltoid.

8. **Skin Creases**: an increased number of skin fold creases around the waist can identify any listing of the upper body towards one side. Possibly indicating tightness of the Quadratus Lumborum.

9. **Iliac Heights**: the iliac crests should appear level, without any rotation. An elevated iliac crest may indicate tightness within the Quadratus Lumborum, whereas a pelvic drop may suggest a weakness of the pelvic stabilisers (Trendelenburg sign), such as the Gluteus Medius or Tensor Fascia Latae.

10. **Gluteal Folds**: the bulk and folds of the gluteal muscles can suggest an under or overuse of the hip extensors. If they are not level this may indicate a tendency to use one more

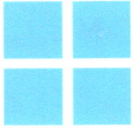

effectively then the other, possibly due to injury.

11. **Genu Varum/Valgus**: bow-legged or knock knees, although a structural deformity, may indicate patterns of muscle weakness and joints susceptible to wear and tear.

12. **Foot Position**: the orientation of the foot can indicate various problems with the foot, knee or hip. If the client/patient is uncomfortable with their feet facing forwards, they can position them to a more comfortable stance. They may turn their foot outwards, suggesting either tightness within the external rotators of the hip or tibial torsion of the tibia. Alternatively, the feet may appear to turn inwards, possibly indicating muscular tightness, tibial torsion or over-pronation.

Side View

1. **Head Position**: the head should be positioned neutrally, displaying no signs of an anterior head carriage. This is associated with the chin jutting forwards or an increase in the cervical lordosis, suggesting either a weakness of the deep neck flexors or a tightness of the neck extensors.

2. **Shoulder Position**: the plumb line should be traced through the deltoid tuberosity, which would indicate a neutral shoulder position. If the shoulders appear anterior to the plumb line it may suggest protraction of the shoulders, which is also a sign of upper-crossed posture caused by tightness of the Pectorals or weakness of the Rhomboids.

3. **Thoracic Spine**: an increased kyphosis at the upper thoracic spine may be a suggestion of an upper-crossed posture or a congenital disease, such as Scheuermann's disease. The thoracic spine may be tender to palpate and the client/patient may have shallow breathing.

4. **Lumbar Spine**: the plumb line should lie through the vertebral body of L4 approximately. Observe the lordosis at the lumbar spine, a loss of lordosis may indicate an over activation of the lumbar extensors such as the Quadratus Lumborum or

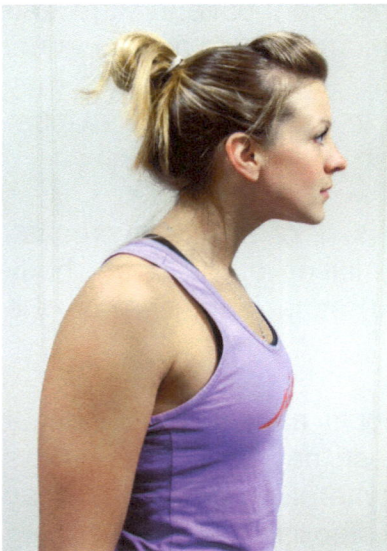

Anterior head carriage or "chin-jutting" is common in todays society

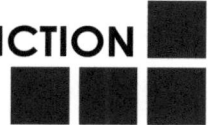

Erectus Spinae muscles.

5. **Knees**: genu recurvatum, a hyperextension of the knees, is often associated with hypermobility either solely in the knees or a generalised hypermobility. If the patient appears to hold a particular knee in flexion though, they may be in pain or discomfort.

The majority of the population in today's sedentary society are walking around with less than perfect postures. The results of the posture assessment may identify certain postural discrepancies. However certain findings may be insignificant. For this reason it is important to identify the relevant information that may need further investigation with the use of other functional tests that will be discussed in later chapters.

Seating Posture

Dainoff (1999) described "sitting" as an erect posture in which the head and the trunk are vertical, the lower legs are bent at 90o at the hips and the knees, and the feet are placed firmly on the floor. Over the past decade, the concept of seated ergonomics has evolved as industrialised countries have become more technologically dependent, which has resulted in more people having sedentary rather than manual jobs.

Posture whilst seated is becoming increasingly important in helping certain populations having a lifestyle free from lower back pain, neck pain, headaches etc. With the stark increase in office based jobs, often demanding up to 8-10 hours sat at a desk per day, and the time spent at desks by children throughout a normal school day, posture, position and duration are valuable considerations to reduce the risks of pain.

Sedentary seated postures develop from birth, as it is one of the first positions we learn as a baby, and with that the ability to control the head, trunk and upper limbs against the force of gravity develops (Wandel, 2000). The seating position itself is generally more relaxing than the standing position due to the loading surface (the gluteal muscles) being greater in size, and

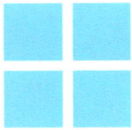

it also allows the muscles in the legs to relax. This translates to meaning that the body expends up to 20% less energy than what it would do standing (Hedge, 2013).

The workplace may have significant effects on the presence of lower back pain, neck pain and headaches, however an appreciation for how detrimental slouching into a soft sofa, or hours playing computer games can have on these complaints is also vital. The ideal goal throughout the day is to maintain the natural curves of the spine during whatever activity is being performed. This will limit any increased demand on the musculature, whether it be the deep neck flexors or the Quadratus Lumborum, to support the loss of curvature. Reducing the static, sustained strain placed on these structures, will aid the prevention of posture-related pain.

Seated posture is not something that needs assessing as part of a Functional Assessment, unless the health and fitness professional feels it may hold some valuable information. The reason why it is not part of the routine is because the posture, as mentioned previously, can be highly subjective dependent upon the environment. This means that clients/patients may modify their posture based on the fact that it is being assessed, as very few people like to feel they are failing, or that the desk they are being assessed at may be different to their set up at work. Figure 23 displays the commonly accepted seated posture and desk set up.

- **Back Support**: should support the natural curves of the spine, including a lumbar support. This will help reduce any strain to the lower back extensors such as the Quadratus Lumborum and Erectus Spinae muscles. If the muscles are held in a constant lengthened state they will inevitably get tight and fatigue. This is in an attempt to maintain the poor posture they are being placed in.

- **Hip & Knee**: the angle of the hips and knees is more commonly advised to be approximately 100-120°, rather than the previously prescribed 90°, as the pressure within the lumbar intervertebral discs will be more equally distributed. The amount of hip flexion available is approximately 60°,

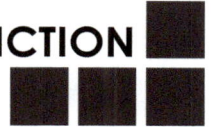

which will obviously vary dependent upon hip mobility among individuals (Schoberth, 1962). If a chair is positioned at a 90° angle, 30° of the flexed movement will be occurring at the lumbar spine, consequently placing the discs under unnecessary pressure posteriorly.

- **Feet Position**: both feet should be firmly placed flat on the ground, or a foot rest if required. The weight should be evenly distributed between the two also to avoid putting undue stress through one side of the pelvis and lower back.

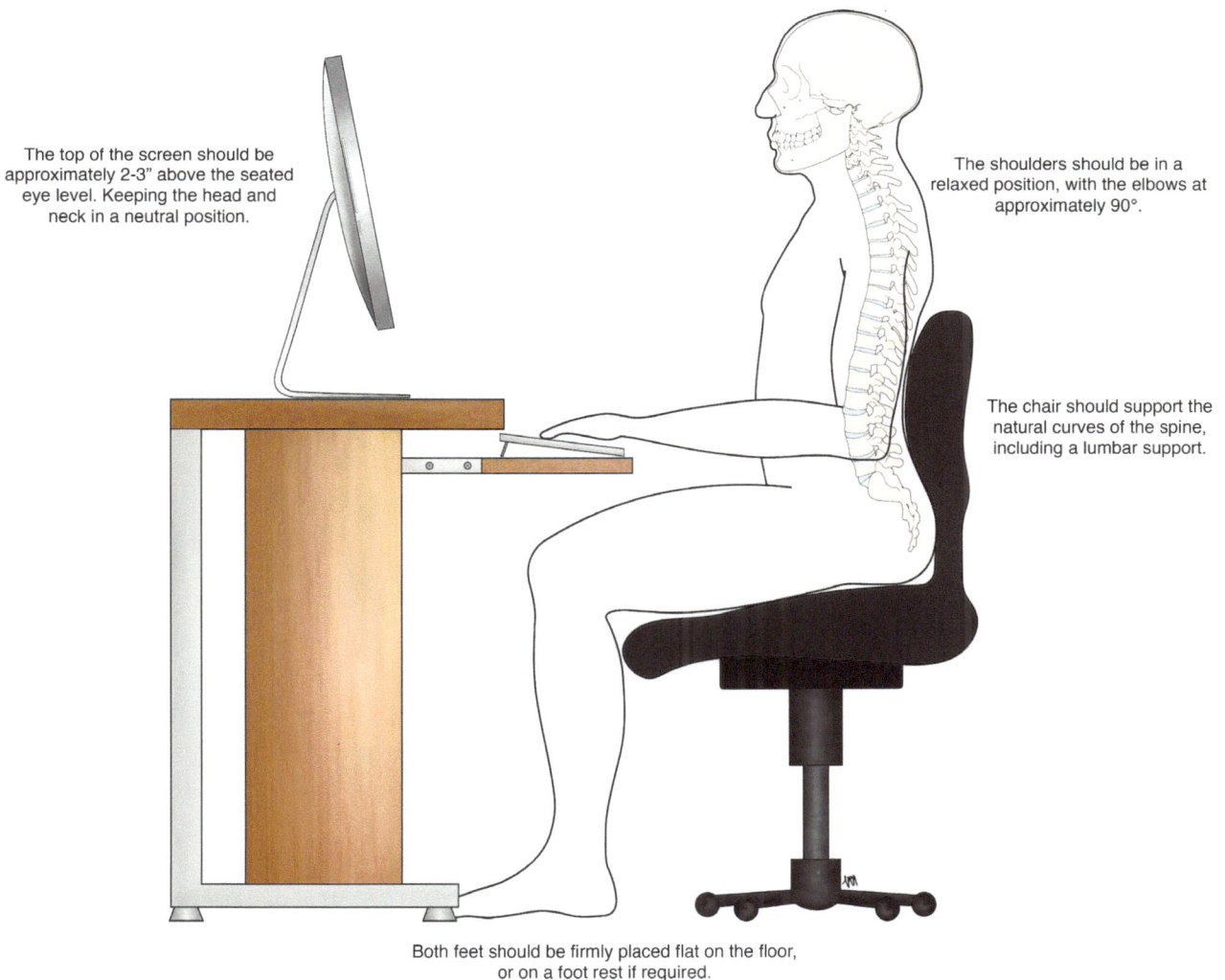

The top of the screen should be approximately 2-3" above the seated eye level. Keeping the head and neck in a neutral position.

The shoulders should be in a relaxed position, with the elbows at approximately 90°.

The chair should support the natural curves of the spine, including a lumbar support.

Both feet should be firmly placed flat on the floor, or on a foot rest if required.

Figure 23: Correct anatomical seated posture

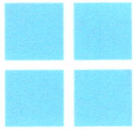

- **Shoulder & Elbow Position**: the shoulders should appear in a relaxed position with the elbows at approximately 80-90°. There should be no evidence of upper-crossed posture or elevation of the shoulders. To limit the possibility of sustaining a repetitive strain injury in the wrists, the keyboard should be placed between four to six inches away from the front of the desk, and centred to the body.

- **Wrists**: carpal tunnel is one of the commonly associated complaints with excessive typing, due in part to the angle at which the wrists are positioned, but also due to the hard surface that the wrists are placed on. For this reason, a wrist rest is often advised to alleviate any pressure on the wrists when resting between typing. It is also advised to place the mouse as close as possible to the keyboard.

- **Monitor Position**: the monitor should be positioned approximately an arms length away from the client/patient, with the top of the screen approximately 2-3" above the seated eye level. This will help keep the head and neck in a neutral position without the over-activation of the neck extensors, thus reducing any excess mechanical stress.

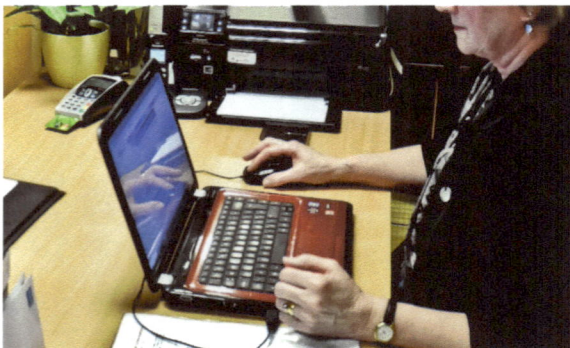

The majority of companies in today's industrialised world, and particularly corporate groups, undertake ergonomic assessments regularly to optimise working positions for their employees. However, it is up to the employee's to enforce the advice from the assessments and from healthcare and fitness professionals. It is very easy for any person to become consumed by the work they are being tasked with. For this reason, the advice is to use some form of subconscious 'trigger' to remind a client/patient to be aware of their posture whilst seated.

Ergonomic assessments can be arranged by compnaies

Below are some 'Postural Triggers' that have been developed with this in mind. The phrases can be placed on a Post-it note or something similar, and positioned within the client/patients peripheral vision whilst sitting at the computer monitor. There are brief instructions for each phrase:

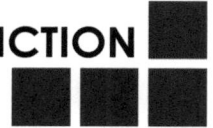

"Draw Shoulders Back" – *sitting up straight in your chair, roll your shoulders forwards as far as possible, and then backwards as far as possible, then find the place mid-way between the two positions. Keep the shoulders low throughout, trying to not let them rise up towards your ears. Hold the mid-way position for 30 seconds.*

"Move Your Head" – *Sitting up straight in your chair, move your head through all ranges of motion in a controlled fashion. Starting with dropping the chin downwards towards the chest, then looking up to the ceiling, look over both shoulders, and finally drop each ear down towards the same shoulder. Repeat the process 3 times.*

"Tuck Your Chin In" – *sitting up straight, place your fingers lightly into the muscle either side of your windpipe, at the front of the neck. Draw your chin backwards, as if trying to give yourself a double chin, until you feel the muscles tighten beneath your fingers. Hold that contraction for 30 seconds.*

"Get Up & Get a Drink" – *As well as giving your eyes a break from the screen, the general consensus is that adequate hydration aids the brain's ability to function efficiently. So get up and get yourself a drink.*

Ultimately the overall goal of reducing the risk of injury is achieved through the use of correct posture, by maintaining the natural curves of the spine, whilst not remaining in a particular position for too long. This will inevitably result in a healthier, more balanced workload between the involved muscles.

Neutral Spine

The constant use of the phrase "maintain neutral spine" by various health and fitness professionals over the years has made it one of the most applicable and generally understood phrases in the battle against lower back pain. On reflection the concept of maintaining a neutral or ideal spinal position may have been around for decades, even centuries. However, the theory was only written about and described in the early 90's. Panjabi (1992),

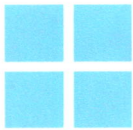

explained how the stabilisation of the spine was very much dependent upon three "subsystems". Firstly a passive subsystem, made up of the vertebrae, discs and ligaments. Secondly, all the muscles and tendons surrounding the joints of the spine that can apply force to the spine, these make up the active subsystem. Finally, the nerves and central nervous system define the neural subsystem, which monitors and directs the stabilisation of the active subsystem upon the passive subsystem.

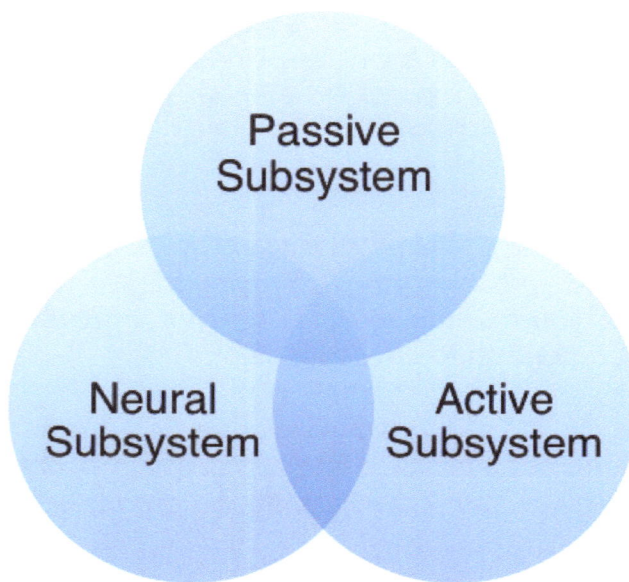

The three subsystems (Figure 24) are interdependent on each other, meaning that if one fails, the other subsystems will compensate immediately in order to reduce the amount of stress on the already dysfunctional subsystem, decreasing the risk of further damage. This may however result in long-term adaptation across the three interdependent subsystems – an aspect that has to be considered when training a client/patient functionally. The client/patient may have had their dysfunction for a period of time, which may result in the true "original" complaint being masked by the compensatory aches and pains.

Figure 24: Panjabi (1992) described three "subsystems" that stabilise the spine

Panjabi (1992) followed on from the original function and dysfunction work, by suggesting the 'neutral zone' was the "region of intervertebral motion around the neutral posture where little resistance is offered by the passive spinal column". He proposed that an increased stress upon the vertebrae, discs and ligaments (passive subsystem) may result in injury to the spinal column, consequently causing possible muscle weakness, instability or lower-back pain.

This implies that in order for the spine to function efficiently with minimal risk by maintaining the physiological boundaries of motion, the spinal stabilising system, made up of the three subsystems, must adjust around its physical demands.

The primary method by which this is achieved is by training the strength and endurance capabilities provided by the active subsystem of the spine. In order for a client/patient to appreciate the neutral zone range, they must first understand how to find, hold and maintain a neutral spine, so that it can be later applied to strenuous, load-based motion.

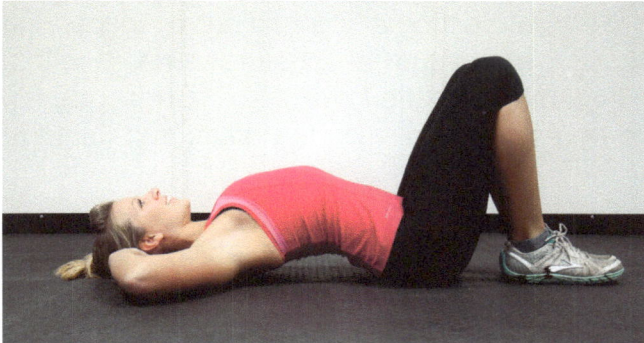

The position of neutral spine needs to be recognised by both the client/patient and the health and fitness professional. Often the most significant aspect of the neutral spine position, much like seated posture, is the position of the pelvis in relation to anterior and posterior pelvic tilt. Images to the left of the page depict how to find the position of neutral spine.

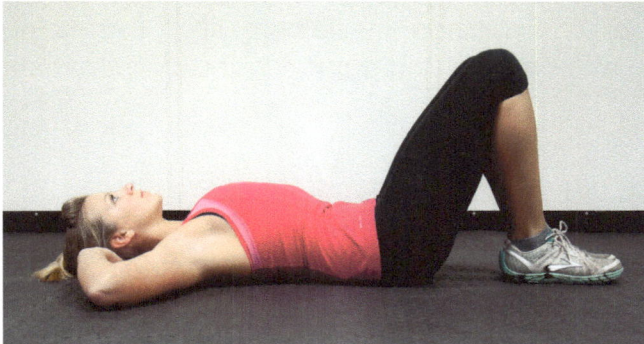

1. Lying supine, with both the hips and knees in a flexed position, and the head rested upon the floor, the upper thoracic kyphosis, shoulders and gluteal muscles should be in contact with the floor.

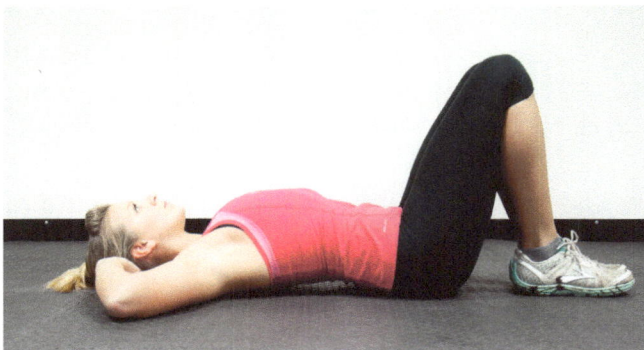

2. The pelvis should be then slowly tilted as far forwards (anteriorly) as possible, increasing the lordosis at the lumbar spine.

3. Then the pelvis should be tilted as far backwards (posteriorly) as possible, flattening the lower part of the back into the floor.

4. Then finally the comfortable position between the two extremes should be found. This position correctly identifies neutral spine.

Finding neutral spine: tilt pelvis forwards (top), tilt pelvis backwards (middle), comfortable neutral spinal position (bottom)

Once the position of neutral spine has been found and an understanding of how to maintain it is achieved, then the position can be adapted to normal and dynamic motions during activities, such as standing up from a seated position,

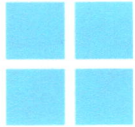

brushing teeth stood over a sink, and even sporting movements such as running. Ultimately, holding the pelvis and spine in a neutral position will encourage the stability and strength of the core and torso muscles to better control the passive subsystem of the vertebrae, ligaments and discs.

Plowman (1992) summarises the importance of maintaining a neutral spine, particularly with sitting and standing, by identifying how a posterior pelvic tilt increases the postural tension within the musculature and ligaments of the lower back. Consequently putting excessive compressive forces on the discs and joints of the spine.

The spine is designed to move in all ranges, including flexion, extension, rotation and lateral flexion. The encouraged use of the neutral spine position during mundane activities such as sitting at a desk, driving a car or riding a bike, will help preserve the spine's ability to move. This will increase its durability, by reducing sustained flexion or extension of the spine, as the client/patient ages.

3.2 Upper & Lower Crossed Postures

Upper and lower-crossed postures provide the basic foundation to muscular imbalance, and will often provide a platform to more unique, specific musculoskeletal dysfunctions. Although muscle imbalance can occur in the absence of either an upper or lower-crossed posture, an already weak, or unbalanced structure as a result of faulty postural position, will often harbour other symptoms as a result of repetitive faulty movement.

An example of this would be patellofemoral pain syndrome, more commonly known as runner's knee, whereby the patella fails to track through the femoral groove due to muscular imbalance between the Vastus Lateralis and the Vastus Medialis Oblique. One potential explanation for this may be due to an anterior or posterior pelvic tilt affecting the anatomical positioning of the hip joint. An excessive anterior pelvic tilt may result in an externally rotated hip joint, and on the reverse side of that, an excessive posterior pelvic tilt might promote an internally rotated hip joint.

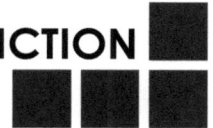

Both of these will affect their respective muscles, causing either a weakness or tightness along the kinetic chain, affecting more and more structures, often in a distal fashion, from the original source of dysfunction as time progresses.

Janda (1988) is credited with the early work on upper and lower-crossed postures. His work is often seen as the pioneering step towards understanding and appreciating muscular imbalance, and has been used by clinicians over the years to predict patterns of tightness and weakness.

Upper-Crossed Posture (UCP)

One of the most common demonstrations of muscular imbalance can be seen in a person with an upper-crossed posture. Its popularity within the society, particularly in developed countries, is a representation of how easily and diversely it can progress. Affecting people from sedentary working postures, eager misinformed gym users and the elderly, this form of postural muscle imbalance is ever-present.

It is simply the weakening and lengthening of the posterior muscle chain including the upper back and neck muscles, with the combined tightening and shortening of the anterior antagonists, such as the Pectorals and deep neck flexors. This results in a postural position often referred to as a 'humpback' or 'chin jutting' posture. Although there may appear to be increased kyphosis, it may not always be structural in nature, as tightness within the pectorals, both major and minor, may cause a dramatic rounding of the shoulders, which will typically exacerbate a functional thoracic kyphosis. This form of kyphosis will often be seen in a person that has a sedentary, desk-bound lifestyle or a gym user avidly partaking in too many chest exercises.

Whereas structural thoracic rigidity is more likely to be seen among the older population, it may have started as a functional thoracic kyphosis that has slowly progressed through the process of degeneration to a rigid structural position. At this stage, the postural position is often irreversible, and may also impair the client/patient's ability to breathe as the sternum may become

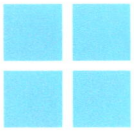

depressed. This means that any identification and consequent training to oppose an upper-crossed posture at a young age can help tremendously in the prevention of the upper-crossed posture developing to a structural problem.

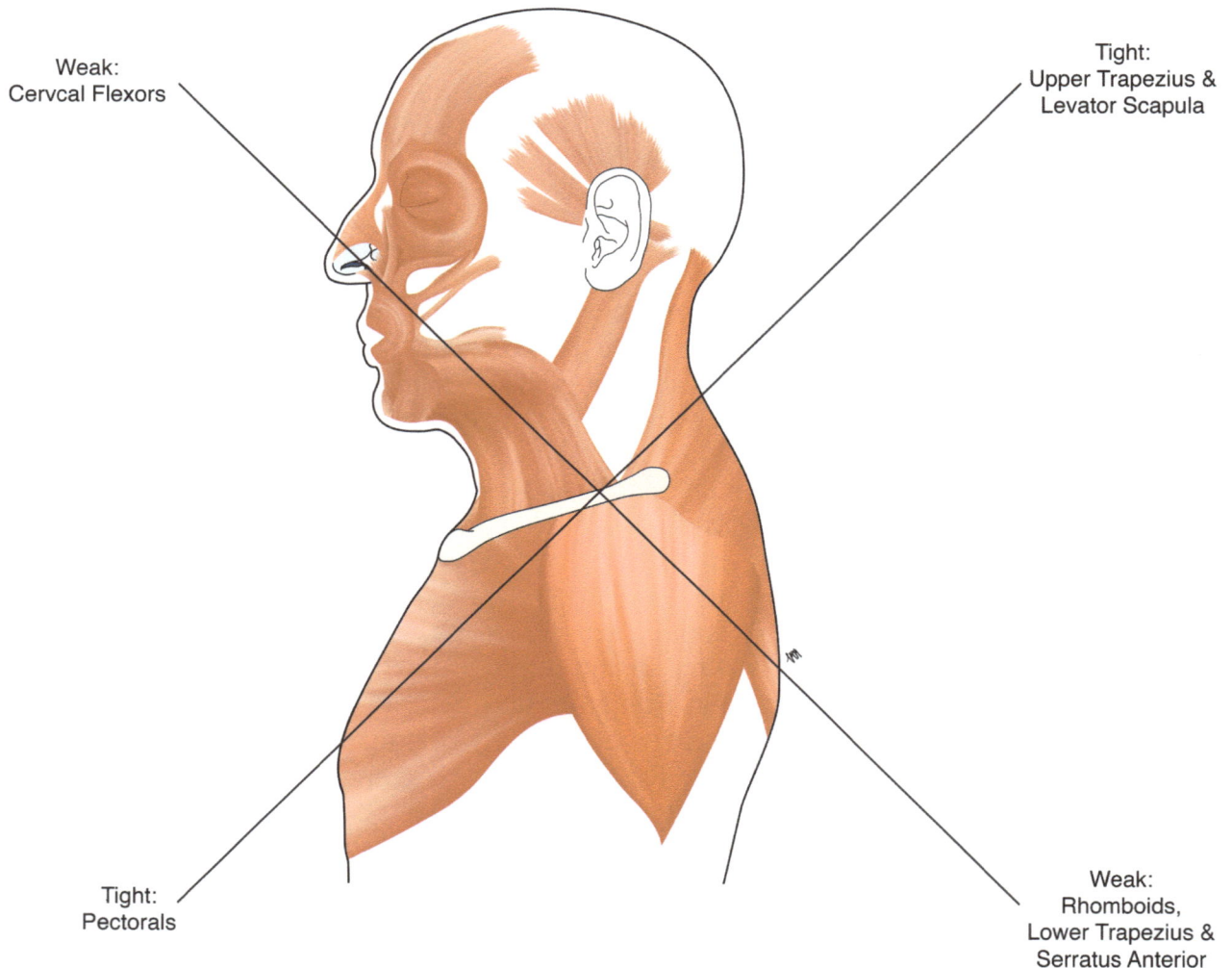

Weak:
Cervcal Flexors

Tight:
Upper Trapezius &
Levator Scapula

Tight:
Pectorals

Weak:
Rhomboids,
Lower Trapezius &
Serratus Anterior

Figure 25: Demonstrates the weak and tight muscles often found with upper-crossed posture

Upper-crossed posture, more specifically can be characterised by short tightening of the Upper Trapezius, Levator Scapulae, Sternocleidomastoid, and Pectorals muscles, combined with a weakness of the deep neck flexors, Lower Trapezius, Rhomboids and Serratus Anterior muscles (Figure 25). Postural changes that can be observed with an upper-crossed posture will include an anterior head carriage, increased cervical lordosis and thoracic kyphosis, protracted shoulders with rotation/abduction and winging of the scapulae.

Janda (1988) suggested that these maladaptive postural changes decrease the stability of the glenohumeral joint. This was based on the thought that the glenoid fossa became more vertical (anatomical position is lateral and mildly superior) as a result of weakness in the Levator Scapulae, thus creating protraction and winging of the scapula. He led on to propose that the loss of stability around the glenohumeral joint forced muscles such as the Levator Scapulae and Upper Trapezius to work excessively in order to maintain the central position of the humerus within the joint.

The rotator cuff muscles control stability at the shoulder, which includes the Supraspinatus and Infraspinatus, Teres Minor and Subscapularis (Honeybourne *et al*, 2000). These will provide little resistance against the stronger muscles such as the Upper Trapezius and Pectoral muscles. Consequently this results in a loss of stability at the joints of the shoulder, caused by an upper-crossed posture.

Due to the location of the origins and insertions of the involved musculature, other joints may be affected, possibly becoming restricted. These include the atlanto-occipital joint, lower cervical joints, cervico-thoracic junction and mid thoracic joints. The client/patient may require some form of manual treatment as well as Functional Rehabilitative Training to improve the mobility at any restricted joints.

Lower-Crossed Posture (LCP)

The anatomical position associated with a lower-crossed posture is much more difficult to observe in general life, as well as being less common than the upper-crossed posture. It involves however, an imbalance in the muscles surrounding the lower back and pelvic girdle. Like the upper-crossed posture, lower-crossed posture is more prominent in developed countries and is often related to poor seated or standing posture.

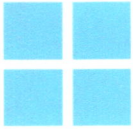

CHAPTER 3.

Weak:
Abdominal
Muscles

Tight:
Erector Spinae

Tight:
Iliopsoas &
Rectus Femoris

Weak:
Gluteus Maximus

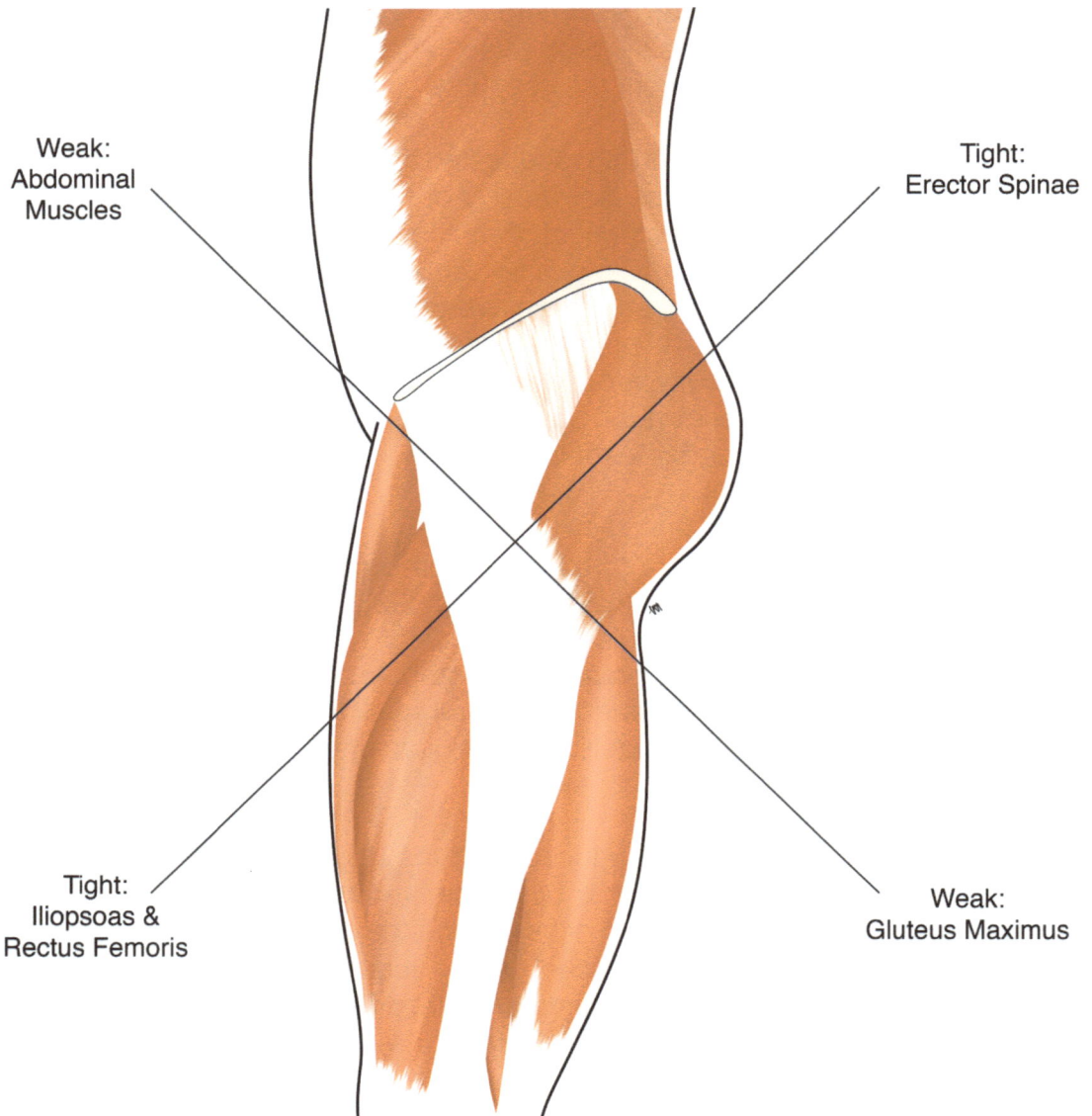

Figure 26: Demonstrates the weak and tight muscles often found with lower-crossed posture

A lower-crossed posture (Figure 26) is defined by tightness through the Erectus Spinae and Quadratus Lumborum, Paraspinals, Rectus Femoris and Iliopsoas muscles, in combination with a weakness of the Abdominal, Gluteus Medius and Gluteus Maximus muscles. This imbalance results in either a posterior pelvic tilt or an anterior pelvic tilt, dependent upon which of the tight groups of muscle are more dominant. A deep and short lumbar lordosis would suggest an imbalance dominated by the

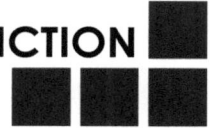

pelvic musculature, such as the Iliopsoas and Rectus Femoris. Whereas, a shallow, extended lordosis would indicate tightness more dominantly in the Erectus Spinae and Quadratus Lumborum muscles.

Janda (1987) identified these two separate variations of a lower-crossed posture, shown in Figure 27. Posture A, demonstrates a lower-crossed posture with an increased lumbar lordosis, anterior pelvic tilt and slight flexion at both the hip and the knee. This increased lordosis and anterior pelvic tilt can increase the amount of pressure placed upon the intervertebral discs, and also place excess compression on the facet joints of the lumbar spine, both contributing factors in the development of lower back pain. Also associated with posture A is an increase in the thoracolumbar kyphosis, which may often cause the Erectus Spinae muscles to become tender. The neck and head position is often not involved.

Posture B is identified by the loss of lumbar lordosis (flat back), as a result of a posterior pelvic tilt. This is most commonly related to the tightness in the Quadratus Lumborum dominating the client/ patients 'normal' pelvic position, as opposed to being dominated by the Iliopsoas in posture A. There may also be an associated upper-crossed posture observed with posture B, including an anterior head carriage and increased thoracic kyphosis (Janda, 1987), as well as possible hyperextension of the knees. There will be marked hypotonicity and reduced mass of the gluteal muscles, particularly the Gluteus Maximus. The dominant activity of the Quadratus Lumborum makes it susceptible to fatigue and spasm, which along with the increased compression on the vertebral discs (Plowman 1992), can cause lower back pain from various origins. The imbalance between the Quadratus Lumborum and gluteal muscles, can leave the lower lumbar and sacro-iliac joints vulnerable to injury due to the unequal strength and force being offered by the two muscles.

The correction of either an upper or lower-crossed posture is a process that may take time and repetition. The muscles involved have probably become accustomed to the position they are in, and although not working as efficiently as they could and placing unnecessary stress on other structures, will prove

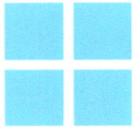

Thoracolumbar hyperkyphosis

Lumbar hyperlordosis

Anterior pelvic tilt

Slight hip flexion

Slight knee flexion

Type A

Head protraction

Thoracic hyperkyphosis

Lumbar hypolordosis

Knee recurvatum

Type B

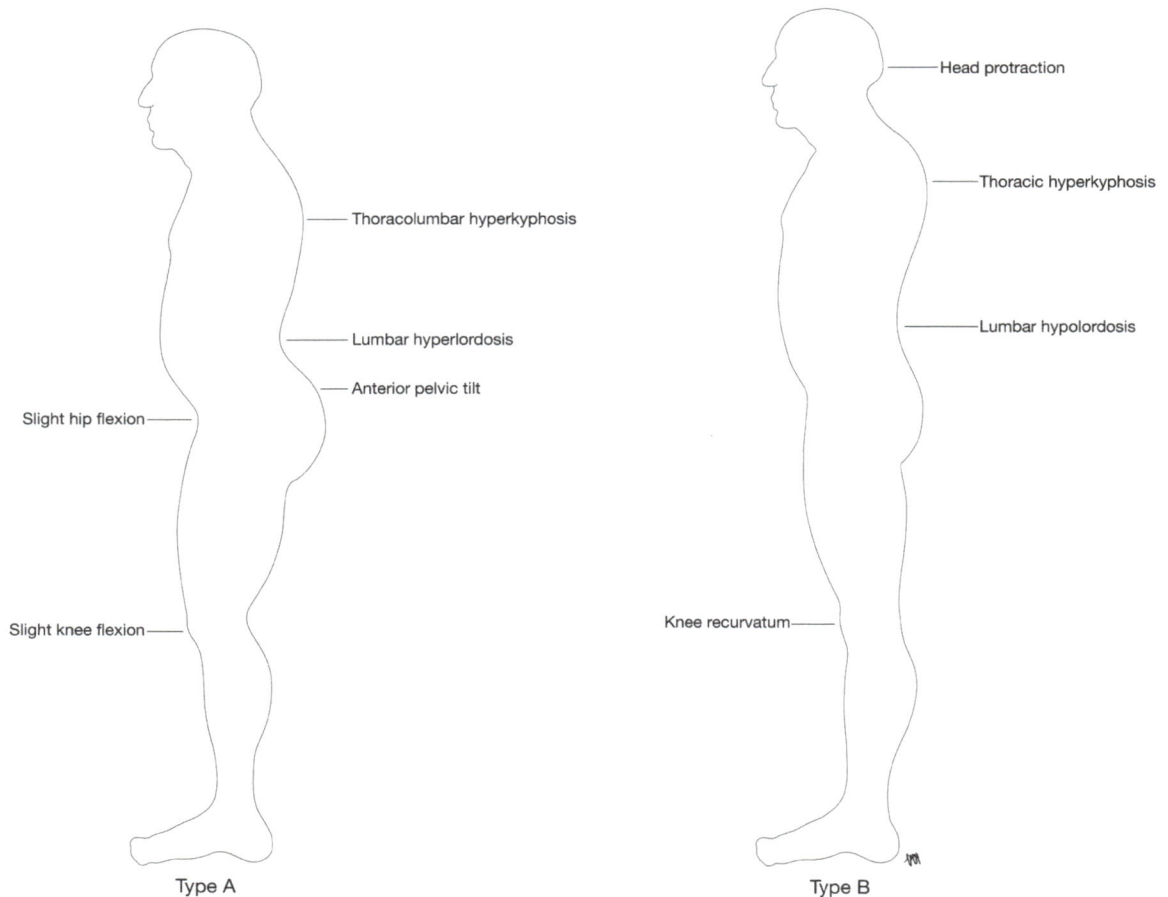

Figure 27: Two variations of a lower-crossed posture, A and B

difficult to correct. It will involve a combination of strength training for the involved weak muscles, routine stretching for the tight muscles involved and persistent motivation for the client/patient. A consideration for the psychological characteristics of the individual will be important, as this form of training is a lifestyle change that will require constant reinforcement.

Upper and lower-crossed postures can take a considerable amount of time until any effects of training are noticed. They develop from poor repetitive positioning or posture in daily life. By encouraging and aiding a change in the poorly accommodated daily movements, such as standing or sitting position, the way in which something is lifted, or a specific repetitive movement, a significant improvement in the work load balance between the involved muscles will be noticed, thus reducing the risk of injury.

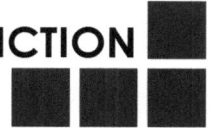

At the end of each chapter, each case study and questions will be relevant to the knowledge acquired in the previous chapter(s).

Case Study 3

A 37-year old male computer programmer presents to you. He has had years of niggling neck and lower back discomfort. He states that he has never really done any serious exercise in the past. He believes that doing something active might help him with his posture, especially with work, where he finds himself sat in front of a computer for hours on end. He has also recently become a father and wants to ensure he is healthy and in good shape so that he can enjoy spending time with his family.

He is a 6'2 and weighs approximately 76kg.

You decide that to understand this client/patient's postural and muscular control, it would be best to first perform a posture assessment. You discover:

- An anterior head carriage
- Obvious rounding of the shoulders
- The right shoulder appears to be slightly elevated
- Thoracic spine appears hyperkyphotic, without any lateral deviation
- There is a loss of lumbar lordosis
- Gluteals bilaterally appear hypotonic
- And you notice a mild flattening of the arches in the feet

The client/patient is keen to get started and appears willing to listen to your advice, as he is "completely new to this".

1. Using all of your knowledge, list all the muscles that you would consider to be weak/underactive in this client/patient?

2. Based on the above findings, would you consider this client/patient to have a postural issue? Please explain your answer.

3. List and explain three exercises that can be utilised to rehabilitate this client/patient?

4. Are there any other lifestyle factors that could be addressed with this client/patient?

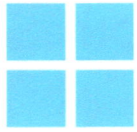

CHAPTER 3.

Notes

4. Core Stability

Learning Objectives

- To understand and appreciate what core stability is, and the muscles that are involved to produce it.
- To understand how core stability is activated, as well as internal and external triggers that stimulate core stability.
- To understand the difference between core and trunk, and their implications.
- To appreciate a difference between strength and stability of the core and/or trunk, with relevant contextual meaning.
- To understand what trunk endurance is, and how to appropriately test it.
- To understand and teach an abdominal brace and hollowing, whilst appreciating a difference between the two.

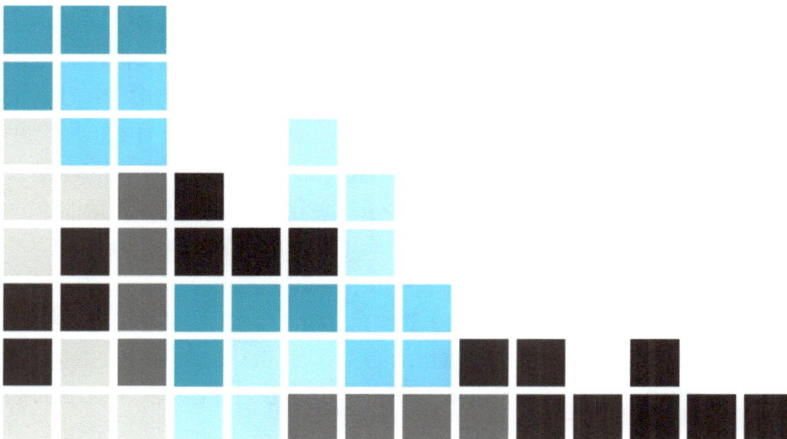

4.1 Core Strength & Stability

Unfortunately the term "core stability" has in recent years started to lose value and merit. It is possible that the concept has become a victim of its own success, as its increased use in varying professions, means that in some of the more misinformed professional arenas, the concept has become involved in its own game of 'Chinese Whispers'. Constantly being passed from one misinformed individual to another, with the concept being slightly modified at each stage. With this having gone on since the original conceptual framework was apparently suggested by Kendall in the early 1950's, it is apparent the more recent generations of professionals qualifying in medicine, alternative therapies, fitness and ergonomics, are becoming increasingly confused with what constitutes the concept of core stability. The over prescription of varying exercises, clinically in the past 20 years, involving static, isometric, plyometric, rotational or contraindicated exercises, identifies how the general perception of core stability training is predominantly misunderstood.

Fundamentally, core stability is the ability to effectively recruit the muscles of the 'core' or trunk together, to provide support and control to the spine and pelvis, especially during movement. (MacKenzie, 2003). The first aspect of that definition recognises that all of the muscles of the trunk should contract together, including the Transversus Abdominis, Rectus Abdominus, Erectus Spinae, Multifidus, Oblique's, the Diaphragm and Pelvic Floor muscles. The combined contraction of these muscles creates an effect similar to that of a corset (Figure 28), increasing the intra-abdominal pressure (Kibler *et al*, 2006). However, Mens *et al* (2006) suggested that a raised intra-abdominal pressure might have detrimental effects on clients/patients already suffering with pelvic pain. It may be difficult to identify true pelvic girdle pain, particularly with the potential of referred pain from the structures and muscles of the lower back, such as the facet joints, Quadratus Lumborum or Erectus Spinae.

The corset-like contraction of the trunk muscles to gain stability of the lower back and pelvis indicates that to achieve stability, there is no flexion, extension or rotation of the spine. However,

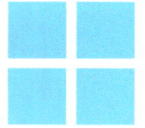

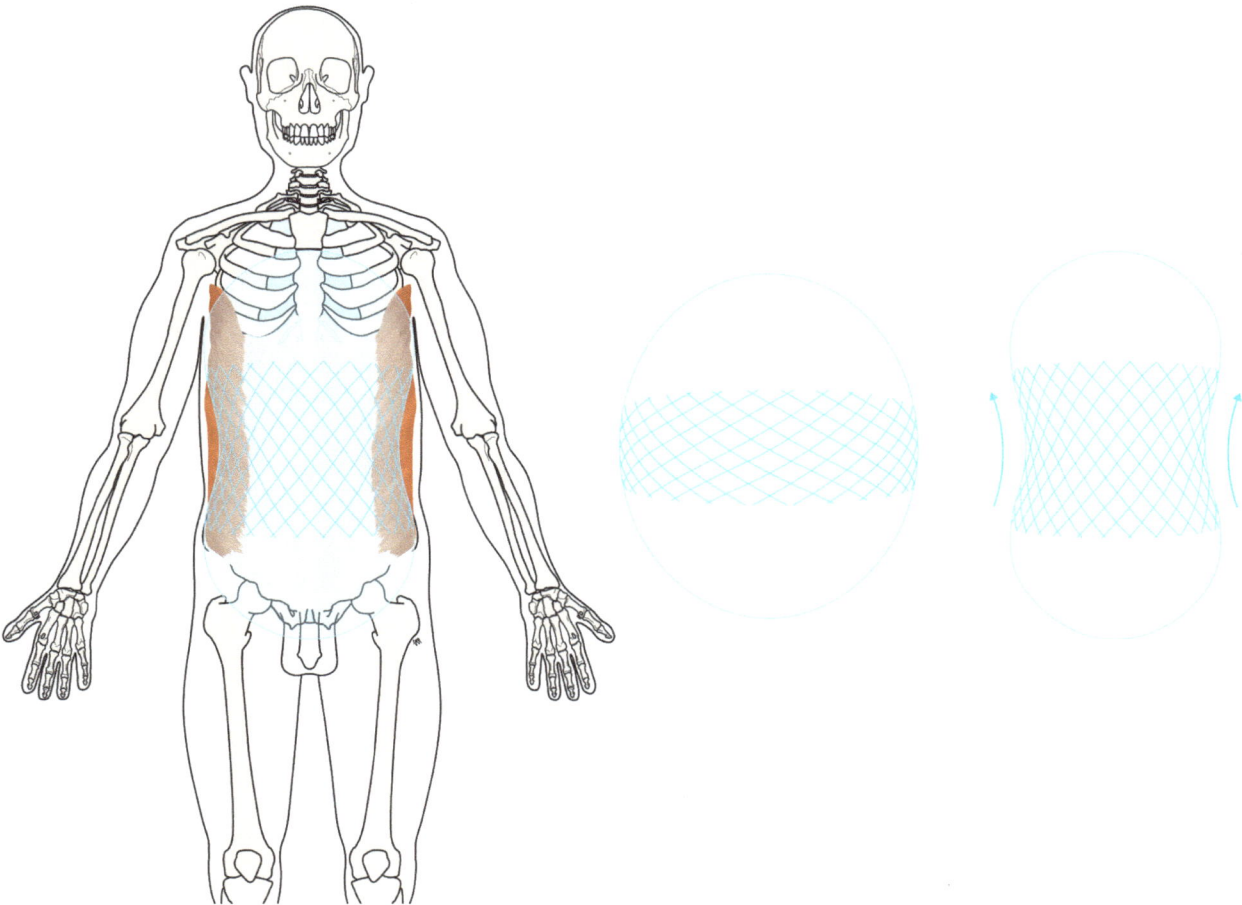

Figure 28: The intra-abdominal pressure is increased by combined contraction of the trunk muscles - acting like a corset

the majority of prescribed exercises for core stability involve either one of these movements or multiple planes of movement. For example, a sit up or dorsal raise involves the spine moving through flexion or extension, respectively. Based on what has already been discussed, core stability involves the co-contraction of numerous muscles, rather than a movement dominated by a single muscle. This suggests that the 'core stabilising' specific part of a sit up or dorsal raise, actually lies in the bracing of the trunk in preparation for movement.

Hodges and Richardson (1996) identified that the muscles of the trunk, more specifically the Transversus Abdominis and Multifidus, activated prior to the prime mover of the limb with movement. Suggesting that the muscles of the trunk act in anticipation of dynamic movement to provide stability to the spine and pelvis, thus to maintain balance. They expanded on this by suggesting it may be a mechanism provided by the central nervous system. This would in fact allude to the theory that the activation of the trunk muscles is very similar to that of an innate reflex, such as the stretch reflex, rather than a voluntary muscle contraction.

A delayed onset in activation of the Tranversus Abdominis has been exhibited in patients suffering which chronic lower back pain when asked to perform rapid arm/leg movements (Hodges & Richardson, 1998). This may be a result of damage to the lumbar fascia, impaired nervous conduction to the muscle, or even a mechanism specifically designed to limit further damage to the lower back (Lederman, 2009).

Based on the evidence suggesting activation timing differences in the Transversus Abdominis being approximately 20Ms (one fiftieth of a second) between asymptomatic and chronic lower back pain patients, Lederman hypothesized that the timings are "beyond the patients conscious control" and thus not susceptible to improvement (Radebold *et al*, 2000). Although he may be correct in identifying that the timings may have a subconscious origin, it is also understood from Learning and Conditional Behaviour (Chapter 2.2), that subconscious control can be modified through learnt experiences.

4.2 Core Activation & Stimuli

The activation of the core muscles to contract and provide stability to the spine and pelvis, as previously mentioned, may be subject to an event similar to a reflex. However, it is commonly theorised that client/patients suffer lower back pain as a result of having poor core stability, but how would this be possible if indeed the stabilisation of the spine is subject to an innate reflex? The core would be constantly contracting to stabilise the spine and pelvis against causes of lower back pain, which according to the NHS (2013), are repetitive movements, such as lifting and bending, and static positions, such as sitting at a desk or driving for too long a period. Thus reducing the prevalence of lower back pain all together.

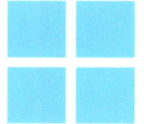

As it is understood, a reflex is an action performed without conscious thought in response to a stimulus, like the stretch reflex during a knee jerk (Figure 29). There are numerous variations of reflexes such as the Withdrawal Reflex, whereby a reflex in response to a damaging stimulus removes the body from potential danger. An example of this can be seen when the hand touches something hot, and the hand quickly withdraws in response to the stimulus.

Another variation of a reflex is the Arthrokinetic Reflex, first identified in 1956. This refers to the way in which the movement of a joint can cause muscle activation and/or inhibition via a reflex (Cohen & Cohen). Although there is evidence that the Tranversus Abdominis and Multifidus activate prior to the prime limb mover, it is still unclear as to whether they activate in response to joint movement of the lower back. This reflex has recently been suggested as having useful implications in understanding chronic lower back pain and improving sports performance. There is also an assumption that whiplash injuries are significantly reduced if a person is asleep during the accident. This would in fact oppose the Arthrokinetic Reflex theory, as there would be joint movement occurring without any activity from the muscles. With theories regarding reflexes' stimuli being explored in forthcoming years, vision and schema may also be other stimuli to consider.

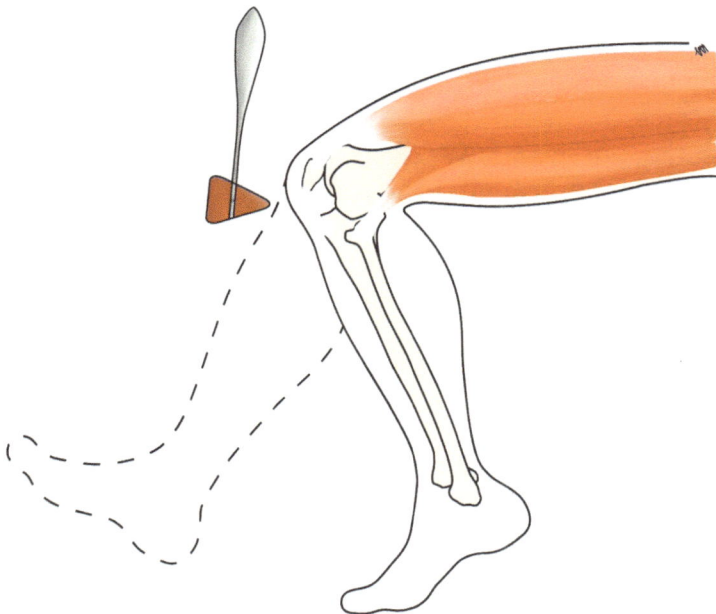

Figure 29: Demonstration of the knee's stretch reflex in response to a stimulus

A visually dangerous or harmful situation may stimulate a protective muscle contraction response, which would inevitably be dependent upon what is deemed dangerous or harmful by the individual. For example, if a punch to the stomach were expected, an individual would perform an abdominal brace to protect him or herself from injury. However, without the visual stimulus of the impact to the stomach there would be no brace and thus no protection against the impact.

CHAPTER 4.

Functionally, addressing what activities or movements the client/patient would consider put their lower back or site of injury at risk is vital in the prevention of reoccurrence. Identify what movement or activity caused the initial injury and what movements or activities are still uncomfortable. It is likely that the spine and pelvis are not stable during those motions, thus identifying aspects to train and improve upon.

Clients/patients who experience lower back pain as a result of seemingly mundane tasks such as brushing their teeth, getting out of the car, retrieving a turkey from the oven, or picking up a child, often do not perceive these actions as harmful, yet they result in acute pain. Of course there might be an underlying weakness or tightness due to either repetitive movements or a sustained position. This may have caused the lower back to become vulnerable to mechanical load and stress, but had the perceptual stimulus of a harmful action been different, the core muscles may have contracted to stabilise the spine and the pelvis, thus avoiding the acute onset of lower back pain. Inevitably it is the client/patients perception of what they deem to be a potentially harmful movement that will require some education, as they can then activate their trunk muscles to stabilise the spine and pelvis in response to the visual stimulus (Skinner, 1938).

> **Key Point**: Clients/patients will usually either present in response to an injury, with the intention of preventing it happening again, or to improve sporting performance.

4.3 Core & Trunk Strength

The argument between which has greater importance, strength or stability, is one that has been long debated within the fitness and medical fields. The two terms are often used interchangeably when explaining the trunk musculature in relation to exercising it. However, there is a definitive difference between the terms:

Strength - The capacity of an object or substance to withstand great force or pressure (Dictionary, 2013).

Stability – A reliable resistance to change, deterioration, or displacement (Dictionary, 2013).

The 'core' trunk muscles, in fact will require both strength and stability to perform optimally for any specific function, in a similar way to how a spider's web is both strong and stable for the purpose of catching its prey. It is important to note though that this strength and stability, again like the spider's web, has a limit. The muscles of the trunk however are capable of increasing its strength and stability through correct use and training.

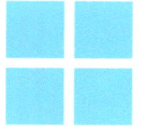

Key Point: "Core" is a loose term used to identify a group of muscles presumed to work together. However, they all work in different capacities depending upon the dynamic movement being performed. Maybe a clearer, more accurate term to use would be *trunk musculature*.

Over time, the purpose or function of the trunk muscles may change. The most obvious example of this is during pregnancy, when a woman's biomechanical function changes dramatically. Following birth, the woman's trunk muscles must then adapt to carrying an ever-increasing mass in various positions and through various motions. With the use of Functional Training, all necessary adaptations can be trained to perform optimally, thus reducing the risk of injury or reoccurrence of injury.

The strength of the any of trunk muscles, like any other skeletal muscle, is purpose specific and is subject to the force it is being placed under (Henneman, 1957). Lederman (2009) questioned the need for 'strength' exercises for the trunk muscles, based on evidence suggesting that there was only a low level ($\leq 5\%$ Maximal Voluntary Contraction) of contraction by the trunk flexors and extensors (including the Rectus Abdominis and External Obliques) during "active standing" and walking (Andersson et al, 1996; Cholewicki *et al*, 1997; White & McNair, 2002). However, Maeo *et al* (2013) identified the most active muscle during an 'abdominal brace' (universally accepted strength exercise for the trunk) was in fact the Internal Oblique muscle (Figure 30), not the Rectus Abdominis or External Oblique. The study suggests that it contracts to 60% of its maximum contraction potential during an abdominal brace.

Lederman also explains that because the Transversus Abdominis, a trunk flexing muscle, is the first anterior muscle to fire in anticipation of movement, does not necessarily mean that it is the most valuable muscle in the trunk. It simply means that it is the first muscle to activate in the chain.

It can be concluded that the term 'core' is a loose term that has been used over the previous decades, in order to group the muscles both superficially and deep to the trunk. It is important

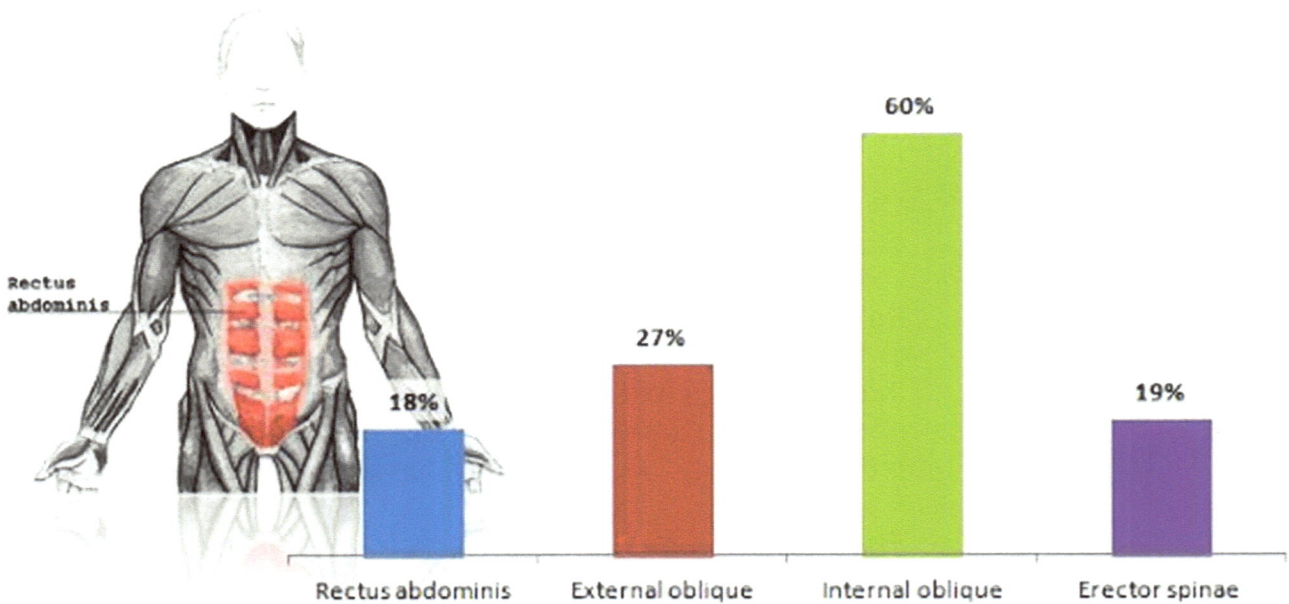

Figure 30: Percentage of maximum contraction in specific muscles during an abdominal brace (Maeo et al, 2013)

that all of these muscles have a degree of strength individually, that can be called upon when the trunk muscles need to activate in an organised fashion to stabilise certain movements and structures. However, it is clear that there is limited evidence to suggest there is a specific and single exercise to strengthen the 'core' muscles. (Figure 31) is taken from the study conducted by Maeo *et al* (2013), and demonstrates the percentage of muscle contraction across numerous exercises in various trunk muscles. It simply highlights that there is not one specific exercise that trains all of the trunk muscles adequately to improve a gross strength across all of the trunk muscles. This suggests a need for variety in exercises when considering how to strengthen the trunk muscles.

In addition to this, it is also very important that the deep muscles (the Internal Oblique for example), as well as the superficial musculature are activated and trained to provide strength increases to all of the trunk muscles. According to the analysis of the exercises above, an effective way of strengthening the deep musculature is with the use of an abdominal bracing exercise. This can be implemented in conjunction with other exercises, movements and postures throughout the day.

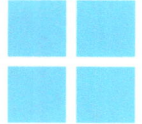

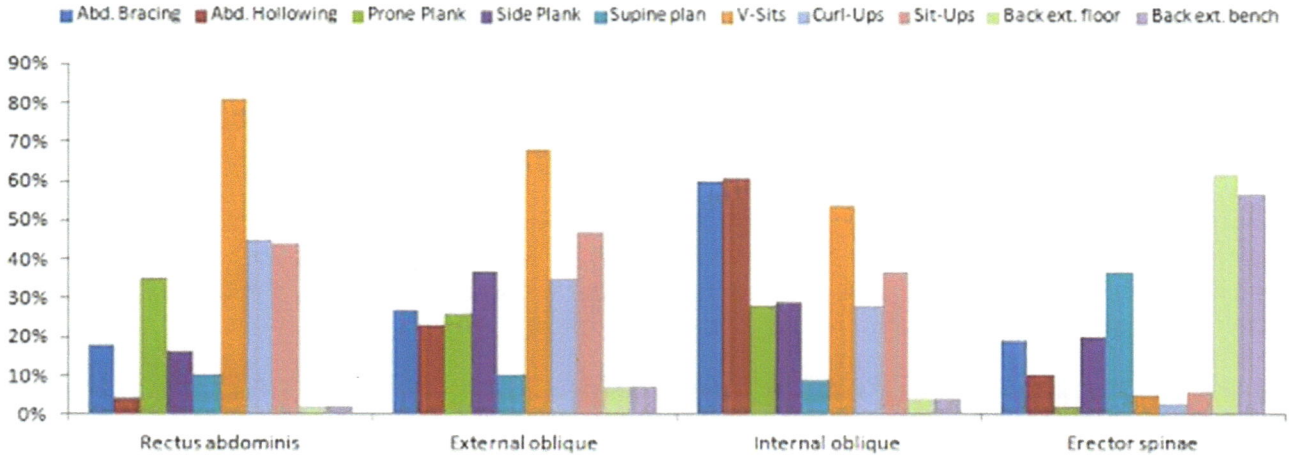

Figure 31: Maximum contraction percentages of various trunk muscles during different exercises (Maeo et al, 2013)

4.4 Trunk Endurance

It is clear from what is understood regarding trunk strength, that there is a continuous low-level contraction of the trunk musculature during mundane tasks such as active standing and walking (Lederman, 2009). This indicates that the trunk muscles must possess endurance properties, such as those held within the Slow Type I fibres, as well as the muscles having Fast Type II fibre properties to perform movements with anaerobic strength and power.

Generally associated with lower back pain, both acute and chronic, is the symptom of muscle spasm or tightness. In 1984, Biering-Sorensen suggested that a lack of trunk muscle endurance was a predictor for lower back pain. However, in a more recent review, the Biering-Sorensen Test was identified as needing more significant research to credit its validity as a predictor for lower back pain. The review did suggest that the test could be used to evaluate muscle performance in client/patients with lower back pain, more specifically before and after a rehabilitation program.

Endurance can be categorised into an isometric fatigue, whereby a contraction can no longer be held, or a dynamic fatigue, which identifies when repetitive work can no longer be sustained (Alaranta *et al*, 1994). Both definitions are important

CHAPTER 4.

> **Key Point**: The Biering-Sorensen Test involves having the client/patient lie prone on an examination table, with the iliac crests aligned with the edge of the table. The lower body is fixed to the table by three separate straps around the ankles, knees and pelvis. The client/patient then folds his/her arms across the chest, and then are asked to maintain the upper body in a horizontal position for as long as possible or for a set time.
>
> Although it is the most widely used test for evaluating the endurance of the trunk extensors, Liebenson (2007) explains that the test is not a 'functional test', and therefore should not be used to examine function. This is completely reasonable, however as part of an Initial Functional Assessment an appreciation for muscular endurance, muscle length and posture are all valuable tools, as well as functionally dynamic tests.

considerations when functionally training a client/patient. For example, a mother that has the constant demands of a toddler to be carried or held would require an isometric contraction to be sustained. However, the dynamic movement of picking the toddler up and putting them down identifies a repetitive dynamic movement.

It is therefore, based on what is understood of these trunk muscles, important for them to be both strong and be able to sustain a level of low contraction to aid the stabilisation of the spine in both an active and dynamic capacity. This will inevitably have a positive effect on preventing the risk of injury, as the trunk is better controlled and coordinated. However, there is no conclusive evidence to suggest that back pain, lower-back or otherwise, can be predicted using the results from universally used "core" strength and endurance tests.

When considering training methods and exercises, there is clearly no one specific exercise that works every trunk muscle to a similar level of activation. This stresses the importance of an approach that involves multiple exercises that work and engage different trunk muscles through different planes of motion. Thus the performance of each individual muscle to work in multiple planes as part of a unit when required, is optimised during various dynamic movements that occur daily.

With optimum performance in mind, every person has an individual activity or need they are required to perform daily, whether that

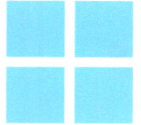

be a sedentary activity such as sitting at a desk or a sporting one such as kicking a ball. Both activities due to their frequent engagement need to be performed as efficiently as possible to ensure sustainability and consistent functioning. This is where a Functional Rehabilitative Training mind-set excels. Having the ability to break down certain movements or positions, and then train each component of that movement or position for strength, endurance and technique will inevitably have a positive influence on the entire movement pattern.

Key Point: The specificity principle used within various training methods identifies that an individual can become skilled at an activity by practicing it. For that reason it is important to break down a movement pattern that is individual to each client/patient and train them to perform each component of that pattern with good form and an increasing load, dependent upon need.

For example, it is impossible to learn speaking French by reading Spanish, although a language is still being learnt; it's the wrong language. This is the reason a power lifter looks physically different to a marathon runner – their training is purpose specific.

Trunk Endurance Test

The trunk endurance test is an acceptable way to actively test the endurance of the muscles involved in supporting the trunk. It challenges the client/patient through various limb movements, and involves the recruitment of different trunk muscles to support the load displacement.

The practitioner is responsible for timing, instruction and the recording of the test. The client/patient will move through timed stages following on from a plank position with instruction from the practitioner. Throughout the entire test it is important that any pain is noted and the test is ended – this in itself can be a useful finding in the Functional Assessment. The lower back, neck and head position should be maintained throughout the test, and if the client/patient is unable to maintain the position after three verbal prompts from the practitioner, then the test should be ended and the time recorded.

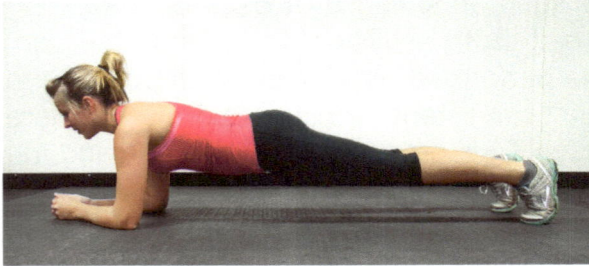

Stage 1 - starting position

Stage 1

The client/patient should be instructed to warm up for 5 minutes on a bike, cross-trainer or an equivalent. They should then, using a mat, assume the start position of elbows and forearms placed on the mat 90° to the shoulder. Then with the hips and knees extended and feet shoulder width apart, they should then raise their body off the mat keeping their lower back, neck and head positioned neutrally.

Once the client/patient is in the correct position, the practitioner should then start the stopwatch and the client/patient should hold the position for 60sec.

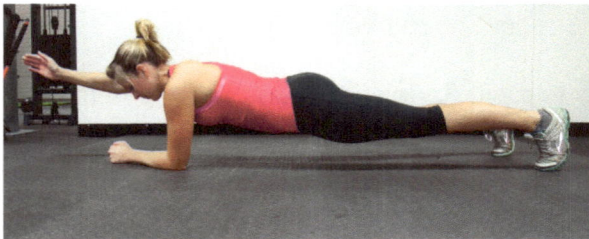

Stage 2 - right arm raised

Stage 2

Without resting after stage 1, the client/patient should be instructed to raise their right arm off the mat and extend it out in front of them parallel to the ground, whilst maintaining the neutral position of the back, neck and head.

The client/patient should then hold that position for 15sec.

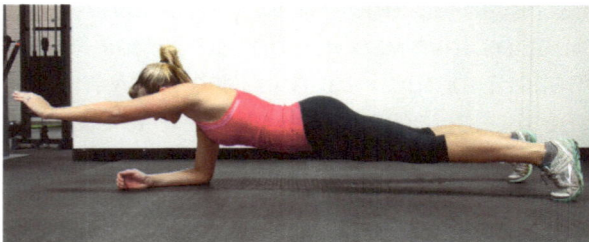

Stage 3 - left arm raised

Stage 3

The client/patient should then return to the start position, and then advance to raise their left arm off the mat, extending it out in front of themselves, again maintaining the neutral position of the back, neck and head.

The client/patient should then hold that position for 15sec.

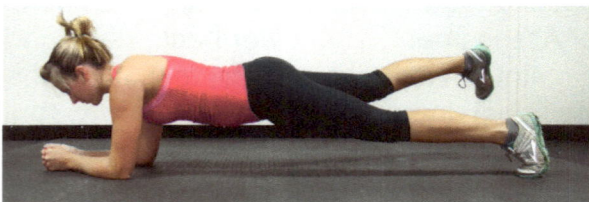

Stage 4 - right leg raised

Stage 4

The client/patient should return to the start position, and then raise their right leg off of the mat, extending it so it is parallel with the ground, maintaining the neutral position of the back, neck and head.

The client/patient should then hold that position for 15sec.

111

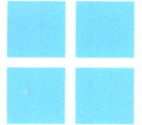

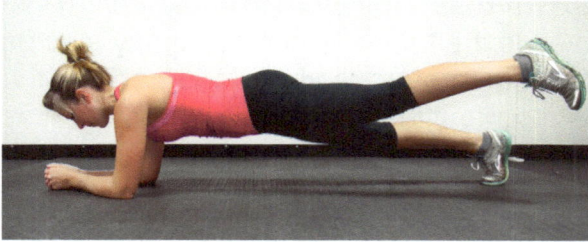

Stage 5 - left leg raised

Stage 5

The client/patient should return to the start position, and then advance to raising the left leg off of the mat, extending it so it is again parallel with the ground, whilst maintaining the neutral position of the back, neck and head.

The client/patient should hold that position for 15sec.

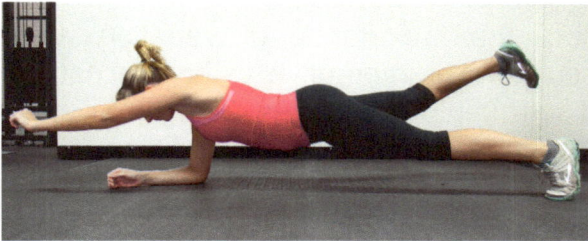

Stage 6 - left arm & right leg raised

Stage 6

The client/patient should return to the start position, then raise their left arm and right leg off of the mat, extending both so that they are parallel with the ground. The back, neck and head should remain neutral throughout.

The client/patient should then hold that position for 15sec.

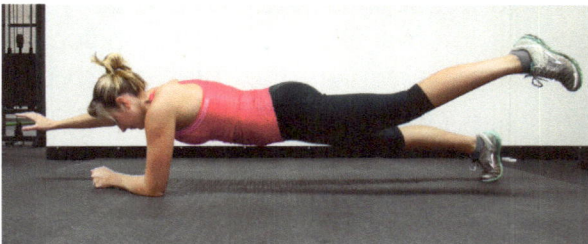

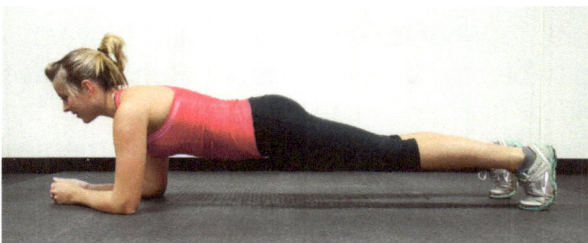

Stage 7 - right arm & left leg raised

Stage 7

The client/patient should return to the start position, they should then advance to raising the right arm and left leg off of the mat so that both are extended and parallel with the ground. The back, neck and head should remain neutrally positioned.

The client/patient should then hold that position for 15sec.

Stage 8 - start position

Stage 8

Finally the client/patient returns to the start position, again maintaining the neutral position of the back, neck and head.

The client/patient should then hold that position for 30sec.

End of test

The results of the test are used as a measure to compare against when the test is performed in the future. The results may also be affected by the client/patients internal motivation to perform the test. For that reason it is important that the practitioner introduces the test positively, thus encouraging the client/patient to complete the test to the best of their ability (Mackenzie, 2003).

4.5 Abdominal Brace

As previously explained, the importance of variation when training the trunk musculature is imperative to having optimal control of the spine and surrounding structures during both active and dynamic movement. It has been identified that there is not one exercise that works all of the muscles equally, but also the 'bracing' aspect that occurs before any movement is important to create the corset-like contraction of the trunk.

As it is understood from current research (Maeo *et al*, 2013), the abdominal brace engages the Internal Oblique more significantly than any other trunk muscle. This makes the Internal Oblique vital to functional movement, as it is the muscle predominantly responsible for the abdominal brace, which occurs prior to any form of active or dynamic movement. This means that not only good form throughout each breakdown of a movement pattern should be trained, but also the endurance of the Internal Oblique, with the use of an abdominal brace, should be encouraged with each movement.

Teaching a client/patient to abdominally brace will inevitably be one of the most valuable tools in Functional Rehabilitative Training. Specific, individual scenarios can be used to explain the importance of the abdominal brace, and how it can be implemented into daily functional tasks. Thus the stress on structures such as the facet joints, vertebral discs, spinal ligaments and tendons, and postural muscles, which are vulnerable to injury, Will be reduced.

For example, a client/patient with a sedentary office-based job will be prone to sitting for a sustained period of time, which is also a risk factor for lower back pain. They may experience this lower back pain when attempting to stand from a seated position. Ultimately, this may mean they are not recruiting certain muscles adequately with proper form. However, initially they will need to understand how to brace their abdomen optimally in preparation to stand up. A scenario like this can be used to indicate why the abdominal brace is important daily. The reason that it is a useful tool is because it is personal to client/patient, and they can instantly relate to using it outside of a training environment.

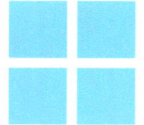

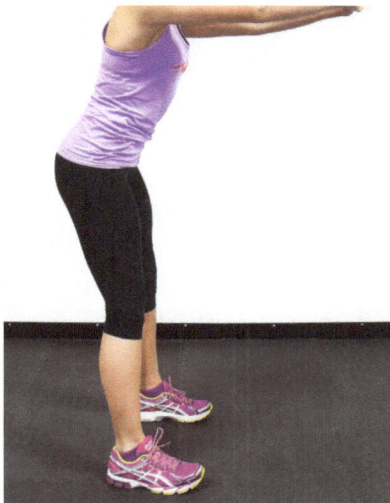

Understanding how to perform an abdominal brace starts by bending forwards at the waist

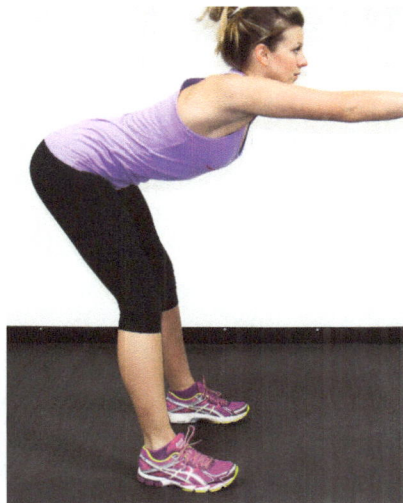

McGill (2004) explains how the abdominal brace is performed:

1. Stand up straight and place one hand on the small of your back and one hand on your abdomen.
2. Bend forward at the waist and feel the lower back (extensor) muscles contract.
3. Come back up to an upright posture and feel them "turn off".
4. Without bending forward, contract the abdominal muscles (as if you are going to be punched – feel them tighten with one hand) and the buttock muscles (as if you are holding in a bowel movement). You will feel the lower back muscles contract with the other hand when you contract your abs and buttocks.
5. Another way to feel the brace is to try coughing or blowing out as if you were going to blow out a candle. You will feel the contraction in the abs, lower back and buttocks.

Once a patient/client is able to functionally utilize the abdominal brace, other aspects of training such as strength and endurance could then be introduced to the trunk musculature. This will help optimise the efficiency of the muscles to work dynamically as a unit, due to the activation of each component in sufficient measure.

4.6 Abdominal Hollowing

Also mentioned in the research by Maeo *et al* (2013) as an effective way to significantly contract the Internal Oblique muscle, is the use of an abdominal hollowing exercise. This involves consciously sucking the belly in towards the lumbar spine, whilst maintaining a lumbar lordosis or neutral spine.

Although the manoeuvre is stated as being an effective way to activate the internal oblique, it also reduces the ability to breath and move with ease and comfort. This is mainly due to the upward contraction of the diaphragm, thus creating space for the contents of the abdomen to become 'hollowed', which consequently will decrease the amount of space available within the thoracic chest cavity. The reduced space within this cavity will have an impact on the amount of expansion available for the lungs, essentially limiting breathing potential, particularly with exertion - when full lung expansion is paramount.

It has been suggested that the abdominal hollowing manoeuvre does provide the least amount of compression to the spine in comparison to an abdominal brace, which provided increased compression on the spine, and a natural non-procedural approach (Vera-Garcia *et al*, 2007). Lederman (2009) expanded upon this work and suggested that a non-procedural approach offered "ideal stability" to the spine. However under load or with functional exertion, the stability that the spine should have available should be optimal rather than ideal. Optimal performance of muscles is often in response to specific training of those muscles. The expectation that is placed upon muscle to adapt, strengthen and improve in performance with appropriate training should also be considered to happen within other similar structures such as tendons and ligaments.

Summary

There is notable evidence to argue against the existence of a 'core' group of muscles that work systematically to reduce the risk of injury to the back by stabilising the spine through a combined contraction. In actual fact, the rationalisation of all the individual

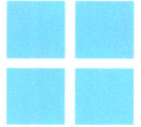

Figure 32: Displays anterior (top) and posterior (bottom) trunk muscles

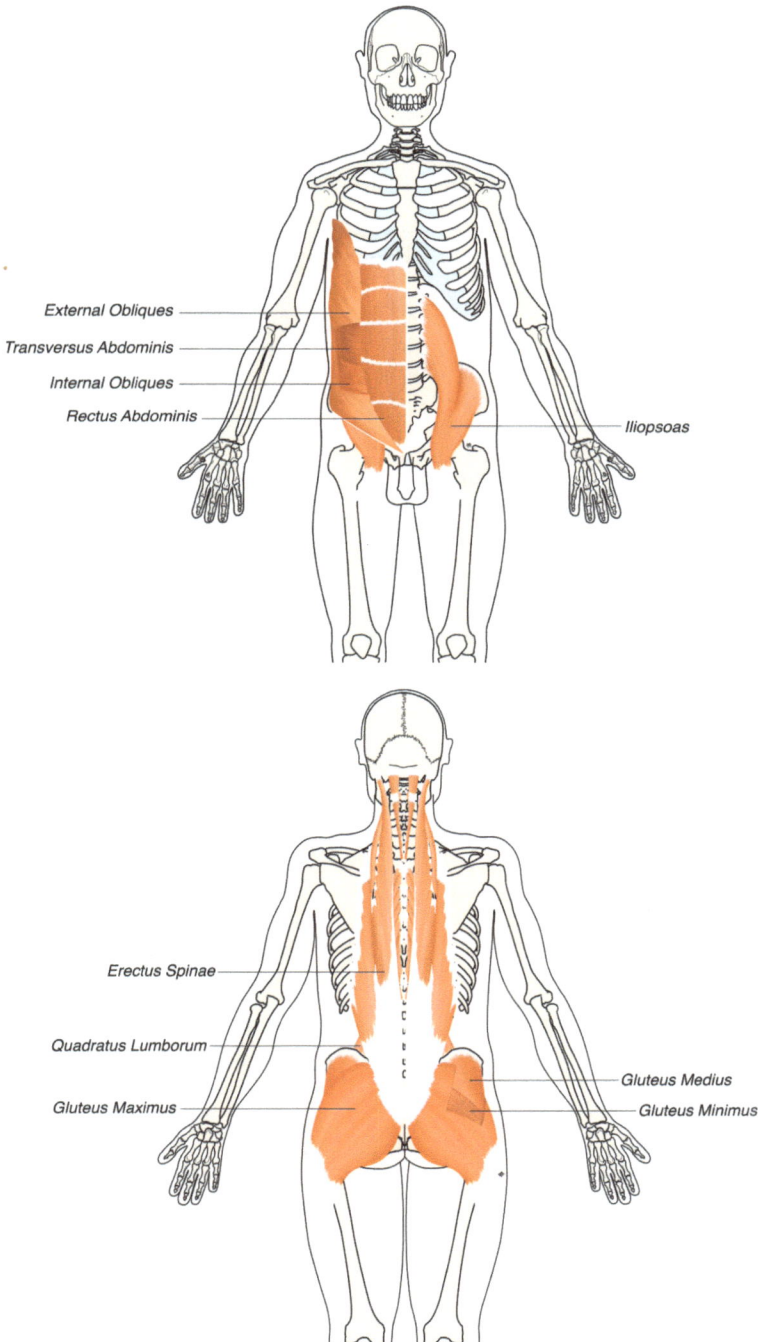

External Obliques
Transversus Abdominis
Internal Obliques
Rectus Abdominis
Iliopsoas

Erectus Spinae
Quadratus Lumborum
Gluteus Maximus
Gluteus Medius
Gluteus Minimus

trunk muscles working in an independent fashion dependent upon the type of movement, the strength required to move, and the perceived risk involved in the movement, is a much more logical conclusion. This proposes a move away from the misleading term of 'core stability'.

However, the more overall contraction of as many trunk muscles (Figure 32) as possible during a single moment, will inevitably add a significant amount of support to the back and pelvis as opposed to the fewer muscles contracting with a reduced contraction during the same moment. So it is important that a client/patient's trunk muscles contract as forcibly as possible as much as possible, and in some situations, on command. This identifies a need variation in trunk exercises, using the abdominal brace as a foundation to isolate the Internal Oblique, with functionally dynamic progressions, which also may require emphasis on the perception of potentially harmful situations.

If each of the trunk muscles is trained to work at its potential and as efficiently as possible, then the assumed benefits will be:

- A balanced, protected spine and trunk with a reduced risk of injury.
- An efficient transfer of power, and support to the limbs, thus improving the body's athletic performance.
- A strong, and well-maintained ability to support sustained postures, such as sitting and standing.

116

At the end of each chapter, each case study and questions will be relevant to the knowledge acquired in the previous chapter(s).

Case Study 4

A 22-year old semi-professional golfer presents to you with bilateral lower back tightness and radiating pain into his right hip region. The pain starts towards the end of the day or after a tough round of golf. As he has only started playing golf within the past 5-years, and is trying to turn professional, he is concerned about the pain limiting his progress. For this reason, he is very keen to resolve the issue, but admits he is not a "natural" athlete and doesn't strike the ball quite as far as some of the other players.

He identifies the discomfort as coming from either side of his spine, which after gently palpating, you notice is relatively tight. After checking his posture you discover:

- Reasonably good muscle tone and upper body posture
- There is a loss of lumbar lordosis
- Gluteals bilaterally appear hypotonic
- Otherwise his posture is considered normal

He fails the trunk endurance test at 17sec during stage 2.

1. Can you identify the origin, insertion and action of the Gluteus Medius muscle?

2. Using your knowledge of exercise prescription and biomechanics, can you suggest three exercises for this client/patient and explain why you have chosen them?

3. Please explain the difference between abdominal bracing and abdominal hollowing, and which would be better suited to this client/patient and why.

Notes

5. Torsional Control

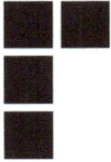

Learning Objectives

- To understand basic biomechanical principles such as force, torque, Newton's Laws, torsion etc.
- To understand the relationship between stress and strain.
- To understand what torsional control is and how it is utilised during exercise.
- To understand and apply logic in order to isolate torsional control from exercises to better enhance the exercise.

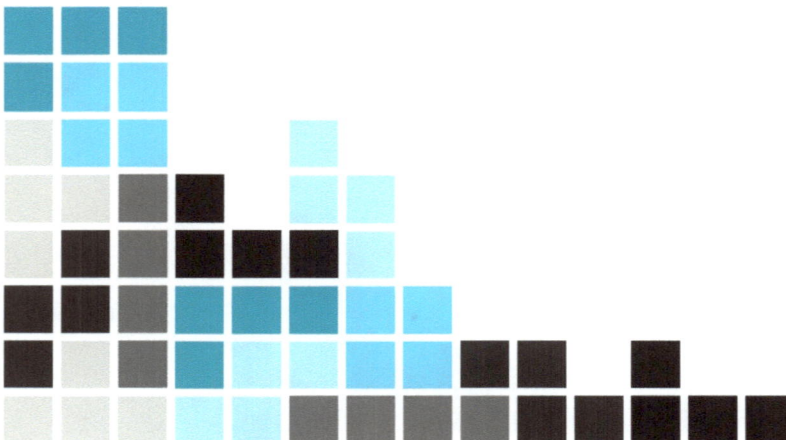

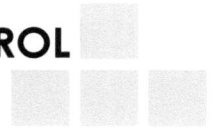

5.1 Torsion & Control

The term torsion is often associated with mechanical engineering rather than biomechanics. However, the biomechanical principle of torsion is not a new concept, it has been researched since the mid-80's. Yang *et al* (1986) assessed the stability of a fused lumbosacral unit under torsional loads, using human cadavers. Research since that point is somewhat sparse, which may be as a result of development and research into the concept of core stability, which is understood to have taken off in the early 90's.

Although there is a lack of supporting evidence and research, this doesn't rule out its validity. The rationale included with this principle is systematically viable. It hinges around moving away from the construct of core stability, and appreciating the ability of the trunk to recruit various muscles independently of each other, subject to load and movement, rather than them acting as a 'group'. Torsional control takes a much more functional, multi-planar approach to trunk stability rather than working through single planes of motion.

To explain and explore multi-segmental torsional control, an inherent understanding of some commonly used biomechanical principles is needed. This appreciation will help generate a greater appreciation for the entire kinetic chain through a breakdown of specific movements and principles.

5.2 Basic Biomechanical Principles

Force is calculated as Mass x Acceleration (F = ma), and it describes the relationship between an object's mass, acceleration and the applied force. It is defined as (Oxford Dictionary, 2013):

"Strength or energy as an attribute of physical action or movement"

Every movement whether it be static or dynamic produces or is stabilised by a force. The muscles themselves generate this with every movement and action.

For example, a static head position is acted upon by gravity and

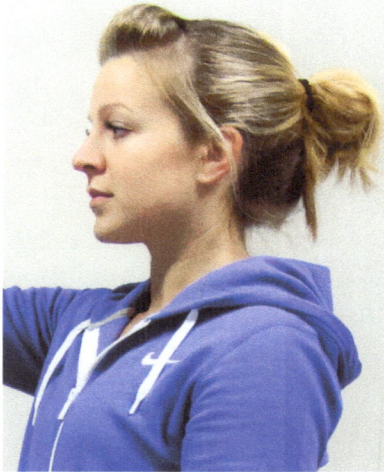

Gravity and the mass of the head is countered by numerous muscles in the shoulder and neck

the mass of the head itself. They both provide an anterior-inferior force that is constantly countered by the contraction of the Levator Scapulae, Upper Trapezius and the posterior cervical muscles. This means that if the acceleration of gravity and the mass of the head are calculated, the muscle force can be calculated to prevent the anterior-inferior pull.

Strength is defined as (Oxford Dictionary, 2013):

"The ability to exert force against a resistance"

There are three different classifications of strength (Mackenzie, 1997), which are:

*   Maximum Strength – the greatest force that can possibly be produced in a single maximum contraction.
*   Elastic Strength – the ability to overcome a resistance with a fast contraction.
*   Strength Endurance – the ability to express force many times over.

For the purposes of understanding strength, *Maximum Strength* is the primary strength classification and can be broken down into two forms, absolute and relative strength.

Absolute strength is the most commonly heard of form of strength, and identifies the maximum amount of force that someone can exert, irrespective of body size or weight. It is often measured with the use of a 1-rep maximum (1-RM) in various exercises. Relative strength is the maximum amount of force that can be exerted in relation to body size or weight. Exercises such as press-ups and pull-ups are often used to measure relative strength. However, they may not be the most accurate measure, as those exercises can often measure endurance rather than strength.

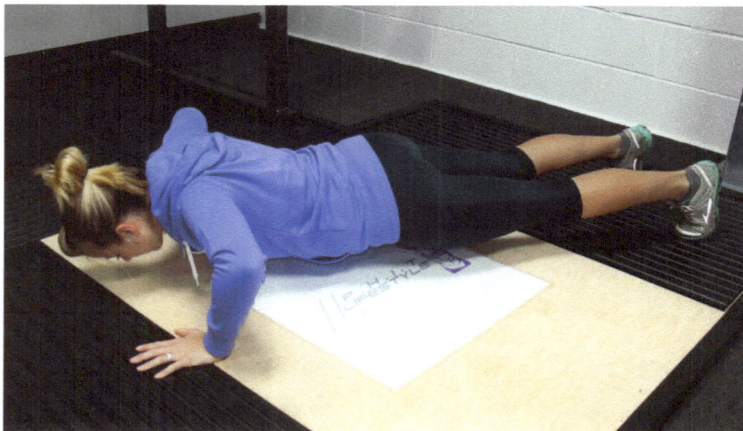

Press-ups are a good measure of relative strength

121

As an example, consider two athletes:

- Athlete 1 weighs 70kg, their 1-RM for bench press is 90kg and they can squat 110kg.
- Athlete 2 weighs 90kg, their 1-RM for bench press is 110kg and they can squat 130kg.

Athlete 2 has the greater Absolute Strength, as they can lift more overall weight compared to Athlete 1. However Athlete 1 has a greater relative strength (Athlete 1 bench pressed 1.3x their body weight and squatted 1.6x their body weight, whereas Athlete 2 bench pressed 1.2x their body weight and squatted 1.4x their body weight). This means that Athlete 1's Relative Strength is greater, and therefore suggests that a person is not "strong" based on how much they can lift.

Stress, in relation to biomechanics refers to (Oxford Dictionary, 2013):

"The measure of an internal load/force placed upon a structure per unit area of that structure"

Essentially the principle of stress is directly applicable to the force/load the ligaments, tendons, muscles and joints are placed under constantly. However it can also be applied to the functional spinal unit (FSU) and its attaching musculature. For example, as the muscles surrounding the spine force the FSU to move, this will inevitably cause the FSU to be placed under stress.

Strain is closely related to stress in biomechanics, and is described as (Oxford Dictionary, 2013):

"The extent of deformation relative to its initial condition"

This simply implies that any force can cause a distortion to an object, resulting in strain to that object. That strain can then be placed on a continuum towards the end result of complete failure, which in human anatomy usually is fracture or rupture, depending upon the structure.

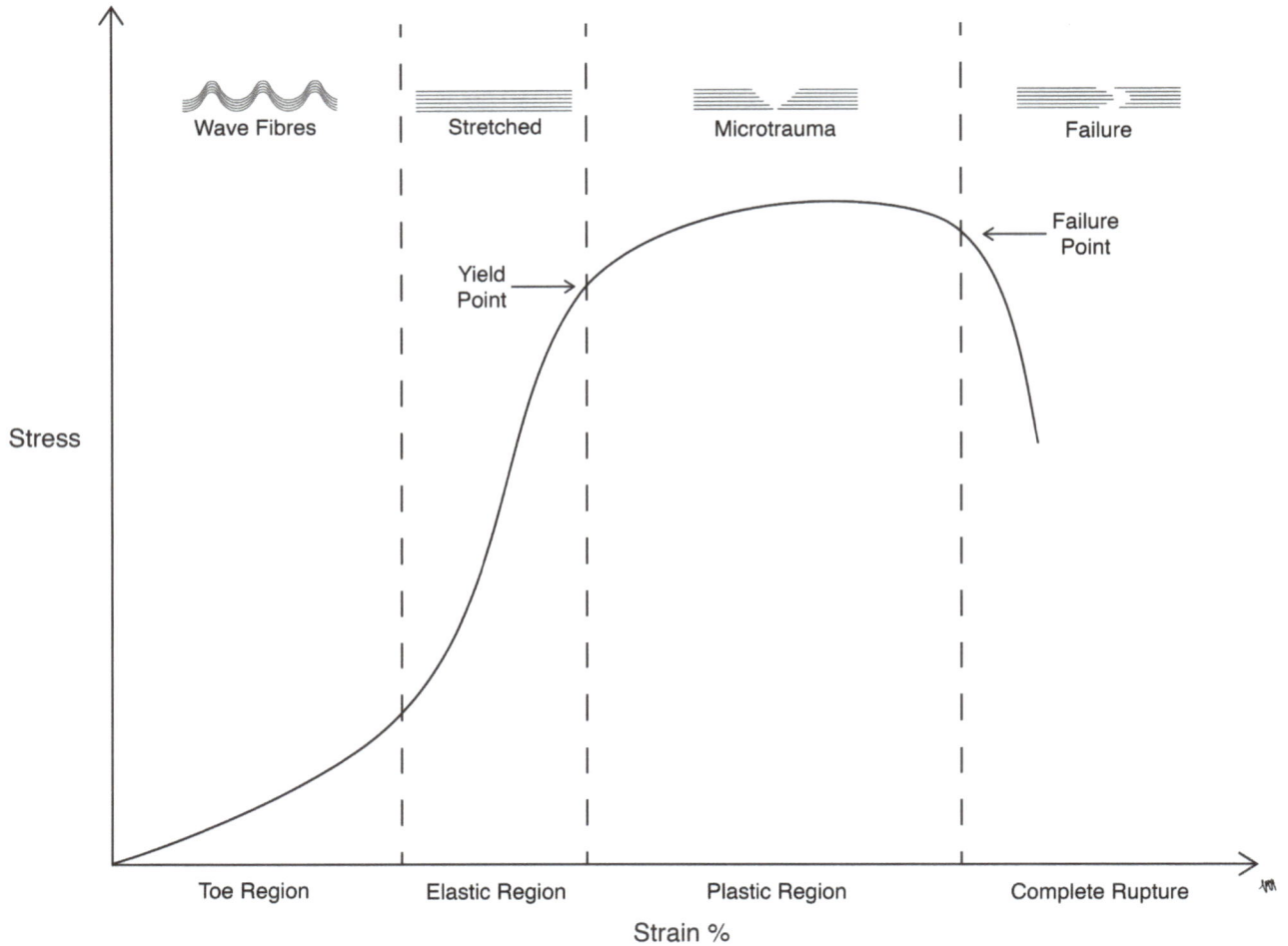

Wave Fibres

Stretched

Microtrauma

Failure

Yield Point

Failure Point

Stress

Toe Region | Elastic Region | Plastic Region | Complete Rupture

Strain %

Graph 2: Graph shows the relationship between stress and strain percentage on tendon stretching

The amount of strain is usually placed into five grades, for example Grade I, Grade II and so on. Each grade coincides with certain signs and symptoms of damage to the structure. Stress and strain can be placed on a chart that depicts the relationship between the two principles and its effects on tendon stretching (Graph 2).

This demonstrates that with increased stress and strain a normal tendon will undergo stretch, micro trauma and then complete failure.

Key Point: A greater speed will be possible with a smaller moment of inertia as the mass is close to axis of rotation.

Law of Inertia states (Honeybourne *et al*, 2000):

"A body continues in its state of rest or uniform motion unless a force acts on it"

This law was formulated by Isaac Newton, and as such is known as Newton's first law of motion. It is essentially a measure of an object or body's resistance to a change in its motion. Law of Inertia does not just consider the mass an object possesses, but also how far the mass is from its axis. Rest can be considered to a have inertia as it is at a constant velocity.

For example, the force would need to be greater to alter the speed/velocity of a 5kg medicine ball compared to a tennis ball, as the medicine ball would have a greater inertia.

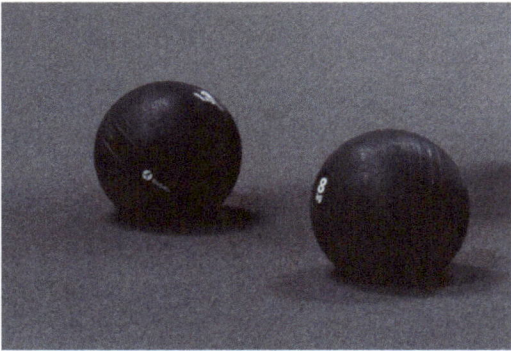

A medicine ball will have a greater inertia than a tennis ball due its mass

Law of Acceleration is Newton's second law, and states (Honeybourne *et al*, 2000):

"The acceleration of an object is directly proportional to the force causing it and is inversely proportional to the mass of the object"

Sporting examples often include a reference to momentum of an object or body, which is a result of velocity and mass. It can be transferred from one object to another, such as a baseball bat and ball (Figure 33), as well as being transferred from one body part to another.

For example, consider a trampolinist performing two somersaults. The first is an open-back somersault and the second is a tucked somersault. It requires far more effort to accelerate the open-back because its mass is distributed farther from its axis of rotation than a tucked. This means that the moment of inertia is greater in the open-back than the tucked somersault, resulting in a slower rotation.

During the late swing phase of gait, these laws also have an effect in moving forward with the lower extremity. Just prior to

CHAPTER 5.

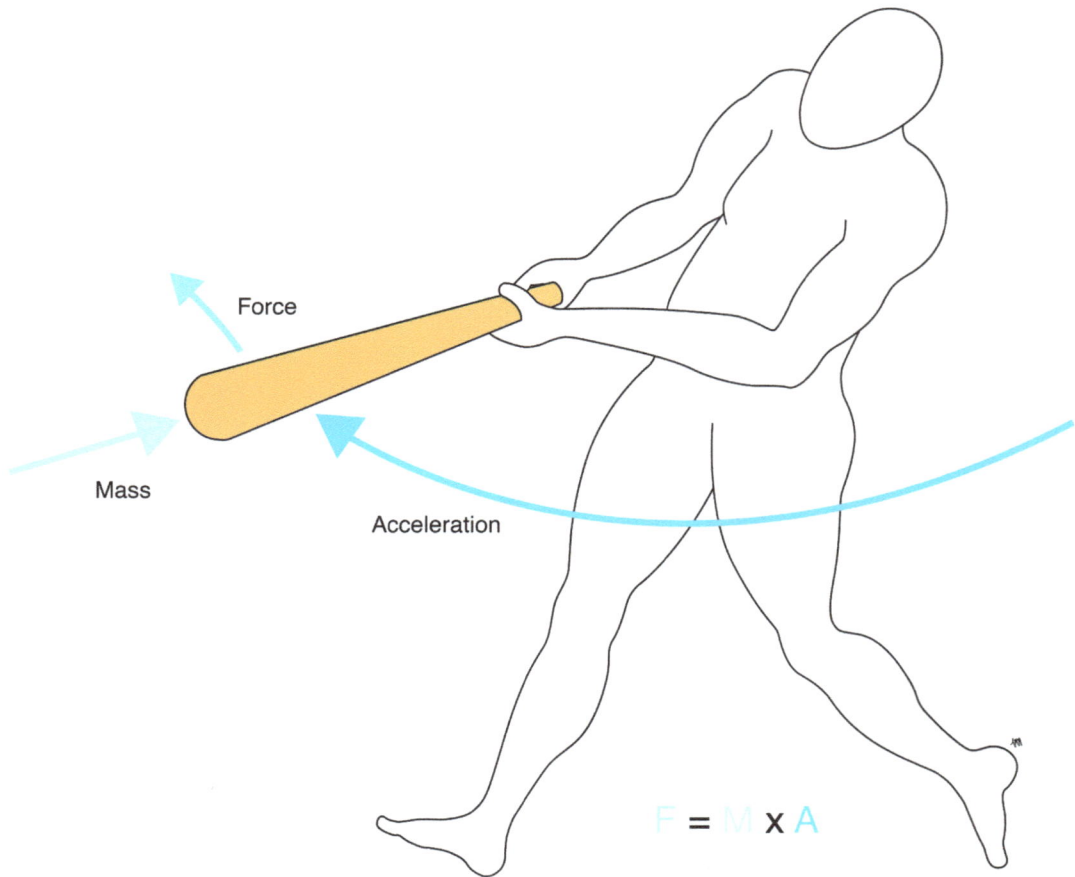

Force

Mass

Acceleration

$$F = M \times A$$

Figure 33: A sporting example that demonstrates how force is equal to the mass of an object x speed of acceleration

heel-strike there are almost no muscles activated that bring the extremity forward, yet it is still proceeding to travel forward in space. This is inertia. To deal with this inertia the body deploys an eccentric contraction of the hamstrings to slow down the extremity to prepare for heel-strike, and to reduce harsh reactionary forces.

Law of Reaction is the third and final law formulated by Isaac Newton and states (Honeybourne *et al*, 2000):

> *"For every action there is an equal and opposite reaction"*

It identifies that when a body or object exerts a force upon a second body/object, the second exerts an equal force back upon the first.

TORSIONAL CONTROL

An obvious example of this is during a sprint race, as the athlete pushes off of the starting blocks, the starting blocks provide an equal force in return to aid the athletes propulsion.

Torque in a biomechanical sense is described as:

"A force that tends to cause rotation"

It is the tendency of a force to rotate an object about an axis, pivot or fulcrum. Just as a force can be thought of as a push or pull, torque can be considered as a twist. So, torque is effectively the measure of the turning force on an object, for example, a bolt or a flywheel. The magnitude of the torque produced depends upon three variables:

- Amount of force
- Angle of application
- Length of the moment arm

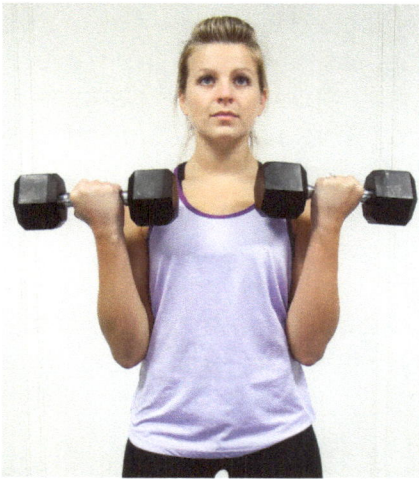

Biomechanically, torque creates movement of the bones (lever) around their corresponding joints, enabling all forms of human movement. The magnitude of torque a muscle can produce will have a direct effect on how great the movement produced will be.

If the goal through training is to increase pain-free range of motion, it is possible to manipulate the variation of torque to maximise the efficiency of moving the lever. For example, a bicep curl is much harder with the elbows fully extended in comparison to them being at 90°. The greatest amount of torque will always be when the force is applied at a 90° angle to the lever.

The bicep curl is often broken down in to a 'Matrix Set' or 21's as it is harder from an extended position

Torsion is the twisting of an object due to an applied torque. It is a term more utilised in engineering than biomechanically. The Oxford Dictionary (2013) defines it as:

"The action of twisting or the state of being twisted, especially of one end of an object relative to the other."

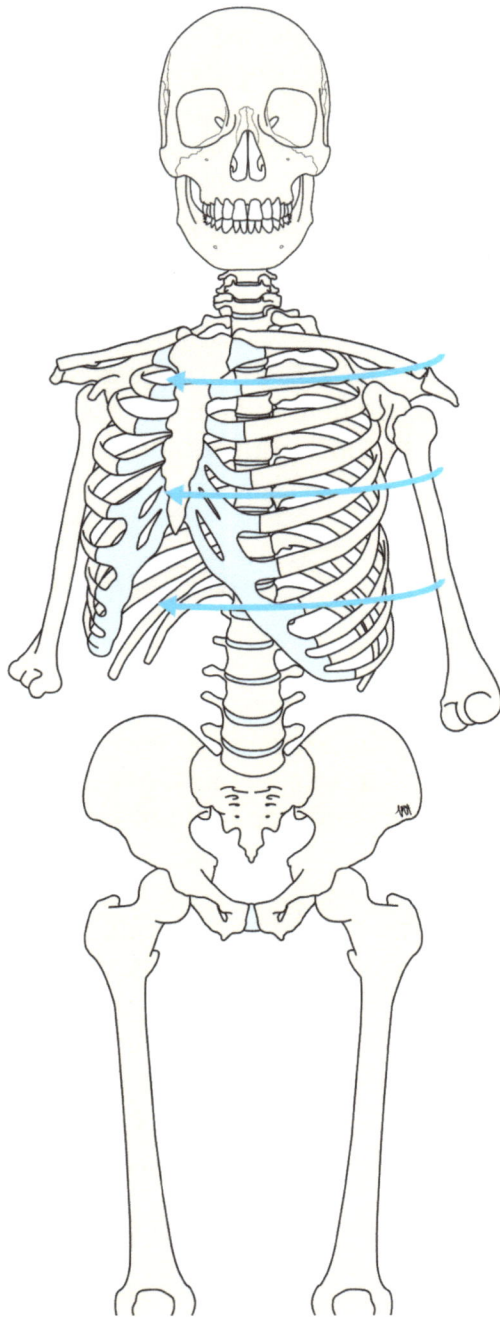

Figure 34: The spine and torso twisitng to create torsion, whilst the pelvis and head remain fixed

Mechanically, torsion is described as a twist being applied to a metal rod, which in essence can also be applied to the shaft of the femur in biomechanics. The rod or femoral shaft however, are rigid objects with very little elastic properties. They still have a point of stress/strain past their available physiological motion, which then puts them at risk of fracture.

This principle can be applied to other anatomical structures also, such as the spine and even the torso as an entire unit. Although the spine consists of multiple individual segments, they are bound together by various ligamentous structures to ensure they move as a complete unit.

The human torso rotates around the axis of the multi-segmental functional spinal unit (vertebrae, joints, supporting ligaments and connective tissue) (Figure 34). The force applied is different from that applied in engineering, as it comes from within the object/torso, with an applied torque generated from the musculature. The musculature of the torso acts upon the spine to increase torque and consequently raises torsional stress. A substantial force could possibly prove detrimental to specific movements and motor patterns or even to the recruiting musculoskeletal systems, especially if these were already weak and vulnerable from previous injury.

A javelin thrower is a good sporting example of the application of both torque and the resulting torsion created. They will generate torque, a measurable force, by recruiting the superficial musculature such as the Latissimus Dorsi, Erectus Spinae, and External Obliques (amount of force). This will drive the extended left arm down through the throw (length of the moment arm), and the angle of application between those multiple points constitutes the variables relative to measuring

TORSIONAL CONTROL

torque. This applied torque results in the torso undergoing a shift towards torsion. If the force created or shift is too dramatic and physiologically not prepared for then the risk of stress/strain considerably increases, as demonstrated by the stress/strain curve (Graph 2).

Ultimately, understanding the physical stress and strain that an individual can place upon this system will help the effectiveness of training it to be stronger and more stable.

It is thought that the theory of torsional control is only relevant with high velocity and high force movements, generated by the initial torque. However, this theory, although very relevant to javelin throwers, sprinters, tennis players, golfers etc., also has implications on the general public; for example, a full time mother getting her toddler out of an obscurely placed cot several times a day, or even a father and son taking turns to start a lawn mower. The theory of torsional control is applicable to the entire population.

It is very much an anaerobic principle. A weakness at any point throughout a particular motor pattern can consequently manifest as pain. This is most likely to occur at a vulnerable structure, such as a muscle or facet joint of the spine.

More general examples that are subject to torsional control in daily activities include:

- Putting on a sock
- Vacuuming
- Getting out of a car
- Picking a baby out of a cot
- Kicking a ball
- A single arm bicep curl

Torsional control considers obsure objects through anaerobic movements

The majority of movements that the human body will perform on a daily basis will require some form of activation from certain trunk muscles, in order to control the spine and maintain the torsional stress placed upon it.

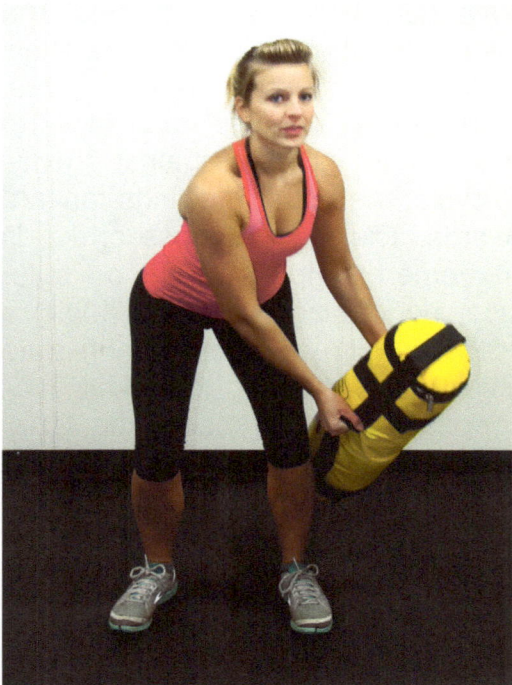

128

5.3 Torsional Control & Exercise

Many patients/clients require Functional Rehabilitative Training (FRT) to help with muscular imbalance or unilateral injuries, such as left sided lower back dysfunction or right shoulder dysfunction. This theory of torsional control can be used not only to strengthen torsional movements (movements that involve rotation of the body by activating certain trunk muscles), but also to aid in the isolation of specific non-trunk muscles, by engaging the trunk musculature separately and limiting the amount of torsion created. Thus, muscles are enabled to work more intensely without the compensatory factors of torsional assistance.

The human body works in a similar fashion to a helical structure, very much like the way commercial buildings are constructed using triangles. This is because the structure adds strength and support to the integrity of the entire entity. The body uses this helical structure by way of agonist and antagonistic muscles, muscles that purposefully work in opposition to each other to provide support by allowing a counter-balance against gravity. For example, during the gait cycle, the left arm swings forward as the left leg swings backwards. The main purpose of this is to provide balance. A more extreme example of this is a single-handed bicep curl. A gym user performing a bicep curl with a heavier weight than their biceps can lift will often demonstrate a rocking motion. This is achieved by recruiting the lower back stabilising muscles of the opposite side to ensure the lift is completed.

> **Key Point**: In this example, although the full range of motion may be achieved, the actual workload accomplished by the biceps muscle itself will be reduced compared to an isolated exercise, with ideal weight and good form. The lower back muscles activate to gain momentum, and thus are overly accompanying the distribution of workload during this example.

5.4 Isolating Torsional Control

The ability and desire of the trunk muscles to want to control the amount of torsional stress occurring around the torso and the spine can also be used to isolate the workload of other peripheral muscles, particularly those of the upper body.

By engaging the trunk muscles in another form of activity or control, they then are redundant in aiding the workload of the muscle being trained (Biceps, Triceps, Deltoids, Pectorals etc.). Manipulating the body's ability to work like a helical structure does this.

Although balance and proprioception are predominantly neurologically driven abilities, the widespread helical relationship between the muscles is the key area that can be utilised to control the body's centre of gravity and stability. This can aid rehabilitative and muscular imbalances immensely.

This process involves:

1. Identifying the muscle that needs to be trained individually without any compensation or aid from any of the trunk musculature.
2. Understanding how the trunk muscles would normally assist during the exercise i.e. does the centre of gravity move more anterior, posterior, or lateral during the exercise.
3. Logically engaging the trunk muscles, which will often include modifying the body's stability or maintaining a close centre of gravity, to enable the target muscle/s to be safely and effectively trained.

Using a lateral raise as an example, both modifying the body's stability and maintaining a close centre of gravity can be demonstrated with the simple inclusion of a gym ball rather than a bench or standing:

> **Key Point**: When using this method of training, it is important to use the same weight for both muscles. The weight selection should be driven towards the strength/ability of the weaker muscle rather than the stronger.

- Firstly, the client/patient should perform a lateral raise sitting on a gym ball using a medium weight, whilst maintaining a neutral spine. The centre of gravity shifting laterally towards the weighted arm can be observed during the exercise.
- The client/patient should then perform the same exercise, but raising off the floor opposite foot to the arm being worked.
- As the centre of gravity attempts to shift more dramatically due to the unstable surface, the client/patient will place a higher demand on their trunk muscles in order to maintain stability.
- The 'distraction' of alternative demand upon the trunk muscles will relieve some of the assistance given to the lateral raise movement, thus placing more specific demand on the Deltoid,

Supraspinatus and Trapezius muscles.

- This specificity placed upon the target muscle will cause a greater recruitment of this muscle and consequently a greater contraction. This larger contraction should result in the better response to training, for example, a faster adaptation to strength training and the muscle becoming stronger.

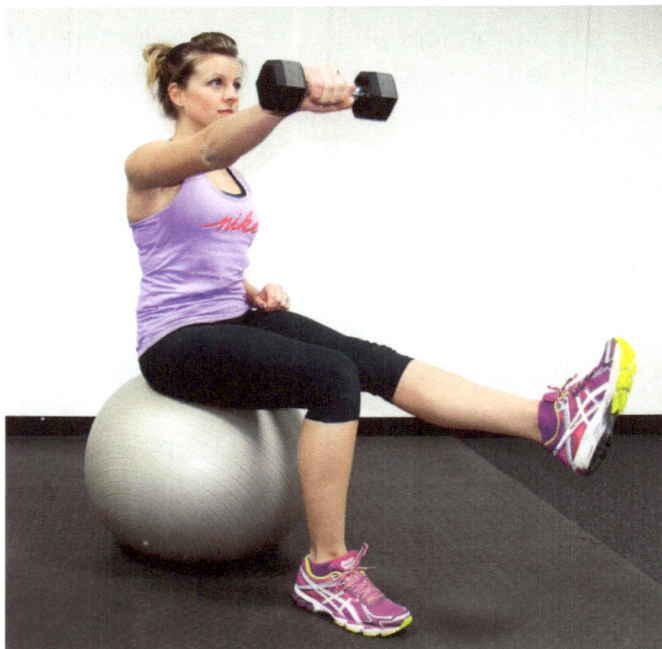

A single arm lateral raise on a gym ball is a good example of how torsional control can be trained

Gym balls, wobble boards and BOSU's are great tools for exploring and varying exercises with respect to isolating the body's natural torsional control.

This method of training is particularly useful when a client/patient presents with an obvious dominance within a certain muscle group from either overuse or inhibition. However the body's ability to control torsion can be used not only to isolate muscles, but the torsional control itself can be trained to strengthen specific daily functional movements.

5.5 Training Torsional Control

The control required to successfully stabilise the vulnerable structures of the spine and trunk under increasing load or repetition, much like any other muscle, demands adequate and correct training.

As the variation in daily activities demanding torsional control is so vast, a key element to training a client/patient, and effectively reducing their risk of injury is in identifying the mechanism of that activity. This can then be used to better understand how to train that movement to be stronger and thus better controlled. The activity may be something very generic, such as walking or putting on socks, however, it may also be something very specific to an individual's lifestyle, such as an awkwardly positioned cot or a sporting action.

The foundation to training a client/patients torsional control is to improve the strength and efficiency of their individual rotational movement. Whilst the trunk muscles stabilise the lumbar spine, the hip and shoulder joints along with the thoracic spine must also be capable of assisting the body's ability to rotate (Dechant, 2010). This aids the stress placed upon the structures in and around the lumbar spine. A good example of this is within a sport that requires a full swing, such as baseball or golf.

During a swing in golf the key emphasis is to turn or rotate through the shoulders and hips to 'wind up' the trunk, in a similar fashion to a wind up toy or yoyo, in order to generate torque. This is often accompanied by the cue of maintaining a strong neutral 'middle' throughout. This forms the basis of all rotational movements, regardless of height, direction, lever or the amount of rotation. This basis can be isolated into three individual components:

1. Straight Arm Rotation – This involves rotating with the arms extended out in front of the body, which alters the centre of gravity due to extension of the levers (arm). During the rotation it is important that an underlying abdominal brace is maintained, however individual trunk muscles will contract with greater force as the movement progresses. A key consideration for this rotational movement revolves around the centre of gravity. As this shifts anteriorly, a greater demand will be placed upon the posterior muscles of the trunk (*Quadratus Lumborum* and *Erectus Spinae*). Consequently, if a weight is added to this movement, it should not be too high, as this movement pattern is more aimed towards form rather than the weight used.

Specific examples of this include picking a baby up out of a cot or during a golf swing.

2. Collected Arm Rotation – This movement pattern progresses on from the first component as it utilises the drive and rotation from the hips as the movement progresses. It also employs a break in the arms before the rotation occurs, causing the arms to be drawn in towards the chest, reducing the load on the posterior trunk muscles. At the end phase of the movement pattern the weight shifts from the centre of the body laterally.

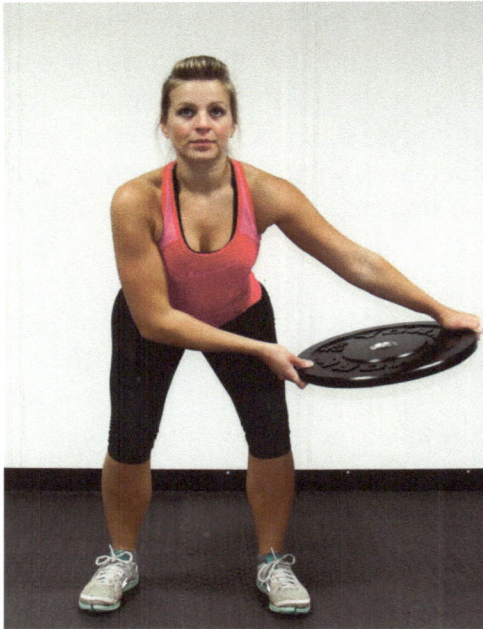

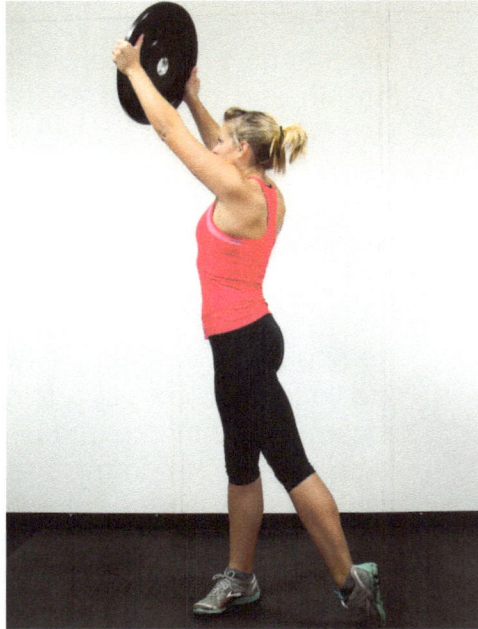

CHAPTER 5.

Straight arm rotatons will cause the centre of gravity to shift anteriorly throughout the movement

At this point as well as the trunk recruitment, it is important that the *Gluteal, Hamstring* and *Quadricep* muscles are used to generate power to stabilise the pelvis as well as the lumbar spine and surrounding structures.

Specific examples of this include placing something on a high shelf or throwing a ball, such as a baseball.

3. Alternating Rotations – This movement pattern utilises aspects from both the two previous patterns. The arms remain straight throughout and the hip girdle muscles provide power and stability at the end stage of the rotation. The client/patient starts in a squat position with their hands between their legs, as the rotation occurs the shoulders, trunk and pelvis move as a unit. This control allows greater force and speed to be used during the movement. Control is key during this pattern, however the effort to move the extended arms from high to low should not fatigue the muscles of the arms, as this is performed via momentum created by the trunk and hips.

Specific examples of this include starting a lawnmower or a pass in rugby.

An important point is that with all these movement patterns, the aim is not to reproduce the rotation or movement performed during the client/patients' activity. The performance of that movement will depend on other factors, including psychological, physiological and environmental. The objective is to teach and train an effective method to move through rotation that may be applicable and transferable to a client/patient's sporting or daily activities.

At the end of each chapter, each case study and questions will be relevant to the knowledge acquired in the previous chapter(s).

Case Study 5

A 30-year old female visits her Chiropractor for the 5th time in a year. Each time, she has come in with the same discomfort, and each time it has resolved instantly with manipulation of her lower back. He has a 12-month old child, which she is constantly picking up to comfort – even during treatment sessions. She has a tendency to favour her right hip when carrying her child.

The Chiropractor has noted that the patient has tightness across the right Gluteus Medius, as well as the left Quadratus Lumborum. Both hip flexors appear tight, but not asymmetrically.

They want to refer this patient to you, so they call to explain what they believe is happening. They explain that the two tight muscles are leaving the joints of the lower lumbar spine vulnerable to restriction – resulting in discomfort. For this reason, they would like the patient to work with you to correct this.

After meeting the client/patient, you realise that they have some gym experience and are keen to "strengthen their back". She explains that the last few episodes of pain have occurred whilst picking her child up from their cot and pram.

1. Can you identify the origin, insertion and action of the Quadratus Lumborum muscle?

2. Using your knowledge and biomechanical understanding, do you think that this client/patient has a weakness or tightness issue? Please explain your answer.

3. Please suggest an isolated unilateral gluteal exercise, as well as a predominantly unilateral lower back exercise that you could prescribe for this client/patient.

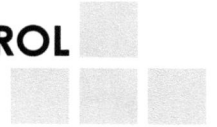

Notes

6. Physiological Adaptations of Training

Learning Objectives

- To firmly understand what is meant by intensity and failure in a training environment.
- To understand different muscle fibres and their adaptations to activity.
- To understand how a muscle changes with regards to physical demand, such as strength and endurance.
- To understand what tempo is and how its affects muscles and training.
- To understand the various types of techniques that can be used to train.

PHYSIOLOGICAL ADAPTATIONS OF TRAINING

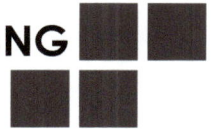

Throughout the fitness industry, experienced and newly qualifying professionals understand a universally accepted idea regarding what number of reps and sets should be given to what type of individual, often dependent upon their goals and time constraints. However little is known about the physiological adaptation that occurs that makes this reasonable hypothesis more of an exercising dogma. The majority of exercise physiology books contain statements such as:

"Performing an exercise between 3-RM (repetition maximum) and 12-RM provides the most effective number of repetitions for increasing muscular strength."

Found in a physiological textbook by McArdle *et al* (1996), it states what is proven to be correct, however there is only theory to support the physiology behind how it happens. Much like the foundation of some alternative therapies such as Chiropractic and Osteopathy, we know these therapies work just not exactly how they work.

It is important that a health & fitness professional understands volume and intensity

Until recently there has been such compelling unity on this understanding, that it has rarely been challenged. However, with new research being published, highlighting the improvements in muscle size and strength with the use of low weight/high rep training programmes as well as high weight/low rep programmes (Holm *et al*, 2008 and Goto *et al*, 2004), it throws into question what physiologically is happening and why we use certain variations.

This aspect of physical training is often referred to as the volume and intensity of training, and should be understood before prescribing training programmes, purely so that the correct adaptations in strength and/or hypertrophy of the correct muscles is optimally achieved. Once understood, exercise selection and the variety of training mechanisms (supersets, pyramids etc.), can be explored to add a different element to the way in which exercise is taught and ultimately enjoyed.

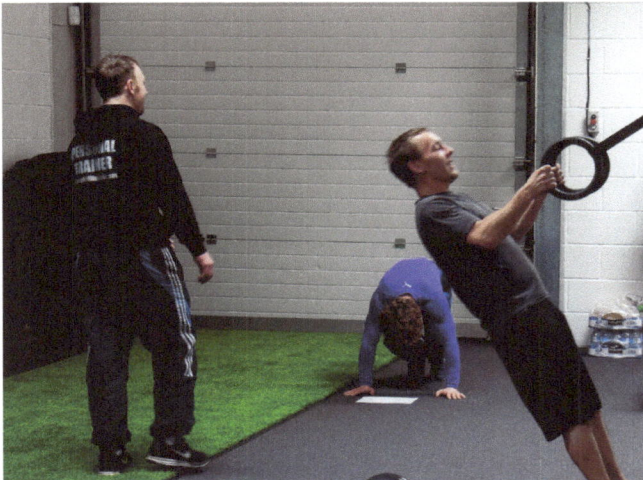

6.1 Intensity

There is a significant reduction in risk of injury to the joints of the body with improved muscular strength and endurance (Corbin *et al*, 2000). Exercise, more specifically resistance training, according to many, has a variable effect on the development of muscle tissue that is often placed on a strength-endurance continuum, dependent upon reps (repetitions of the exercise) and the respective weight loads (low, medium or high). This continuum is expressed in many ways, and will be discussed in the following. An example of such a continuum is displayed below (Figure 35):

Rep Range for Power-Endurance Continuum

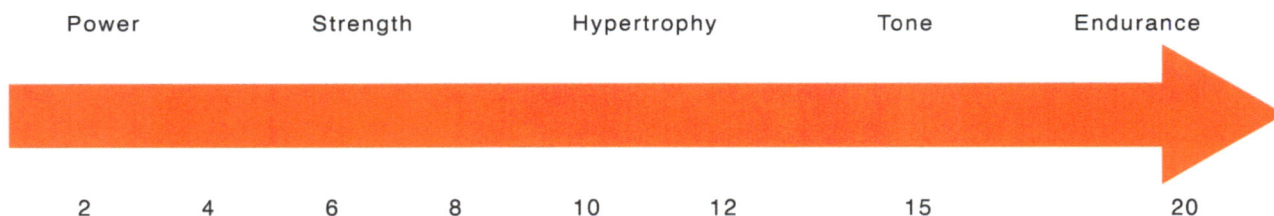

Power	Strength	Hypertrophy	Tone	Endurance

| 2 | 4 | 6 | 8 | 10 | 12 | 15 | 20 |

Figure 35: Rep ranges for power-endurance continuum

Ultimately, the health and fitness community is in search of a physiological understanding as to how many reps need to be performed to stimulate an increase in muscle size as opposed to muscle strength or endurance or even power, and how that process happens.

Intensity is an important part of training, as choosing either a low or high intensity to perform an exercise can, and very often does, underpin the general approach to a Functional Rehabilitative session. It can be defined as the amount of effort produced compared to the amount of effort maximally possible (one-repetition maximum or 1-RM). A percentage of the 1-RM is often worked out to determine the intensity of an exercise, for example 85% of 1-RM is an estimate of what resistance could be tolerated for six repetitions before failure. An

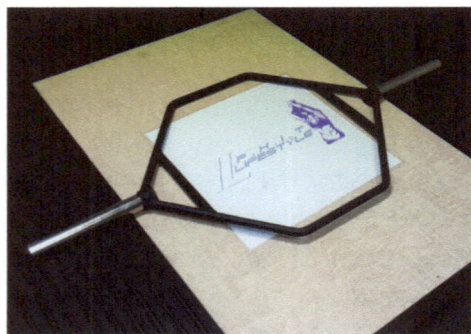

Resistance training can have a variable effect on muscle tissue

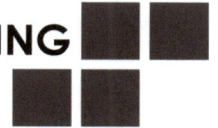

estimate of reps based on a percentage of the 1-RM is shown in Table 4, according to three individual sources, along with the average from all three together. This table can be used as a guide, if attempting to train at a specific intensity level based on 1-RM percentages.

Reps		1	2	3	4	5	6	7	8	9	10	11	12	15
	Brzycki	100	95	90	88	86	83	80	78	76	75	72	70	
% 1-RM	Baechle	100	95	93	90	87	85	83	80	77	75		67	65
	dos Remedios	100	92	90	87	85	82		75		70		65	60
Average % 1-RM		100	94	91	88	86	83	82	78	77	73	72	67	63

Table 4: shows the percentage of 1-RM results from three inidividual studies (Brzycki, 1998; Baechle et al, 2000; dos Remedios, 2007) and an average from all three

6.2 Failure

Failure is the sensation felt when physically no more effort could be exerted to perform another repetition of an exercise. This sensation will often be momentary, and some believe that training to failure should occur within every set. However this is seen as an aggressive approach to training and is probably better suited to training for power and explosive strength, due to the physiological effects occurring within the muscle fibres.

Initially it is important that all clients/patients have an appreciation of the sensation of failure, hence it is recommended that with Functional Rehabilitative Training, clients/patients be only pushed to failure on the final set of the exercise. If they still have not reached failure, five repetitions on from their original repetition target, get them to stop. This merely identifies that they can work harder and that information should be noted on their programme ready for the next session. Pushing a client/patient to failure excessively beyond the post-repetition target, may risk injury, but also it may risk demotivating them as they may feel beyond their perceived limits, and that the trainer is being too

CHAPTER 6.

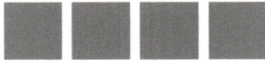

forceful. The advice would be to use the situation positively, and explain that they could have either used more resistance or more repetitions to work closer towards failure – where the positive muscle adaptations occur.

6.3 Muscle Fibres

In 1957, Henneman suggested the 'size principle', which explained that in order to move a load the muscle motor unit (groups of muscle fibres) recruits the smaller fibres initially, and then the medium sized fibres and finally the larger fibres are activated. This idea stemmed from the belief that the body naturally reduces the risk of fatigue by stimulating the slow, fatigue-resistant fibres before the fast, strong and less fatigue-resistant fibres (Honeybourne *et al*, 2000). The consideration for what type of recruitment (slow/fast, aerobic/anaerobic etc.) is required for an individual's functional movement pattern will eventually become a subconscious process. Table 5 identifies the various characteristics of the three different muscle fibre types.

Characteristics of Muscle Fibres	Slow Oxidative Fibres (type I)	Fast Oxidative Glycolytic Fibres (type IIa)	Fast Glycolytic Fibres (type IIb)
Structural			
Fibres per motor neurone	10-180	300-800	300-800
Motor neurone size	Small	Large	Large
Type of myosin ATPase	Slow	Fast	Fast
Sarcoplasmic development	Low	High	High
Functional			
Aerobic capacity	High	Moderate	Low
Anaerobic capacity	Low	High	Very High
Contractile speed	Slow	Fast	Fast
Fatigue resistance	High	Moderate	Low
Motor unit strength	Low	High	High

Table 5: demonstrates the different characteristics of muscle fibre types (Honeybourne et al, 2000)

Slow Oxidative Fibres (type I) – Otherwise known as slow twitch muscle fibres, due to their contractibility being slower compared to that of the type II fibres. The neuromuscular impulse is slow due to the myelin sheath surrounding the muscle being thin,

141

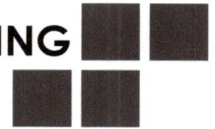

thus reducing the amount of insulation available, and essentially keeping the muscle cool. This allows the muscle to be able to contract at a low rate for a longer period of time, and along with the combined advantage of an increased number of mitochondria and more blood capillaries, these fibre types don't produce quite as much fatiguing by-products as fast fibres. This consequently makes these fibres more suited to aerobic work, where enzymes, when activated with oxygenated blood, will break down fat and carbohydrates into water and carbon dioxide. (Honeybourne *et al*, 2000).

Fast Oxidative Glycolytic Fibres (type IIa) – These fibres are known as fast twitch fibres which can contract more quickly than the slow twitch fibres. This is due to a thicker myelin sheath surrounding the muscle, which also allows the muscle to contract with a lot more force. The increased force production stems from the increased number of muscle fibres within each motor unit. The type IIa fibres are unique in the sense that they also have oxidative qualities, which means they can utilise aerobic respiration as well as anaerobic. Anaerobically, carbohydrates are broken down to pyruvic acid to produce energy, however this process, although it can release energy quickly, also produces a rapid build up in lactic acid. This acts negatively on the enzymes synthesis and causes the muscle to fatigue quickly (Honeybourne *et al*, 2000).

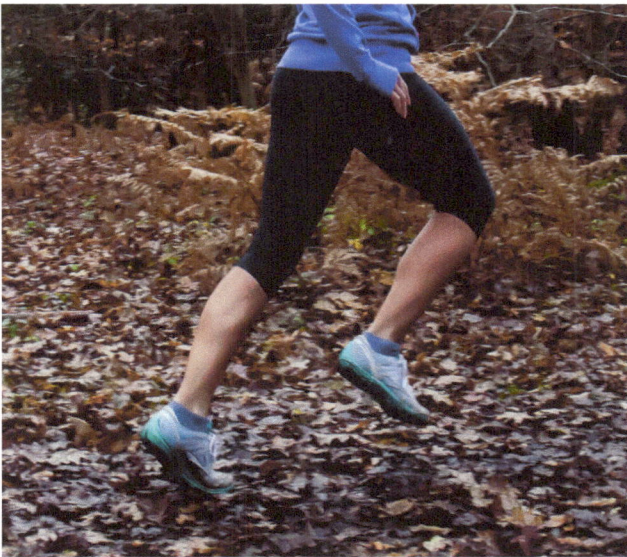

Fast twitch fibres generate a quick contraction with greater force than slow twitch fibres

Fast Glycolytic Fibres (type IIb) – A step up in the force and speed of contraction compared to the previous two muscle fibres. These fibres are large, very well insulated and can release energy very quickly. This allows the contraction to be a lot quicker. In comparison to the slow twitch fibres they possess few mitochondria, thus making them predominantly anaerobic fibres, as the energy breakdown system is also quick. This results in the high production of the by-product, lactic acid, increasing the amount of fatigue in a shorter period of time (Honeybourne *et al*, 2000).

Consideration for fibre types will help guide a Functional Rehabilitative Trainer's understanding of what it is they are trying to achieve for their client/patients. Utilising the slow oxidative fibres will mean avoiding high intensity type work, such as sprints or high load exercises, and will often suit client/patients in need of developing a postural endurance for a sedentary lifestyle. Whereas, the high intensity, high load training may suit specific movement weaknesses or clients/patients involved with sport.

6.4 Muscle Hypertrophy, Strength & Endurance

Regardless of what an individual's goals are with training, the key principle is hypertrophy. Often related directly to the increase in muscle size as a result of increasing size of the cells, however, literature suggests hypertrophy happens in two different forms (myofibril and sarcoplasmic) to stimulate the synthesis of skeletal muscle proteins (West *et al*, 2009).

The theory of myofibril hypertrophy infers that the actin and myosin protein filaments increase in number, resulting in a direct increase in strength as well as a marginal increase in the actual size of the muscle itself. This is based on the principle that the increase in number of filaments will directly lead to an increase in the number of potential cross-bridges being formed between the muscle proteins, allowing for an ultimately 'stronger' contraction.

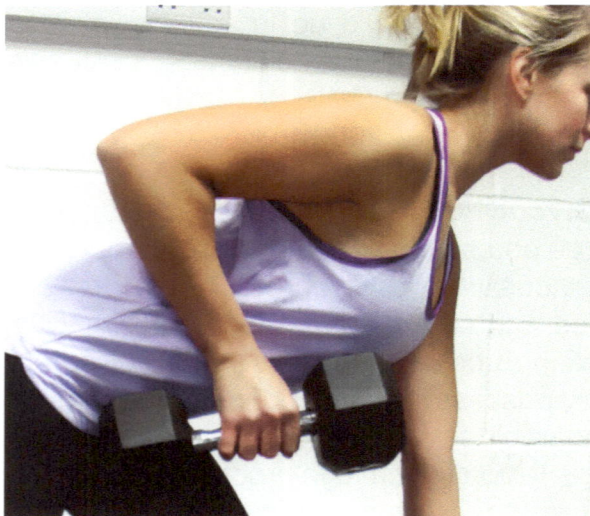

Sarcoplasmic hypertrophy suggests the sarcoplasmic fluid within the muscle cells increases with minimal increases in muscular strength. It must be clarified that although these theories have held substantial merit within the fitness community, there is still a need for more research, particularly for sarcoplasmic hypertrophy.

Although the research remains inconclusive, particularly towards the theory of sarcoplasmic hypertrophy, there is still literature that has identified whether heavy load/low rep training can result in significant strength gains in comparison to low load/high rep

Hypertrophy occurs in two different forms - myofibril and sarcoplasmic

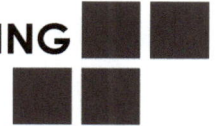

training, regardless of subcellular activity.

Originally, the suggestion that heavy loads increased muscular strength whilst higher reps built endurance is credited to the work of DeLorme (1945). His work demonstrated that increasing the load rather than the number of repetitions developed strength improvements.

A study by Anderson & Kearney (1982) tested the effects of high weight/low reps (6-8reps), medium weight and reps (30-40reps) and light weight/high reps (100-150reps) resistance training. Each group was tested for maximum strength, known as 1 rep maximum (1-RM), relative endurance (number of repetitions with 40% of their 1-RM), and absolute endurance (the number of repetitions completed with 27.23kg) over nine weeks. Table 6 displays the results from the study.

Training Group	Change in Max Strength	Change in Absolute Endurance	Change in Relative Endurance
Heavy Weight & Low Reps	20.22%	23.58%	-6.99%
Medium Weight & Medium Reps	8.22%	39.23%	22.45%
Light Weight & High Reps	4.92%	41.30%	28.45%

Table 6: demonstrates changes in strength & endurance over a nine-week period (Anderson & Kearney, 1982)

The results support DeLorme's work, although they also demonstrate a significant increase in strength within all three training groups, and an increase in absolute endurance within all three groups. The percentage of improvement does appear directly proportional to the original theory of heavy loads increasing strength more than lighter loads, and low loads improving endurance more than heavier resistance training. There is an improvement in strength and endurance across all three training groups, which suggests that hypertrophy may not be either myofibril or sarcoplasmic, but potentially both.

Similar studies have been conducted using lower rep ranges than Anderson & Kearney (100-150reps) for the high-rep training

group, and similar results were found (Stone & Coulter, 1994). This adds credence to the belief that all forms of resistance training improve both the strength and endurance of the muscle motor unit, but greater improvements in strength occur with a combination of heavier loads and a lower number of repetitions, whereas greater improvements in endurance appear more prominent with lower loads and a higher number of repetitions. These are considerations any health and fitness professional should have when prescribing exercise programmes. The decision of what type of load and how many repetitions to suggest should be led by the client/patients goals and objectives.

In terms of different subcellular adaptations to varying numbers of repetitions, there appears very little conclusive evidence. This is an area that will inevitably become more established in the future as technology advances. Based on the information present though, what appears to be the case is that myofibril hypertrophy is the apparent end result of micro-trauma to the muscle following the use of consistent resistance training. The sarcoplasmic hypertrophy that is often discussed is the acute effect of training, which contributes towards the feeling of being 'pumped', the acute swelling effect within the muscle after being worked.

To explain the varying differences between muscle development or hypertrophy in, for example a power-lifter performing high load/low rep (2-4reps) exercises and an average gym user looking to tone up using medium loads/medium rep (12-15reps) exercises, muscle micro-trauma has to be considered, along with the ferocity of how the micro-trauma occurs.

The power-lifter due to the heavy load, according to the size principle (Henneman, 1957) will cause greater damage to all the muscle fibres, including long fibres, which are the last to be recruited. In theory, following the micro-trauma the muscle fibres will repair themselves and add to the amount of fibres (myofibril hypertrophy) to ensure that the specific muscles adapt to the load they are being placed under. This principle is known as Wolff's Law (Wolff, 1986). The average gym user however will be causing less significant damage to the longer fibres, by using a medium

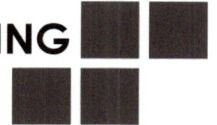

load, directly resulting in the amount of micro-trauma being reduced to the overall amount. They will have had to perform several repetitions (12-15reps) for the muscle to recognise that the load is greater than everyday resistance. These scenarios will directly influence the amount of tissue repair that will occur due to micro-trauma, and that will result in a varied response to myofibril hypertrophy dependent upon both, how and what load the specific muscles are adapting to.

This principle also applies to the number of sets that are selected. In order for muscles to respond in a positive way, it is important that they are subjected to a reasonable amount of work dependent upon what is to be achieved. The general consensus is that the amount of sets to be used will usually follow an inverse relationship to the amount of repetitions. This means that as the amount of repetitions increase as the amount of sets reduce. This is represented on a modified Strength-Endurance Continuum in Figure 36.

Rep & Set Range for Power-Endurance Continuum

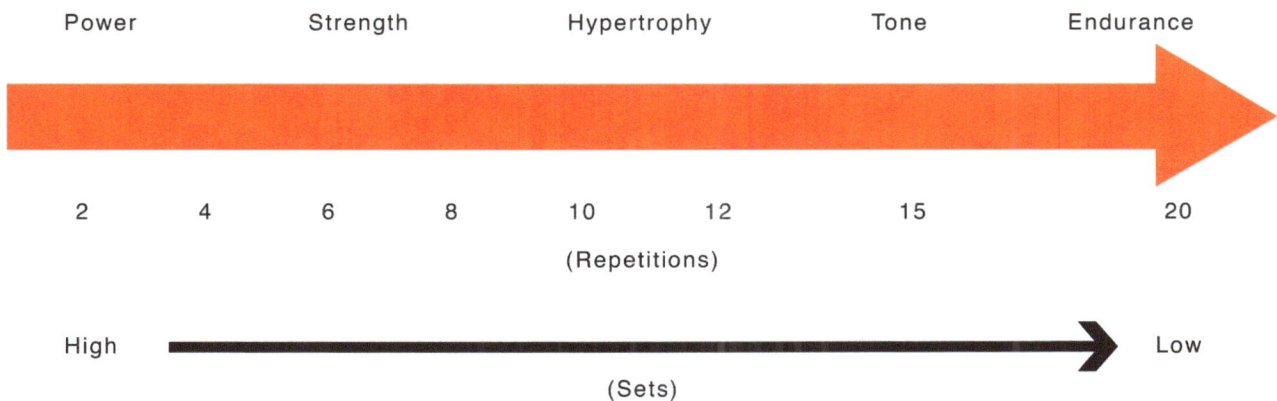

Power	Strength	Hypertrophy	Tone	Endurance

2	4	6	8	10	12	15		20

(Repetitions)

High →→→→→→→→→→→→→→→ Low

(Sets)

Figure 36: Shows a modified Power-Endurance Continuum, which loosely identifies the recommended reps and sets for certain goals

Initially it is advisable to start a client/patient with two sets of an exercise, performing twelve repetitions with each set. Based on the increasing experience of the client/patient, this may be subject to change, but primarily a beginner may not recover adequately

before their next resistance session. Quality of training should always be emphasised rather quantity with resistance training, and that is sometimes lost with moderate muscle soreness.

6.5 Tempo

In relation to resistance training, tempo refers directly to the pace at which a repetition is performed, with explicit consideration for the amount of time for rest, pause, and eccentric and concentric contraction. It has been suggested that different variations in tempo can have a direct effect on the muscles' ability to improve power, strength or hypertrophy (Miller, 2013; Pryor *et al*, 2011).

Four numbers, for example **21X1**, usually represent the expression of tempo on a resistance programme.

- **Phase 1 – The first number (2)** identifies how many seconds the eccentric part of the movement lasts. For example, lowering the bar during a bench press.
- **Phase 2 – The second number (1)** again indicates the seconds the movement is paused in the position where the muscle is stretched, when the bar is at its lowest position before being raised.
- **Phase 3 – The third number (X)** correlates to the actual lift, or concentric phase of the movement. An X suggests the movement should be performed as fast as possible.
- **Phase 4 – The fourth number (1)** is the time the movement is paused before performing another repetition. For example, holding the weight above the chest during a bench press.

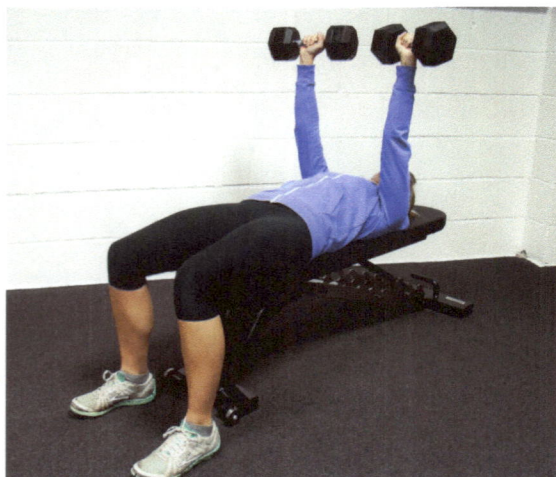

Phase 4 represents the pause during an exercise, such as a bench press

As mentioned in the previous section, all goals (power, strength, hypertrophy etc.) regarding resistance training are achieved through micro-trauma to the muscle fibres. However the amount of micro-trauma due to load selection will directly impact whether the muscle repairs to accommodate muscle mass or a need for increased muscular strength.

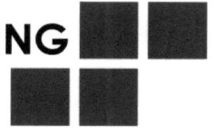

For this reason, tempo is an important consideration, although much like a lot of this topic, not an exact science with room still for more research. In an attempt to isolate the most 'valuable' phase of a repetition, the process of micro-trauma is incredibly significant. It is believed to occur most prominently with the eccentric phase of the repetition, as the fibres are forcibly separated due to a force greater than the muscle is adapted to, causing myofibril tearing (Proske & Morgan, 2001). This suggests that a longer eccentric phase and eccentric pause (**3211**) would cause a significant, but controlled amount of micro-trauma to the muscle fibres to supplement the development of strength and hypertrophy.

Munson (2013) explains how Malachy McHugh, a biomechanics researcher, believes the theory of micro-trauma is inaccurate due to a muscle tear or strain being a true injury to the muscle, rather than an after effect of resistance training. Alternatively McHugh argues that the muscle fibres lose their normal organised structure, which in itself is a rather vague expression. It appears at this stage that there is disagreement regarding the terminology for the process, by which it can be agreed that sarcomere damage occurs, rather than the actual cellular process itself. Proske & Morgan (2001) state that there are two "generally agreed" upon signs of damage to a muscle immediately after eccentric contraction, disrupted sarcomeres within the muscle and damage to the excitation-contraction coupling system. The most pertinent part of this argument should surely be which of these happens first, rather than the interchangeable terminology. Current understanding cannot firmly identify which of the two processes happens first, similar to a "chicken and egg" scenario. All that is known is that both occur during exercise, more so during the eccentric phase of the workload.

A shorter eccentric phase and pause would initiate a stretch reflex within the muscle, as demonstrated in Figure 37. The stretch reflex is a protective, innate response of the muscle to prevent excessive damage caused by excessive stretching. As understood from the musculoskeletal receptors section, muscle spindles respond directly to a stretch within the muscle. The reflex that happens in response to that is very quick as the

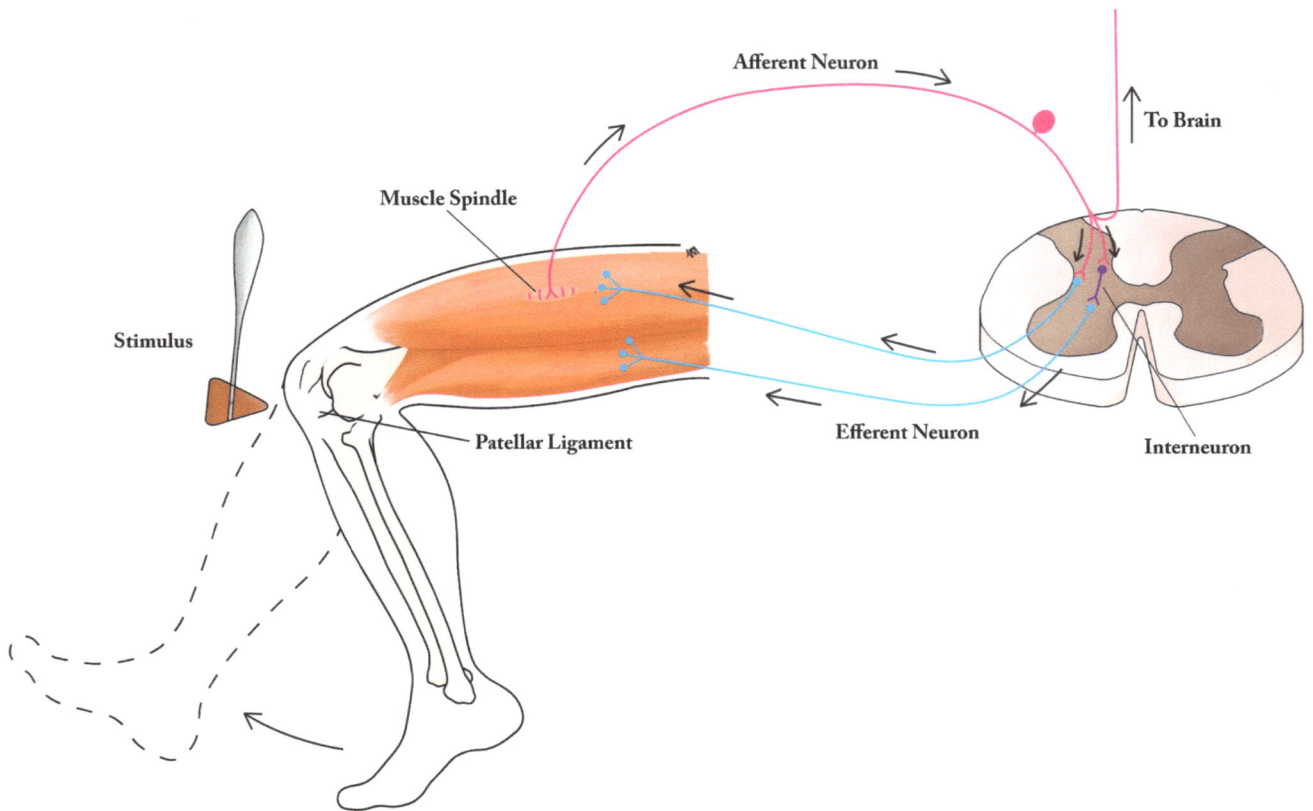

Figure 37: Demonstrates how the knee jerk reflex is stimulated through the nervous system via the muscle spindle

impulse is immediately sent to the spinal cord rather than the brain, and then the response to contract the muscle is instantly sent back. This reflex occurs in various forms such as in postural control, where leaning to one side, will result in a stretch reflex contraction of the opposing muscles to counter the movement, or more significant to resistance training, when a muscle is placed under an abrupt heavy external load, for example, throughout the quick eccentric lowering (**1X1X**) of the bar during a bench press. The stretched and supporting muscles during the bench press (Pectorals and shoulder stabilisers) would contract due to the stretch reflex, whilst simultaneously inhibiting the antagonist muscle (Latissimus Dorsi).

Resistance training with a quick lowering phase will inevitably stimulate the stretch reflex within the muscle. Understandably, this form of training will often better suit client/patients using heavy loads with low reps, as the physiological adaptations will be greater towards improving power and explosive strength.

149

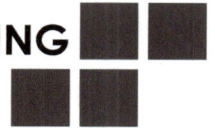

With the information available, it is reasonable to hypothesise that different tempos will therefore specifically target different responses in increasing power, strength, hypertrophy etc. For example, a slower tempo through Phase 1 and a pause and Phase 2 (**3211**), where the muscles are eccentrically loaded and lengthened, will work more effectively for strength and hypertrophy gains. Whereas a faster tempo (**1X1X**) would suit training driven towards increasing power, as the fast pace through eccentric contraction would induce a stretch reflex at the muscle and more aggressive damage to the muscle fibres.

Initially of course, the client's/patient's ability and experience of resistance training will be relatively unknown. Even if they claim to be the most experienced weight lifter in the gym, they may demonstrate poor form or may not have moved away from fixed resistance equipment. For this purpose it may prove helpful to introduce all new clients/patients to a generic reps and set range with a generic tempo. This will help gauge, based on an accumulation of experience, how to progress each individual client/patient within their own ability and goals.

A basic recommendation would be using two sets of twelve repetitions with a balanced eccentric and concentric loading phase (**2121**), which would be expressed for example like this:

Squat 2 x 12 (2121)

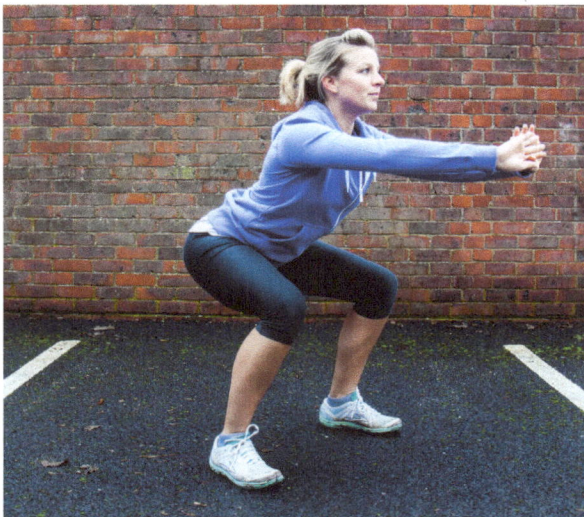

As the client/patient is progressed through their sessions, there are many other considerations that a Functional Rehabilitative Trainer may subconsciously or consciously recognise, such as a faulty movement pattern, incorrect breathing technique and the ability to alter minor details in function with instruction. It is advised that the client/patient is not advanced in terms of tempo until these aspects of Functional Rehabilitative Training are satisfied, so that there is a limited risk of reoccurrence of the original injury or complaint.

A squat commonly has a faulty movement pattern, which can be corrected

CHAPTER 6.

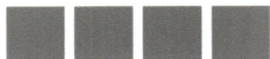

6.6 Advanced Training Techniques

Training techniques are an imperative tool when designing, customising and making resistance training enjoyable. Ultimately from what was discussed earlier regarding Wolff's Law, there is no one ideal way to train. The muscles will merely adapt to their physical demands if a method of training is sustained for a period of time, so it is important to add variety. Different training techniques such as the ones discussed in this chapter are very much open to experimentation. This will challenge a Functional Rehabilitative Trainer's imagination, making training a creative and gratifying experience. The key principle is that there is no one correct way to train with regards to resistance; it is much like how a healthy diet should be, balanced and varied.

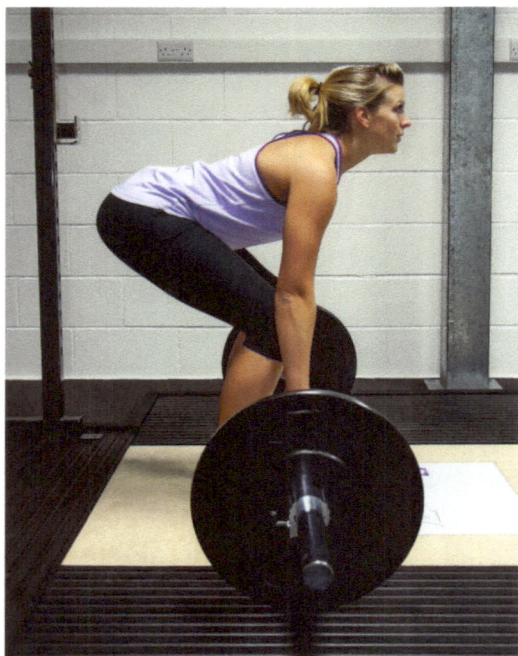

Good form is also a learnt skill, throuh the process of repetition

The term 'muscle memory' is not a term that is used to describe the process of muscle adaptation, as the two processes are distinctively different. This is important to mention, as throughout various texts the two terms are used interchangeably, and it is key to this chapter that an appreciation of the difference is accepted. 'Muscle memory' is a synonym often used to explain motor skill acquisition through repetition, which could be affiliated to the process of learning known as operant conditioning (Chapter 2.2). Examples of such are skills like throwing, riding a bike and even driving. Muscle itself does not have the ability to hoard reels of memory for every fine and gross motor action, the action is only stored through the process of repetition. That repetitive action is then stored within the part of the brain associated with habits and skills. However, muscle adaptation highlights the muscles ability to undergo micro-trauma, and then repair its structure to withstand a heavier force.

A number of techniques are now in circulation in an attempt to increase the intensity of resistance training and to add diversity to the way in which training is possible. The idea is that the increase in intensity will increase the rate of progression. However, from what is currently understood from the previous chapter there is only so much damage that resistance training can do to a muscle

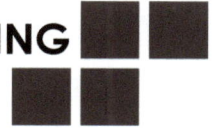

before it fails, which essentially highlights that there is a limit to how quickly muscle adaptation can occur.

Drop Sets or Strip Sets

This technique involves continuing an exercise with a lower weight once muscle failure has been reached with a heavier weight. A key component of this technique is to reduce the rest period as much as possible between sets to ensure the damage to the muscle fibres, particularly the larger type IIb fibres, is significant – this correlates with the understanding of the size principle by Henneman (1957).

Drop sets can be done using a variety of equipment (dumbbells, barbells and machines), however as the key aspect is to limit the amount of rest to as short as possible, machines are the easiest type of equipment to use. Resistance can be changed by the moving of a pin, as opposed to a barbell where several different weights would have to be prepared to effectively reduce the rest periods. Using barbells is possible, although changing plates can also consume time and may only prove effective with two spotters to help change plates quickly. The starting weight is down to personal choice as is the amount of sets that are performed.

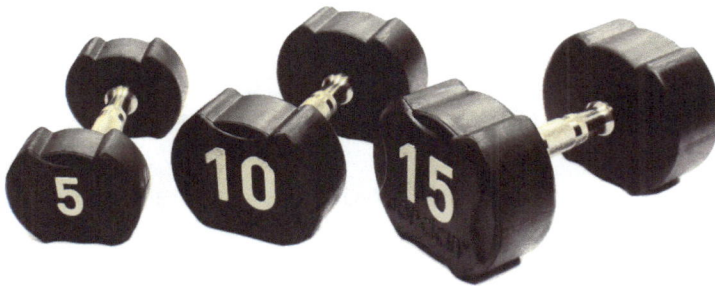

Dumbbells can be used easily during a Drop Set

An example of a drop set is to perform a barbell bench press, having two spotters either side of the bar. Set the weight at a 10RM (e.g. 60kg), and perform as many reps as possible until failure with good form. When failure is reached, the two spotters take off 5kg each (10kg total) and then the process is repeated with minimal rest between sets until failure again. Weight drops should be distinct (60, 50, 40, 30 etc.) until either the bar alone is left or the target number of sets is reached.

CHAPTER 6.

■ ■ ■ ■

Pyramid Sets

The Ascending Pyramid technique uses a progression from a light load/high rep set to heavy load/low rep set in subsequent sets, although the opposite, going from heavy load/low reps to light load/high reps is referred to as a Reverse Pyramid. Unlike a Drop Set this technique has rest periods between sets to allow the muscle to relax and take on fresh oxygenated blood, whilst disposing of any deoxygenated that will add to muscle fatigue.

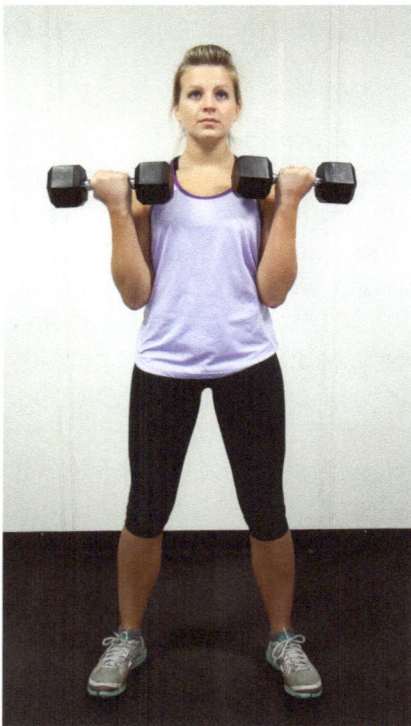

Pyramids, particularly ascending, are good to use with the very first exercise of a routine as the light load/ high reps acts almost as a warm-up for the joints and muscles. When used in this way, it may be best to use a compound exercise such as a bench press, lat pull-down or squat, rather than a tricep rope extension, bicep curl or leg curl.

An obvious pitfall of using Pyramids is that as the muscle fatigues throughout the sets, the weights increase, meaning that the muscle is at its weakest during a key stage where the adaptation to an increased load occurs. The size principle is limited by fatigue, resulting in less of the longer (type IIb) fibres being recruited. Ideally this technique would suit a beginner in an attempt to perfect technique with increasing resistance.

A bicep curl can be used easily to perform an Ascending Pyramid

An example of an Ascending Pyramid set would be a bicep curl with the dumbbells being pre-arranged to make them accessible and available. The exercise should be performed with a rest period between sets of 30-60sec, with each repetition performed at a controlled tempo, such as **2121**. This will encourage good control throughout the exercise accompanied with a sufficient recovery period before increasing the load. Again, form is crucial and if it is compromised the resistance used for the next set should be re-considered. An Ascending Pyramid may be written like:

Set 1 – 12 reps   Light Weight (e.g. 8kg)
Set 2 – 10 reps   Light/Medium Weight (e.g. 10kg)
Set 3 – 8 reps   Medium Weight (e.g. 12kg)
Set 4 – 6 reps   Heavy Weight (e.g. 14kg)

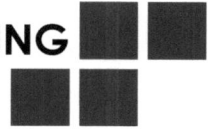

PHYSIOLOGICAL ADAPTATIONS OF TRAINING

Burn-out Sets

This technique is usually employed at the very end of a routine due to its intensity and the damage that it causes the muscle fibres, and consequently the sheer fatigued state the muscle finishes in. It can be performed using anything from 15 reps to 100 reps, although they have to be performed in one solid set or as few sets as possible.

If the intended Burn Out Set is going to consist of more than 40 reps, then it is advisable to select a weight that will allow for 15-20 continuous reps without stopping. The stops however should be brief and probably no longer than 10-15 seconds. This will allow the muscle pain to diminish slightly and for the client/patient to catch their breath. If longer than the 10-15 seconds then the client/patient should finish the set and readdress the starting weight for the next session.

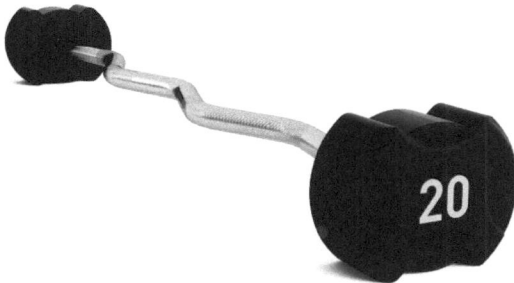

A good example of when a Burn Set is best utilised is at the end of a bicep workout. A full workout should have been performed up until the Burn Set, where the intention is to cause as much damage to the muscle as possible, for this purpose the exercise example is a preacher curl, with full range of motion. A total number of 40 reps is the target, with a weight causing failure around 20 reps (12kg). The entire 40 reps should be completed with as little rest between failures as possible, but also with smooth and controlled form. Once this is significantly compromised, the rest periods should be utilised.

Preacher curls can be used effectively in Burn-out sets

Heavy Singles

This is a form of training that works well for client/patients that are trying to increase power or explosive strength. It works well because it is performed as "single" reps with a heavy load, however the load should not be the clients/patients 1RM, as there will be a number of sets to complete. The number of sets can often vary from 4-10, and the decision will primarily be an

154

CHAPTER 6.

■ ■ ■ ■

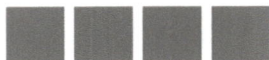

individual one depending on goals, time limits and programme design.

The heavy load will cause a near-maximum recruitment of muscle fibres (size principle), including the type IIb fibres, needed for anaerobic work such as powerlifting. It best suits compound exercises or exercises that use large muscle groups (Pectorals, Latissimus Dorsi, Glutes etc.). Because of its intensity during one movement, it may have greater effect to utilise as many muscles as possible. Limiting the amount of rest between sets will restrict the amount of muscle recovery, for this reason rest between sets should be restricted and kept to between 30-60sec.

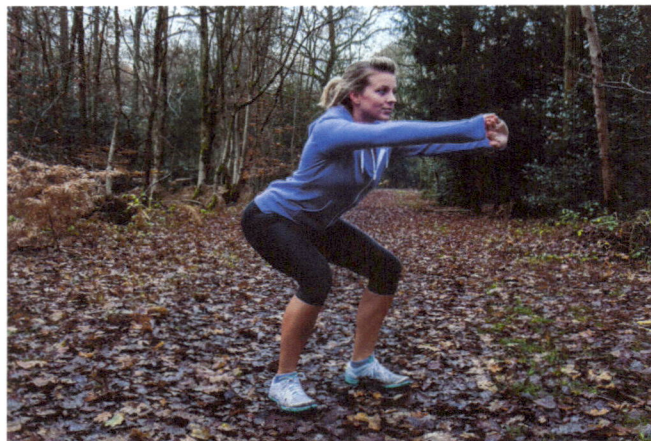

Heavy Singles work really well with power exercises such as a squat

Performing only one single repetition per set enables a greater emphasis to be put on form and load. It is a very useful way to train if the client/patient is working towards powerlifting competitions, as their form over 10 sets with a heavy loaded single repetition will encourage muscle adaptation, making a single lift during competition more habitual.

A reasonable exercise to use with this technique is a squat. The bar can be loaded to roughly 90-95% of 1RM, and then, ideally with a spotter, the client/patient performs one repetition of a squat with good form and control to a possible tempo of **11X0**. Rest for 30sec and then repeat, until the desired number of sets are completed.

Supersets

This is one of the most common forms of training, mostly due to its ability to reduce the general workout time and maximise muscle fatigue. Its key feature is the minimal rest period not only between sets but also between exercises, as this techniques utilises two exercises simultaneously without any or as little rest as possible, making it rather intense but manageable. Over the years there have been many variations suggested:

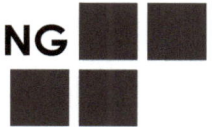

- **Antagonist Superset** – working two opposing muscle groups. For example, Bicep Curl + Tricep Pushdown
- **Compound Superset** – using a compound exercise and an isolation exercise together. For example, Bench Press + Pec Fly
- **Isolation Superset** – two exercises concentrated to one muscle group. For example, Tricep Rope Extension + Skull-crushers
- **Pre-Exhaustion Superset** – a modified compound superset, where the muscle isolated exercise is performed before the compound exercise. For example, Leg Extensions + Squats
- **Post-Exhaustion Superset** – opposite to the previous superset, where the compound exercise is performed before the isolated exercise. For example, Squats + Leg Extensions

Again, much like the majority of technique selection, it very much depends on what goals are trying to be achieved. For instance, a client/patient whose gym visits are fairly sporadic may not be best suited to a split-body training programme, as they may only work one body-part potentially once a month. For this person using both an agonist and antagonist would ensure they are using the basic, larger muscle groups within every workout. However, a dedicated exerciser, who trains three to four times a week maybe best suited to either a compound/isolated or a two-isolated exercise superset.

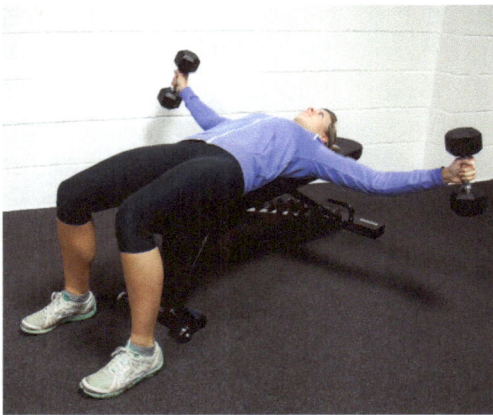

Pec fly is a good exercise to include in a Superset

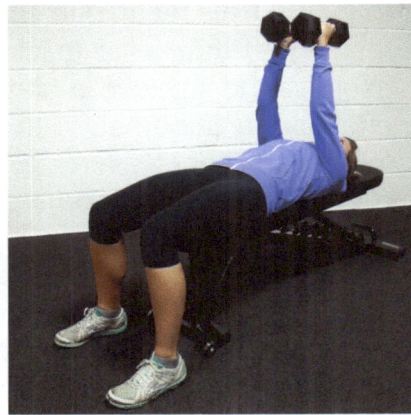

Repetition ranges for supersets follow the same principles set out in the beginning of this chapter, although the resistance that will be used will need to be reduced to account for the increased amount of muscle fatiguing agents (carbon dioxide, lactic acid etc.) that will be produced. Supersets are also of benefit to clients/patients aiming to lose weight. This is because the intensity of the technique will raise the heart rate

CHAPTER 6.

considerably, providing an increase in oxygenated blood to the type I muscle fibres, which in turn will stimulate the enzymes to breakdown carbohydrate and fat.

An example of how supersets can be used is to prepare two sets of weights, one set for a Bench Press and the other for a Pec Fly. The client/patient will perform:

Bench Press 3 x 12 (e.g. 24kg)
Pec Fly 3 x 12 (e.g. 10kg)

Both should be performed at a tempo of **2121**, with good technique and control. Failure, as with all resistance training, is when the technique is considerably compromised due to exhaustion or fatigue. Working to failure, and not beyond, reduces stress that could potentially be put on other structures unnecessarily. The load can always be reduced if the client/patient appears to be struggling significantly throughout the superset. They should be instructed however to move from one exercise to the other with as little rest as possible between sets. Towards the end of the final set they may also require a spotter, due to the muscle fatigue.

Tri-sets

An expected progression on from Supersets is to use Tri-sets, where three different exercises simultaneously are used, rather than two. This technique carries all the hallmarks of the Superset technique, as it is a quick and easy way of including several exercises to achieve a state of muscle fatigue greater than the effects of a Superset. With the obvious increase in intensity due to the additional exercise, this technique is recommended for clients/patients with some past resistance training experience.

This technique can also be used in various formats like Supersets such as antagonist, compound, isolation, and pre and post-exhaustion Tri-sets. The main advantage of this technique is to allow for a greater use of imagination with exercises, specifically by the way in which exercises are selected and used together to reach a sensation of muscle fatigue. An interesting dimension available with Tri-sets, is for example adding an exercise for

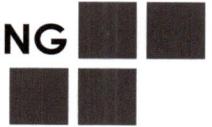

the 'secondary' muscle. In a chest programme, the 'secondary' muscle would be the Triceps.

With this scenario in mind, the concept of a Compound Superset for the pectorals could also involved an exercise for the Triceps. This would mean the Tri-set would have three separate weight stations set up, so that the exercises can be performed one after the other with as little rest as possible. The first exercise would be a Bench Press, the second a Pec Fly and finally the third could be Skull-crushers. This arrangement gives the primary muscle, the Pectorals, a mild recovery period during the Tricep exercise. It may be written like:

Bench Press 3 x 10 (e.g. 20kg)
Pec Fly 3 x 10 (e.g. 10kg)
Skull-crushers 3 x 10 (e.g. 10kg)

Each exercise should be performed at a tempo of **2121**, again with good form throughout. As with a Superset, the client/patient should move between exercises with relative sharpness to limit the amount of recovery within the muscles.

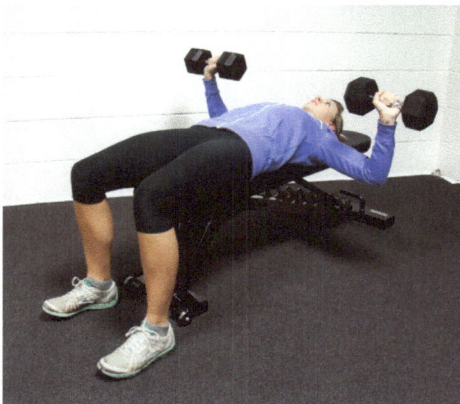

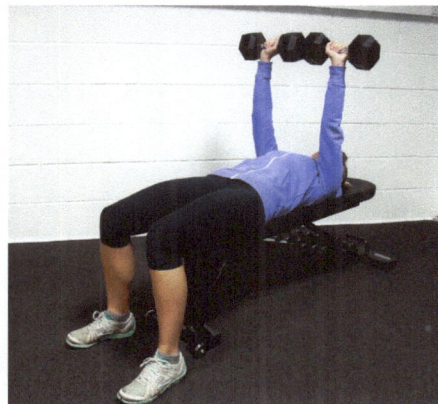

Bench press can be integrated easily into a Triset

Tri-sets offer a little more room for experimentation compared to the conventional Superset technique, although it is advised that before constructing a functional programme involving high intensity training methods, the Functional Rehabilitative Trainer has trialled the individual aspects of the programme first. This will give the trainer as much feedback about the exercises they are prescribing as possible.

Giant Sets

This technique is another advancement, this time on from Tri-

CHAPTER 6.

sets and consequently Supersets. Essentially Giant Sets add one additional exercise to the overall set, to make four exercises instead of the previous three used within a Tri-set. The approach to using this technique is mildly different as all the exercises will be focused around one muscle group specifically, as opposed to agonist and antagonist muscles. The intention behind this is to elevate the metabolic rate, thus encouraging the breakdown of fat, and the damage to the muscle fibres, by incorporating a greater amount of work within a smaller timeframe.

Much like the previous two styles, Giant Sets create a shorter workout period, although this fact should not be taken lightly. The sheer intensity of this technique is definitely not recommended for beginners, and should be approached only when good form and breathing is demonstrated throughout a normal set range, and either a Superset or Tri-set has been performed in the past. Each set should be difficult to perform, eliminating any aerobic approach to this form of training, which will result in greater production of fatiguing by-products (carbon dioxide, lactic acid etc.).

The transition between exercises should be short (10-15sec maximum), and if the resistance is too heavy then it should be changed during the Giant Set. It is likely during the first few sessions that the resistance selected will be either too heavy or too light. This is only because performing at the required intensity for this technique will alter what load can be maintained as the muscle dramatically fatigues. Following the initial sessions, muscle soreness in the days following will be considerable. This is such an important consideration, as a client/patient may have a manual job or sporting commitments that may be impaired if muscle soreness is too intense.

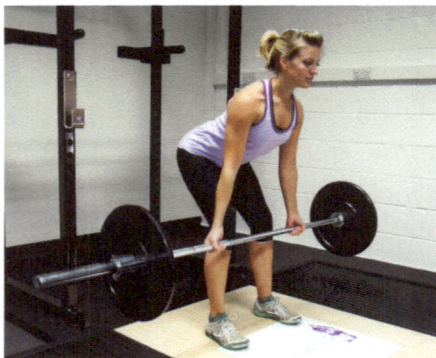

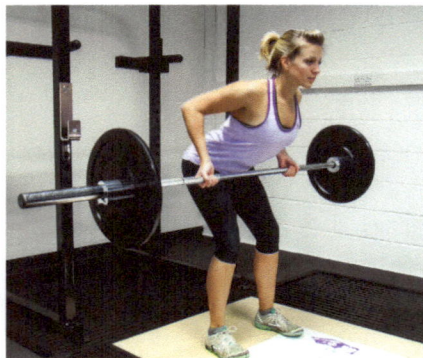

A bent-over row can be easily utilised in a Giant Set

An example of how a Giant Set could be utilised is during a back workout. Including exercises that target different parts of the back

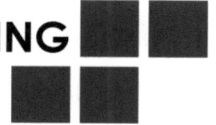

such as a Deadlift, Bent-over Row, Pull-ups and a Straight-arm Pulldown, will work the targeted muscles from various angles. Form and control should be emphasised throughout the entire set without compromise. The reason for this particularly with Giant Sets, is due to the high intensity of the set itself, any poor form along with inevitable muscle fatigue will put vulnerable structures at risk of injury. This example may be written like:

Deadlift 3 x 12 (e.g. 40kg)
Bent-over Row 3 x 12 (e.g. 20kg)
Pull-ups 3 x Failure
Lat Pulldown 3 x 12 (e.g. 40kg)

The tempo should be similar to that of a Superset and Tri-set (**2121**), and any variations or adaptations to exercises or resistance should be recorded ready for the next session.

Negative Sets

This style of training is very often used to cause as much micro-trauma to the muscle fibres as possible, by overloading the muscle during the most traumatic phase of the movement (the eccentric phase). For this reason Negative training is usually performed at the very end of a workout.

The technique is performed using a heavy weight - there is a lot of varying information and opinion around regarding what is considered 'heavy'. The general consensus is to start by using a clients/patients 1RM and then to increase the weight if the number of repetitions is completed easily. Negative sets take full advantage of the size principle, by recruiting all three possible fibre types throughout the most damaging aspect of movement. This accentuates the effects of muscle adaptation to increased loads, which will inevitably encourage gains in strength.

Each repetition should only be performed in the eccentric phase, for this reason it is recommended that a spotter be used for this technique. The spotter's role is to return the resistance back to start of the eccentric phase with as little aid from the client/patient as possible. Each repetition should also be slow and controlled,

CHAPTER 6.

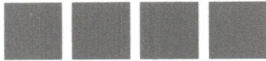

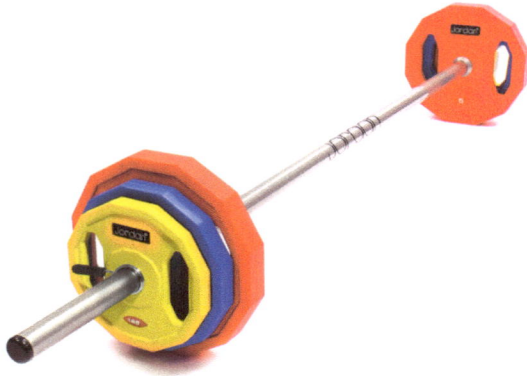

A barbell bench press is an exmple of a ideal exerise for Negative Sets

essentially working against gravity and pushing against the falling weight, and should take between 3-6sec.

An example of how Negative Sets can be used is at the end of a chest workout. Using a Barbell Bench Press with a spotter set the weight at the client/patients 1RM. They should then take control of the bar and lower the bar in a controlled manner at a 5sec tempo. Once the bar reaches the end range of motion, the spotter should lift the bar back to the top of the movement, and then another repetition can be performed. Negative Sets can be expressed like:

Barbell Bench Press (Negative) 3 x 6 at 1RM

Breakdown Sets

Based on the understanding from the Rep and Set Range Continuum, the theory behind Breakdown Sets is to isolate the workload done by all three different fibre types (type I, IIa and IIb), to maximise the amount of work the muscle does in one training method. This technique is performed in a similar fashion to a Superset – with minimal rest between exercises, and uses like a Tri-set, three exercises. However, each exercise is performed with a different load and repetition range, for instance the first exercise is performed for possibly 5reps with a heavy load (86% 1RM), the second is performed for 10reps with a medium load (73% 1RM), and the final exercise is performed for more than 15reps with a lighter load (>63% 1RM).

This will enable the muscle to adequately work through a strength, hypertrophic and endurance capacity, promoting an overall approach to resistance training.

As mentioned, this is to be performed much like a Superset or Tri-set, with minimal rest periods enforced. The number of sets recommended is between 2-4, thus promoting as much muscle fatigue across all capacities as possible. There is scope for a degree of experimentation in the way the technique is prescribed,

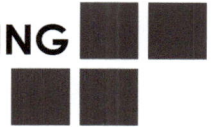

for instance, whether the exercises given are all compound or isolated, or a variety, and in which order they are performed. It is recommended that the client/patient start with the heaviest of the three loads, however this can be modified if desired to vary the training routine.

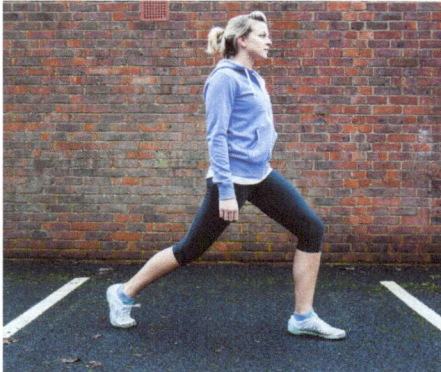

Static lunges are a useful exercise to include in a Breakdown Set

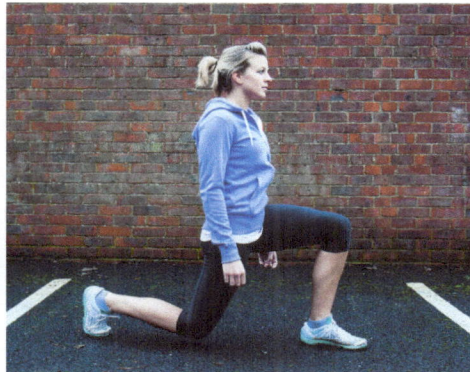

An example of how this technique can be used is within a leg workout, using exercises such as a Barbell Sumo Squat, Static Lunges and Plyometric Squat. The weights would again have to be pre-arranged, so that the exercises could be moved between with relative ease. Form is important, particularly during the final set of each of the exercises. Any use of plyometric training, especially within a technique with limited rest periods, should be approached with caution, as it will also raise the heart rate significantly. The client/patient should have some water available.

This could be expressed like:

Barbell Sumo Squat 3 x 5 at 86% 1RM
Dumbbell Static Lunges 3 x 10 at 73% 1RM
Plyometric Squats 3 x 20 at >63% 1RM

CHAPTER 6.

▪ ▪ ▪ ▪

At the end of each chapter, each case study and questions will be relevant to the knowledge acquired in the previous chapter(s).

Case Study 6

A 15-year old boy wants to start training with you. He has recently been selected for the regional athletic team after some hard training in the gym. He now wants some expert guidance, and his mum and physiotherapist agree that he is skeletally mature enough to train properly.

His disciplines vary between javelin, 400m and 100m, and he seems to perform well in all three. He has no injuries, although he is treated regularly for muscular soreness. He explains he has been using mostly machines for the past 18-months, as well as regular cardio training. Power and strength are his primary goals, however he doesn't want to lose speed.

He wants to train five days a week, and "will probably do another hour" as well as time with you. This is because he doesn't have many friends outside of school, and also wants to be selected by the national team.

After a quick assessment, you identify:

- He is 6'1
- Has a slight upper-crossed posture, and an associated anterior head carriage
- He has more of a mesomorph body-type, but obviously is still muscularly immature
- During the trunk endurance test he fails 21sec into stage 5
- Otherwise, he is a fit and healthy 15-year old

1. Using all of your knowledge and biomechanical understanding, please suggest a general 45-minute routine for this client/patient. Consider all aspects of training.

2. Are there any psychological concerns that you have regarding this client/patient based on what you know about them? If so, please explain.

3. Can you identify the origin, insertion and action of the hamstring muscle?

4. Stretching should be a vital part of any teenager's training programme. Can you suggest a routine for this client/patient?

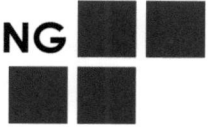

Notes

7. Gait Analysis

Learning Objectives

- To understand what gait is, and the different phases through gait.
- To understand what a gait analysis form should display, as well as an ability to systematically assess gait using the form.
- To have an appreciation for various discrepancies as well as normal findings during gait analysis.
- To understand what is meant by pronation and supination.
- To understand and appreciate the differences between various running techniques with respect to an individual.

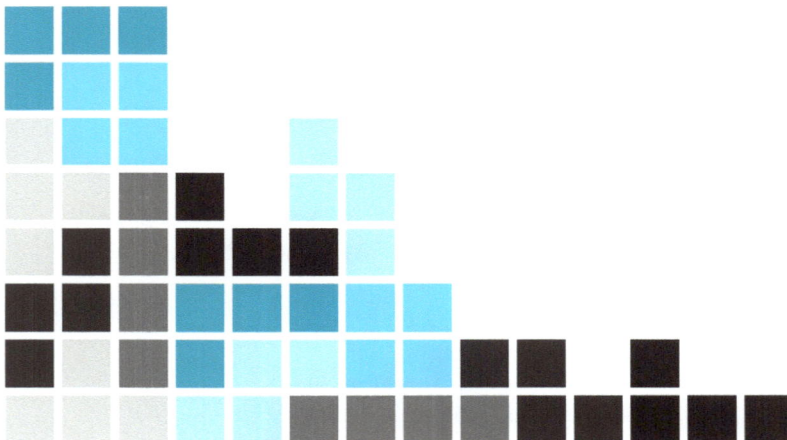

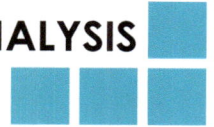

Gait analysis is the measure and observation of the mechanical factors affecting joint loading, orientation and neuromuscular function during walking and running.

It is commonly observed throughout a trainer or orthotic fitting that the assessor has a primary focus on the lower limb – particularly in the orientation of the foot and ankle. This focus, for this purpose is completely adequate. However, the biomechanical analysis of a person's full Gait Cycle can be used to identify much more than the direct implications to the foot and ankle. If used correctly it can be an important tool in assessing biomechanical abnormalities and potential weaknesses throughout the entire body that could be predisposed to injury.

The NHS (2012) explains that the average person walks between 3,000 - 4,000 steps everyday. Even over a single day, that is a significant amount of steps to take with a faulty kinetic chain or muscular imbalance, and that is without the consideration for improper footwear, single strap bags and young children wanting to be picked up throughout the day. It is easy to understand why assessing Gait can be paramount in identifying the potential for injury not just at the feet and ankles, but also at the hips, back and even the shoulders.

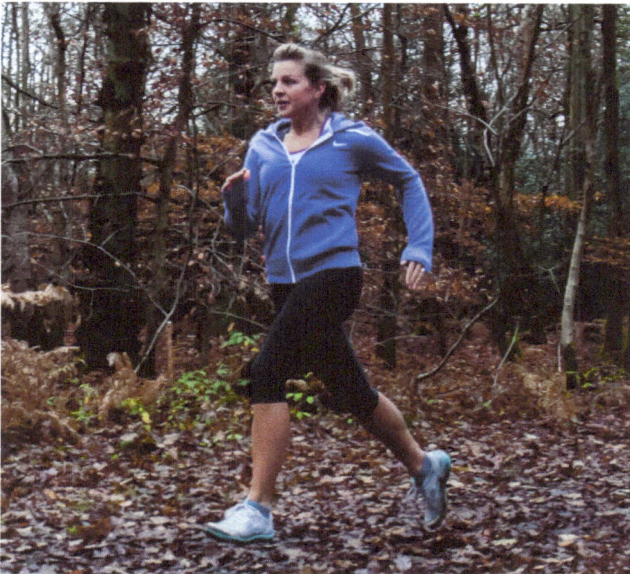

The gait cycle has both a complete stance and swing phase

The Gait Cycle is a continuous repetitive pattern of either walking or running, and it has two main phases of movement – the stance and swing phases. A full complete Gait Cycle should include both a stance and swing phase from 'Heel Strike' to 'Heel Strike' of the same leg.

The stance phase should account for approximately 60% of the Gait Cycle during walking, and describes the period whereby the foot is in contact with the ground. The swing phase identifies the period during the cycle where the foot is off of the ground, which accounts for the remaining 40%. These two phases are made up of smaller, more distinctive phases (Figure 38) as described by

CHAPTER 7.

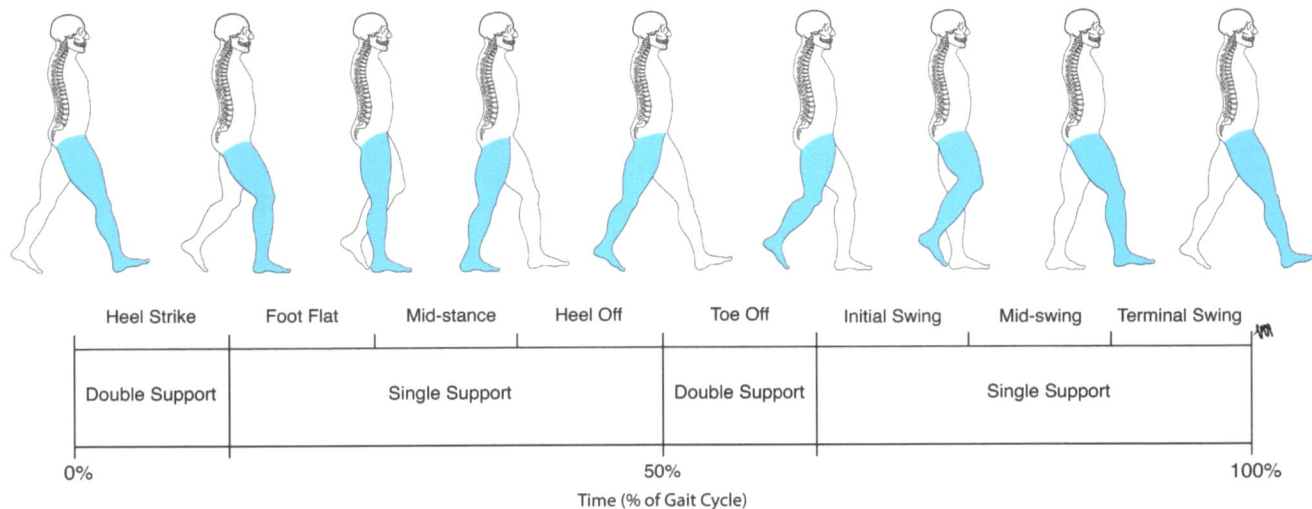

Heel Strike | Foot Flat | Mid-stance | Heel Off | Toe Off | Initial Swing | Mid-swing | Terminal Swing

Double Support | Single Support | Double Support | Single Support

0% | 50% | 100%

Time (% of Gait Cycle)

Figure 38: the various stages throughout the gait cycle

Schultz *et al* (2005):

- **Heel Strike** is a short period that begins as the heel makes contact with the ground, and also provides the first instance of Double Support – where both feet are in contact with the ground, which is unique to walking. The hip will appear at approximately 30° flexion with the knee in full extension, as well as the ankle being dorsiflexed.
- **Foot Flat** is a phase where the foot starts to roll into pronation as the ankle and foot joints absorb the impact. The hip joint moves into extension as the knee flexes – which like the foot and ankle absorbs shock, but also propels the body forward.
- **Midstance** is supported solely by one leg. The hip and knee both move into extension as the ankle joint becomes neutrally positioned, which provides the maximum amount of contact with the ground as well as providing additional propulsion.
- **Heel Off** begins when the heel leaves the floor. The majority of the body weight at this phase is distributed across the metatarsal heads, however Double Support is also provided at this phase as the opposing heel strikes the ground. The hip extends to approximately 15°, as the knee begins to flex and ankle platarflexes.
- **Toe Off** as the name suggests, this phase begins as the big

167

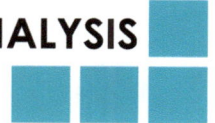

toe leaves the ground. The hip starts to return to its original flexed position, as well as the knee flexing to approximately 40° in order to bring the foot through the swing phase without scuffing the toes.

- **Midswing** is the final stage before the cycle repeats itself. The hip flexes to its original 30° as the knee extends and the ankle becomes dorsiflexed.

When considering the gait cycle during running, a greater proportion of the cycle is dedicated to the swing phase. This is due in large part to the shorter period of time the foot is in contact with the ground. There is also no Double Support throughout a running gait cycle. In fact there is a phase where neither foot is in contact with the ground, which is known as the flight phase.

The process of assessing gait can be broken down into four key components depending primarily on the patient/client, but also on the judgement of the assessor. Walking and running are obviously the main variables, as gait can change dramatically between both. Other components are walking/running with and without trainers.

Assessing gait should always be client/patient specific and the reason for doing so should be key consideration throughout. Asking a client/patient to run when they have pain or discomfort with walking is unnecessary. For example, the assessment done on a client/patient that gets hip pain whilst running will be different to that done on the client/patient who experiences pain at the base of their heel when walking from meeting to meeting. Every individual functions in a way that is both unique and specific to them.

7.1 Gait Analysis Form

A form to assess gait analysis has some fundamental elements that should be included. This structure will give the assessor guidance through the assessment but also aid the assessor's ability to feedback the findings to the client/patient in a methodical way.

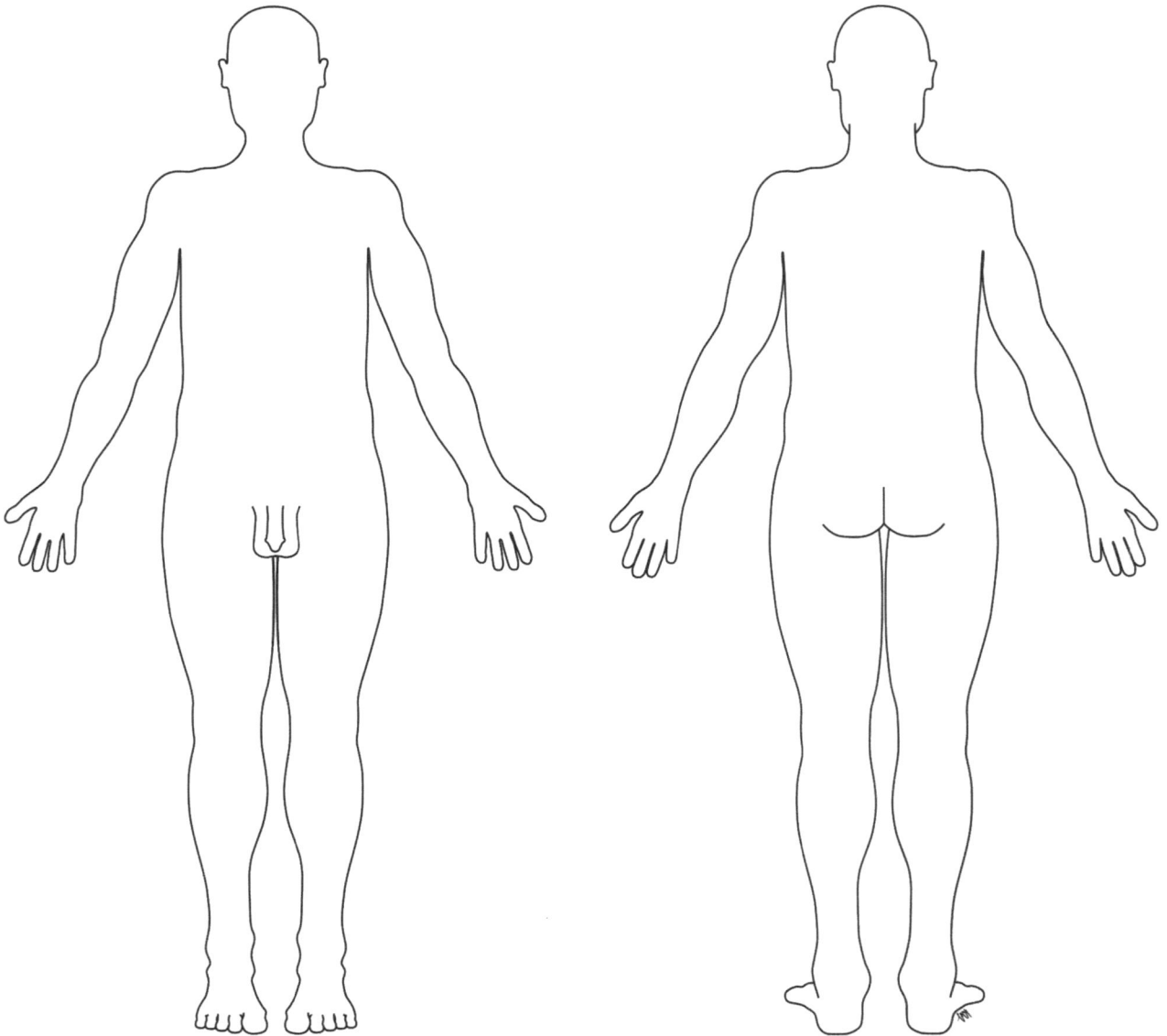

Figure 39: displays a blank anterior and posterior human body

A blank diagram of the human body (Figure 39) will allow space for tight muscles to be drawn on or highlighted, and offers a valuable visual aid when explaining findings.

The form can then be laid out in whatever fashion is comfortable to the assessor. It will need space to record findings of the assessment itself; an example has been included below (Table 7). The form is then designed at the discretion of the assessor to

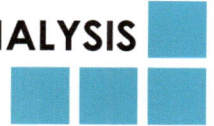

Gait w/out Shoes - Walk	Gait w/out Shoes - Running
Head & Trunk: Posture	Head & Trunk: Posture
Shoulder Complex: Swing, Posture, Tension	Shoulder Complex: Swing, Posture, Tension
Hips & Legs: Level, Movement	Hips & Legs: Level, Movement
Knees: Deformity, Movement	Knees: Deformity, Movement
Ankles: Calcaneus, Strike, Movement	Ankles: Calcaneus, Strike, Movement
Foot & Hallux: Arches, Toes, Movement	Foot & Hallux: Arches, Toes, Movement

Table 7: demonstrates an example table that can be used to systematically record findings

include such things as recommendation on orthotics, referral to another professional or even relevant exercises. The form should be easy for the assessor to transition through, whilst having plenty of space to record findings of the Gait Analysis.

The analysis part of the form should be clear and include relevant sections or steps of the assessment for the purpose of guidance, but also feedback. Below, each section within the table has been broken down to explain what could be observed.

CHAPTER 7.

Head & Trunk

Observation of the way a person holds their head and upper body can indicate many things:

Anterior Head Carriage: this finding is ever more present within the population, especially alongside sedentary postures. Commonly the head will sit slightly forwards away from the midline (plumb line), indicating either a weakness of the deep neck flexors or an overcompensation of the neck extensors due to kyphotic posture (upper-crossed posture).

Lateral Deviation: commonly this finding will be related to either torticollis (involuntary muscle spasm of Scalenes or Sternocleidomastoid) or whiplash associated symptoms. The client/patient may even complain of an uncomfortable night's sleep or that they 'cricked' their neck.

Thoracic Rigidity: the ability of the thoracic spine to extend contributes greatly to the efficiency of the lungs and ribcage to expand during breathing. It may not be evident straightaway that a client/patient has rigidity within their thoracic spine using just a gait analysis alone. Signs that can be observed include rounding of the shoulders, leaning forward through the trunk, and an increased kyphosis – all can be precursors to thoracic rigidity. These observations/signs can then be focused on using Wall Angel Test (Chapter 8.4) to assess the rigidity of the thoracic spine.

Upper-crossed Posture: this is another prominent finding among the sedentary population, and more increasingly common in the gym environment. This is due in large part to a high number of men, particularly young men, participating in heavy weight training without consideration for stretching. Upper-crossed posture is a combination of several findings including anterior head carriage, extension of the upper cervical spine, rounded shoulders and a hyperkyphosis. Upper-crossed posture is most commonly caused by muscular imbalance rather than the structural integrity being compromised. However, importantly a person can have thoracic rigidity without having upper-crossed posture.

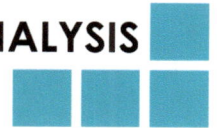

Shoulder Complex

Shoulders can hold some of the most significant findings when considering the implications of the kinetic chain on the upper body during gait, as well as individual mechanical dysfunctions. Shoulders may display some dramatic asymmetry, this in itself can be a finding, but it commonly is observed as an asymptomatic, normal finding within a client/patient. However, it should not be quickly dismissed.

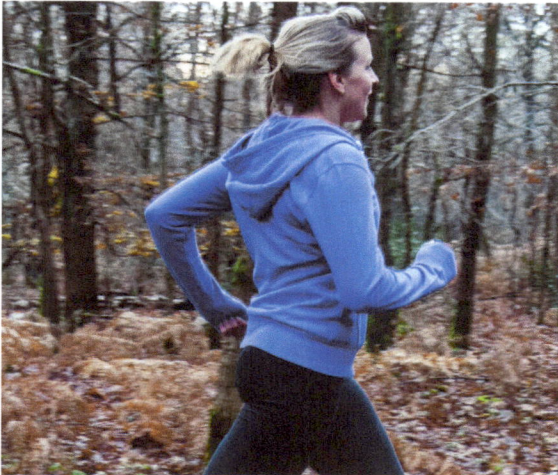

The shoulder complex should be observed during the gait cycle

Rounded Shoulders: as well as being a significant sign in the identification of upper-crossed posture, rounded shoulders can also present as a finding in its own right. Most commonly they are associated with tightness in the pectorals or weakness in the Rhomboids and Lower Trapezius muscles. This finding can be appreciated from a side view, with the centre of the humeral head being anteriorly placed away from the plumb line.

Reduced Shoulder Swing: the shoulder swing is an important part of gait as it aids counter-balance to the action of the legs, but also helps develop momentum and consequently power through the stride. If one shoulder appears to have a reduced swing then the biomechanics of the gait may be impaired, with numerous other joints and muscles compensating for the strain. Upon recognising that there is a reduction in swing on one or maybe both arms, it is important to observe the rest of the body for any abnormal gait patterns. A compact bilateral arm swing will often indicate a cautious gait, either due to the client/patient feeling unbalanced or to protect an injury.

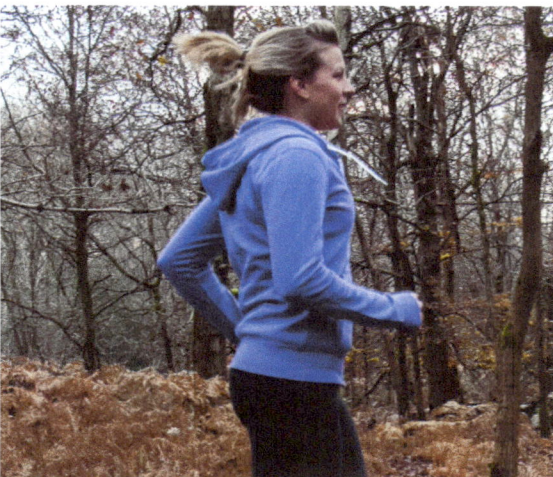

A reduced shoulder swing can significantly alter the gait cycle

Raised Shoulders: the shoulders will appear shrugged and the general gait will look rigid. This is often a defence mechanism that the body will acquire, most commonly in response to injury such as whiplash or sleeping awkwardly. Firstly ask the client/patient if they are aware they are doing it, they may be doing it out of habit or they may even be able to tell you why they have adopted it. If they are unable to identify a possible reason for their shoulder/s being raised, then observe the rest of the kinetic chain through gait for any abnormalities that may help explain why they have accommodated it.

Hips & Legs

This component of gait analysis is especially important to understand, as it comprises numerous pivotal joints within the gait's biomechanics. The observation of the hips and legs may display some significant muscular imbalance and weaknesses that potentially could be predisposing to numerous injuries. It is also important to consider other components such as the lower back and knees that could be compensating for weakness and imbalance at the hips and pelvis.

Hip Drop: otherwise known as a Trendelenburg gait, it is a sign of neurological weakness or inhibition of the Gluteus Medius. It is recognised by the tilting of the pelvis downwards on the side of the swinging leg. This means that the stance legs' gluteus medius is weak or inhibited as it is failing to stabilise the pelvis in a neutral position during gait. Although the term Trendelenburg gait is specifically used for *neurological* weakness, there is an air of discrepancy in its use to suggest a functional weakness or imbalance of the Gluteus Medius muscle. A catwalk-styled gait will be observed in clients/patients that do not use either Gluteus Medius muscles.

Pelvic Rotation: if in fact the pelvis is rotated, the rotation possible at the sacroiliac joints has recently been rumoured to be minimal, possibly of nothing more than 5° on each side. This means that definitive signs of true pelvic rotation will be difficult to observe, especially through clothes. However, the appearance of pelvic rotation may be apparent – it is likely that any rotation is associated with both the lumbar spine and musculature or a scoliosis. This may result in a rotated pelvic appearance due to the Coupling Principle (Chapter 1.5) of the facet joints; whereby the facet joints rotate as well as laterally flexing either towards or away from the direction of rotation. This is dependent upon the orientation of the facet joints. Acute muscle spasm or restriction

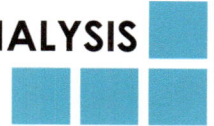

within the facet joints may also result in the appearance of a pelvic rotation.

Reduced Hip Extension: if a reduction in hip extension is observed, it is important to first understand whether the reduction is being caused by a problem functionally or structurally. More commonly clients/patients will have a functional weakness or muscular imbalance either because the Gluteus Maximus is weak, the hip flexors are tight, or the Erectus Spinae or Hamstrings are overactive. To confirm a suspected finding, tests such as the Modified Thomas Test (hip flexor tightness) and Hip Extension Motor Pattern (Gluteal and Hamstring activation) can be very helpful (see Chapter 8.8). Structural abnormalities such as hip dysplasia, slipped upper femoral epiphysis or osteoarthritis will need further medical investigation such as an x-ray or MRI.

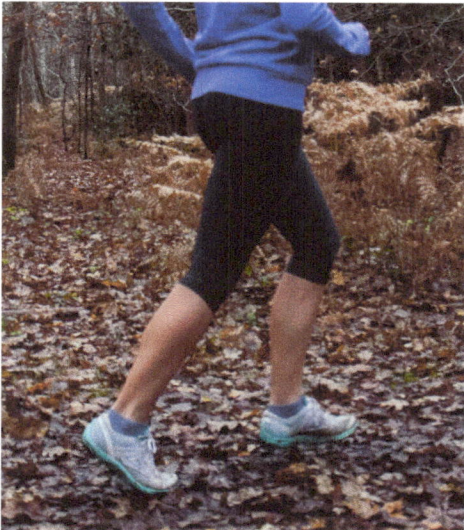

Reduced hip extension is often related to inactive or weak glutes

Increased Hip Flexion: is usually recognised as a compensatory mechanism. It is also known as a high-steppage gait, and is quite common among clients/patients that suffer with neurological weakness of L5 nerve root. This is due to a neurological weakness of the dorsiflexors of the foot, which causes the client/patient to excessively flex the hip in order to bring the swing leg through the gait cycle without scuffing the foot/big toe – which may potentially cause them to trip and fall.

External Hip Rotation: more commonly found in men rather than women, possibly due to a greater amount of elastin within female musculature. External rotation of the hip can be interpreted by observing the positioning of the feet along with the tone and/or bulk of the Gluteal muscles, particularly the external hip rotators (Gluteus Maximus, Medius and Piriformis). The foot position in a client/patient with an externally rotated hip is known as *Too Many Toes* sign. In a client/patient with a neutrally positioned hip, 2 – 2½ toes should be visible from a posterior view during gait, any more than this may suggest an excessive amount of external rotation at the hip. Often an increase in hip external rotation is due to tight, hypertonic or hypertrophic muscle, such as the piriformis or Gluteus Medius muscle. Palpating these muscles will give a better understanding as to which, if any, is causing an increase in rotation.

Internal Hip Rotation: similar to hip extension, this can be caused by both structural discrepancies as well as functional imbalances. However, distinguishing between the two may prove difficult using just gait analysis. A common cause of excessive internal rotation is congenital hip dysplasia, which is a condition that is caused by the head of the femur not fully forming through childhood. This causes the ball and socket joint of the hip to be fairly shallow. Assessing the hip range of motion for a lack of internal hip rotation alongside a positive *Drehmann* sign – a compensatory movement of external rotation of the hip when the hip is flexed, may indicate a structural problem. This would have to be examined and investigated by a medical professional. Functionally, either restriction of the joint capsule or tightness of the internal rotators of the hip muscles is ordinarily the primary reason for an increase in internal rotation – assessed again by passive hip range of motion, observing especially for any reduced movement throughout adduction, abduction and extension.

Knees

Clients/patients may often present with a structural deformity of the knee (Figure 40), or the structures surrounding the knee joint, such as the muscles, tendons and ligaments, may be aiding other biomechanical weaknesses throughout gait. An example of this is the additional work placed upon the Hamstrings during a high-steppage gait, which may place additional strain on the muscle's insertion around the knee joint. When assessing the knees it is important to remain observant to the biomechanics of the hips as well as the knees, as the two are often closely associated.

Genu Valgum: also known as knock-knees (Figure 41). When standing the knees will touch but the feet will not. It is an irreversible deformity of the lower extremities that can lead to muscular imbalance and consequently compensatory pain at the knees throughout gait. The pain can often be avoided with a regular stretch routine for the muscles of the lower extremity.

Genu Varum: also known as bowed legs (Figure 41). When

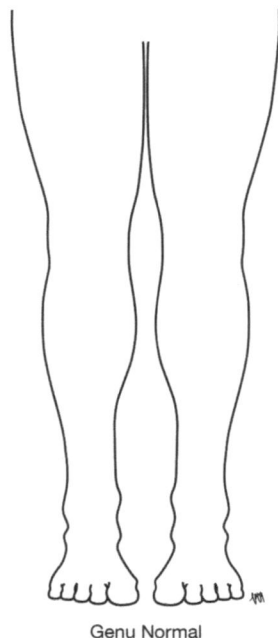

Genu Normal

Figure 40: demonstrates normal knee posiiton

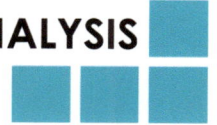

standing with the feet together the knees will not touch. As above it is irreversible and can often cause muscular imbalance throughout the kinetic chain and especially in the lower extremities.

Genu Recurvatum: also known as back knees. The knees will appear hyperextended and thus have a naturally increased length in the hamstrings. Clients/patients that present with hyperextension of the knees are often hypermobile, which should also be a consideration when assessing and training an individual with hypermobility. Potential muscular imbalances and biomechanical dysfunctions often occur at the knee and continue up the kinetic chain towards the hips and lower back as other muscles attempt to compensate for the lack of stability at the knee joints.

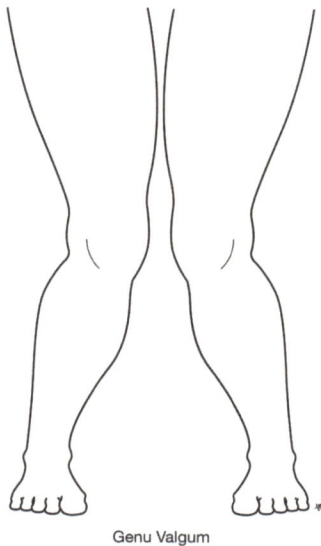

Tibial Torsion: is a twisting of the tibia that will cause the foot to appear as if it is turning inwards, which will often present very similarly to an increase in external hip rotation. This means that it can often be confused with a structural or functional problem at the hip joint due to the orientation of the feet. There are two tests to help distinguish between tibial torsion and excessive external hip rotation. The first is performed with the client/patient standing, both feet should be facing forwards, and then the orientation of the patella can be observed. With tibial torsion the patella will appear straight, but there may be a marked bowing of the tibia or the client/patient may report discomfort whilst maintaining their feet to face forwards.

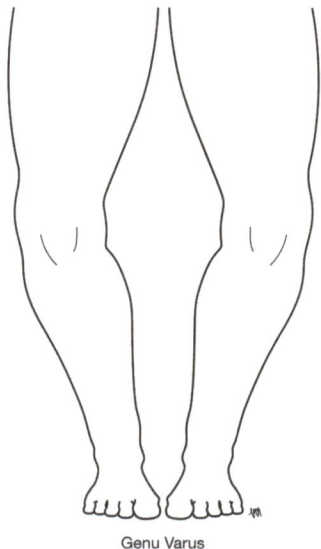

The second assessment is to have the client/patient seated and importantly with their feet off of the floor, the orientation of the ankle joint line can then be compared with the joint line of the knee. A medical professional should always confirm tibial torsion; the correct protocol if tibial torsion is suspected is to refer to a musculoskeletal professional.

Ankles

Together with the feet, the ankles are inevitably the most important part of the gait cycle. They can often be excessively analysed for this reason without regard for the biomechanics of the kinetic

Genu Valgum

Genu Varus

Figure 41: demonstrates valgus deformity (above), and varus deformity (below)

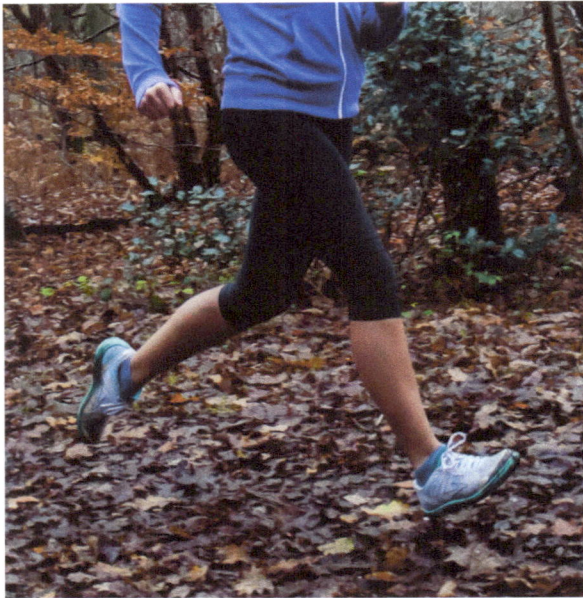

The way the foot strikes the ground is an important aspect of gait analysis

chain superiorly to the feet and ankles. This is most commonly demonstrated during an assessment for running trainers. With the numerous stabilising ligaments at the ankle susceptible to injury from an early age it is understandable why this can be crucial to analyse, and should also coincide with an understanding of previous and current injuries to the feet and ankles.

Heel strike: the heel strike is arguably the most vital aspect of the walking, and in some circumstances the running gait cycle. It is the first aspect of the stance phase and is important for two primary reasons. The first is related to the loading of the body's weight through all of the joints of the ankle and foot, which then reduces the amount of compensated shock and force through other more proximal joints such as the knee and hip, thus reducing the risk of injury. The ankle joint is also a highly ligamentous structure that is responsible for a considerable amount of proprioception. The heel strike through the gait cycle allows the greatest amount of time for the ankle and foot to absorb information regarding its position in space, as well as its surroundings (curbs, stones, terrain etc.) – a fundamental attribute that significantly reduces the risk of injury.

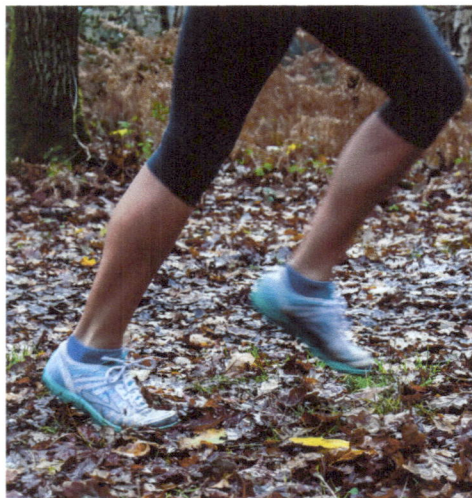

Calcaneal movement during toe off may suggest an issue with gluteal control

Calcaneal Movement: as the foot comes through the final stage of the stance phase (the Toe Off), as opposed to the calcaneus tracking neutrally through the swing phase of gait, it may track initially either internally or externally. This is known as either calcaneal inversion or calcaneal eversion, respectively. A subtle and mild calcaneal eversion is an ideal finding in a normal gait cycle as it identifies the foot is working through pronation, and thus recruiting the glutes. This process stores energy and enhances the lower limbs' ability to accelerate through propulsion.

Limited Dorsiflexion: this finding is often relative to the client/patient's range of motion bilaterally, with any asymmetry suggesting a potential limitation in dorsiflexion at the ankle

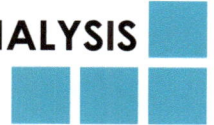

joint. For example, someone may have a tight Gastroc complex bilaterally, however it may not necessarily suggest a restriction in dorsiflexion. During the mid-swing phase, the foot will be dorsiflexed sufficiently so that the big toe does not catch the floor. If there is a limitation in dorsiflexion of one of the ankle joints, it may be observed that the client/patient will either swing their lower limb around a lateral axis, or to excessively flex the hip – mimicking a high-steppage gait, thus avoiding tripping on the toe through the swing phase. A way of testing for limited dorsiflexion is to assess the talar joints movement using a Step Down Test (Chapter 8.10), during which the client/patient may complain of a pinching sensation or restriction in the anterior aspect of the ankle.

Stability: throughout childhood, children may suffer from an inversion or even an eversion sprain of the ankle. Due to the nature and orientation of the ligaments surrounding the ankle joint this will often result in the ligaments tearing, and in more serious circumstances resulting in an avulsion fracture of the malleolus – the bony tip of either the tibia or fibula. The ligaments at the ankle joint have a significant responsibility with regard to the bodies' ability to maintain balance. Due to these reasons it is possible that an ankle may be observed as being unstable. If instability in the ankle is recognised, it is perfectly reasonable to ask the client/patient whether they have previously injured it, or even if they recognise the instability on a daily basis. Ligamentous strains or tears, will not only affect the length of the ligaments due to the scar tissue and regenerating fibres, but also the proprioceptive qualities of the ligaments is likely to be impaired, which will contribute towards the joint's stability. This should be an important consideration with rehabilitative training.

Foot & Hallux

The foot and hallux (big toe) are the final biomechanical structures along the kinetic chain before the force and energy of the gait cycle is transferred to the ground. If there is an obvious dysfunction or muscular imbalance around these structures, it could potentially be compensated for higher up the chain. The longer the period of time something is compensated for, usually the more structures become involved. This means that instead of one biomechanical issue, several start to develop, which can often make rehabilitation and recovery a lengthy process. The findings that can be observed by looking at the foot and hallux can often be reasonably obvious (Figure 42), however it is possible to become fixated on a specific area and forget the rest of the biomechanics. There can be a stark and significant difference between a client/patient with or without shoes on, as well as between walking and running.

Over-pronation: also known as dropped arches or flat feet. Over-pronation can happen for a number of reasons including poor muscle control, displacement of the navicular, damage to the anterior talo-fibular and posterior talo-fibular ligaments (ATFL & PTFL), and even laziness. It is rather difficult to interpret whether the cause is structural or functional as there may be an involvement from both aspects. Commonly, people will have had 'flat feet' since childhood and this is often maintained due to a lack of knowledge and understanding regarding its implications.

Often a client/patient will ask upon it being identified, "if it is not painful or causing any problems, then why fix it"? Depending upon the individual and their daily functional needs this statement may be perfectly valid. However, with the average person taking around 3000-4000 (NHS, 2012) steps per day, it is arguable that a problem may develop over time – adding to the adage that prevention is better than cure. Professional athletes, gym users and even regular walkers would benefit from improving an over-pronation issue. Over-pronation can put the kinetic chain under great stress, especially with running, making it much more susceptible to injury.

On examination, a noticeable deviation of the calcaneus (heel bone) will be observed. This should coincide with a flattening of the longitudinal arch of the foot. With the client/patient standing naturally for them, the assessor should be able to palpate a gap between the longitudinal arch and the ground. A diminished or absent gap would suggest a flattening or drop of the arch.

Over-supination: also known as high arches or clinically as

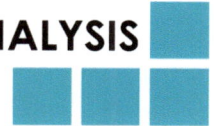

pes cavus, which directly translate to 'foot cave'. This directly relates to the space between the longitudinal arch of the foot and the ground representing a cave-like structure. The excessive elevation of the longitudinal arch, caused commonly by tightness in the muscle and tendons in the dorsum of the foot, can also cause the toes to be become contracted into a clawing position. The dorsum of the foot is often tender and uncomfortable due to the hypertonic and rigid state of the muscles in the foot. This will place excessive stress upon the metatarsal heads, especially throughout the toe off phase of gait where the stress is concentrated specifically over the first metatarsal.

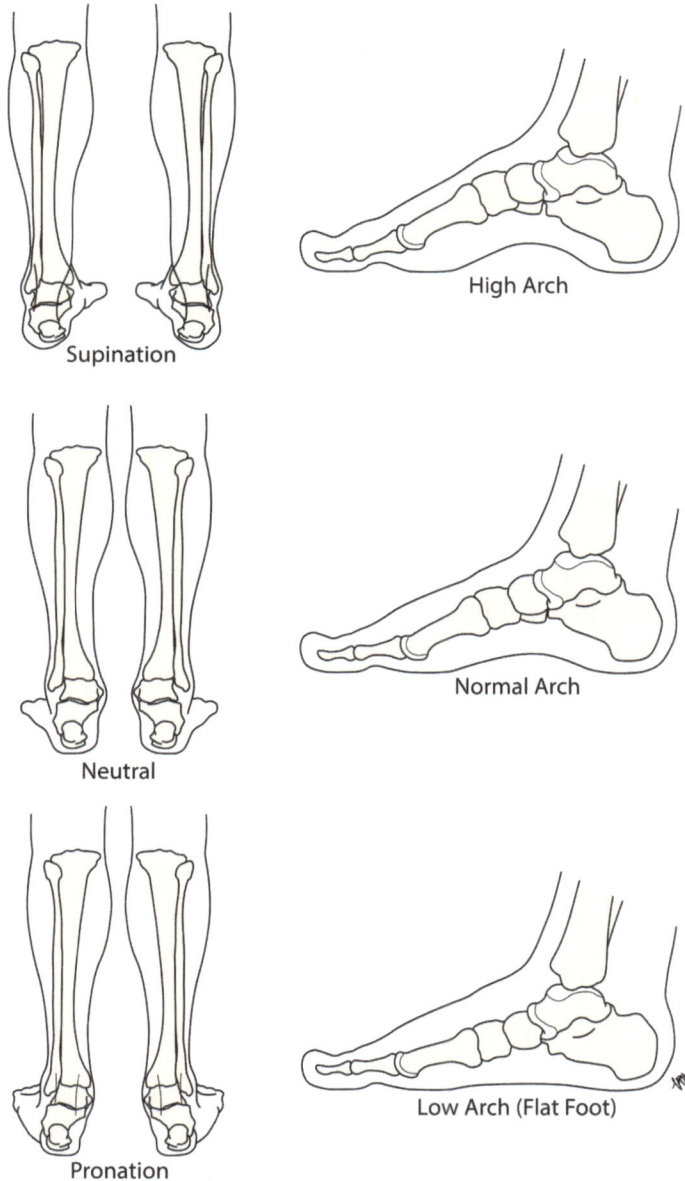

The rigid nature of the foot restricts its ability to pronate following the heel strike, which places the ankle under a greater risk of injury, such as inversion sprains. As well as the risk of sprains, the constant and increased force being directed through the metatarsal heads will increase the risk of injuries such as metatarsal stress fractures and Morton's Neuroma.

The prevalence of over-pronation is greater than over-supination, suggested to be at a ratio of about 9:1 (Austin, 1994). Proper assessment, fitting and selection of trainers and shoes can dramatically improve the risks associated with both.

Figure 42: foot position with supination, neutral & pronation

Hallux Rigidus: the fixation or 'rigid' nature of the hallux (big toe) that can often be observed during the toe off phase of gait. Observation will reveal a limited extension of the big toe. It is thought to relate to wear and tear of the metatarsophalangeal joint (MTP) from either an acute trauma, or repetitive use. At the toe off phase of gait, either pushing off the ball of the foot or exaggerating knee flexion (high steppage) to bring the big toe through without scuffing may compensate for hallux rigidus. It may be painful to extend due to degenerative changes. The client/patient should be asked to actively flex and extend the big toe without weight bearing to assess true range of motion of the big toe.

Talus Neutral

This involves assessing the talus firstly for its natural position, and then for its neutral position. It can help identify whether any flattening is either functional or structural. The client/patient is instructed to stand naturally with an even distribution of weight across both feet. In this position, the assessor should be able to palpate the dome of the talus on both the medial and lateral aspects with their thumb and index finger. When the talus is neutrally positioned, the dome of the talus should be equally palpable on both the medial and lateral aspects. If it is not equal, instruct the client/patient to invert their feet as far as possible, and then evert them as far as possible, and finally they should be instructed to find the position mid-way between the two extremes – this will usually bring them to approximately talus neutral. Small modifications can be made to correct if the client/patient is not exactly equal.

A functional over-pronation is indicated by an ability to maintain talus neutral whilst maintaining a gap between the longitudinal arch and the ground, in a client/patient that naturally has a flattened arch. If the client/patient is unable to maintain a gap between their longitudinal arch and the ground, it is likely they may have a structurally dropped navicular or other anatomical variation that restricts their ability to raise their arch from the ground.

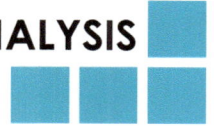

7.2 Running Techniques

The increase in running events throughout the year, such as marathons, charity events and even triathlons, have led to a dramatic increase in the number of people seen daily out 'pounding the pavement'. Besides the obvious health benefits of regular exercise, running also carries a sense of freedom and stress relief that is not often associated with other sporting activities.

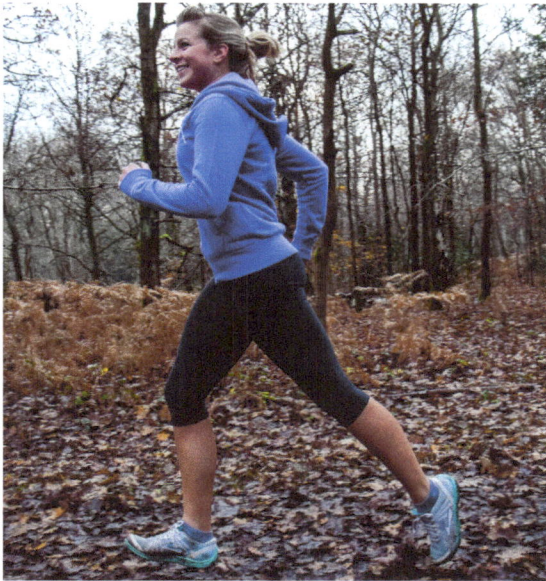

Running provides numerous benefits to both physical and mental health

The past decade has seen a rise not only of the trainers that are available (traditional, supportive, minimalist and even barefoot), but also the techniques that can be adopted by runners. This increase has provided a greater awareness of options available to runners, which could have led to its modern popularity. People are able to hold an identity within a community with the use of colour, style and technique, without being ostracised or out-casted. However, through the haze of new options and theories, the prevailing questions loom. Which is the right trainer to wear, what is the best technique, and is there any significant research to suggest either way?

In truth, the research into these topics does not count for a great deal of the decision process. The choice on trainers, style and technique is more often than not decided upon by exposure to an acceptable trend or theory. This is in part due to the general population's perception of current research being rather controversial, not to mention the academic style of writing deterring even the most research conscious of people. In short, this topic is more often than not determined by advertising and marketing techniques rather than current supported research.

Across the world, regardless of culture or fashion, the running community most recently has become divided over running technique. It seems everyone is quick to have an opinion on the topic – which often mirrors his or her own technique. Technique, more specifically identifies the foot strike, the way which the foot initially makes contact with the ground during running. The three categorised types of foot strike include:

- Heel Strike - The heel strikes first and rolls onto the forefoot
- Neutral Strike – The strike occurs somewhere between the forefoot and heel with both effectively landing at once
- Forefoot Strike – The ball of the foot strikes first and pushes through the big toe

When exploring whether there is in fact a 'correct' technique, an understanding and appreciation for each technique is paramount. This way an informed opinion can be formulated based firstly upon the correct biomechanics and kinetics, and also the client/patients demands and needs. Every runner is unique and will have an individual goal, whether that is to get fit or to run a marathon.

Heel Strike Running

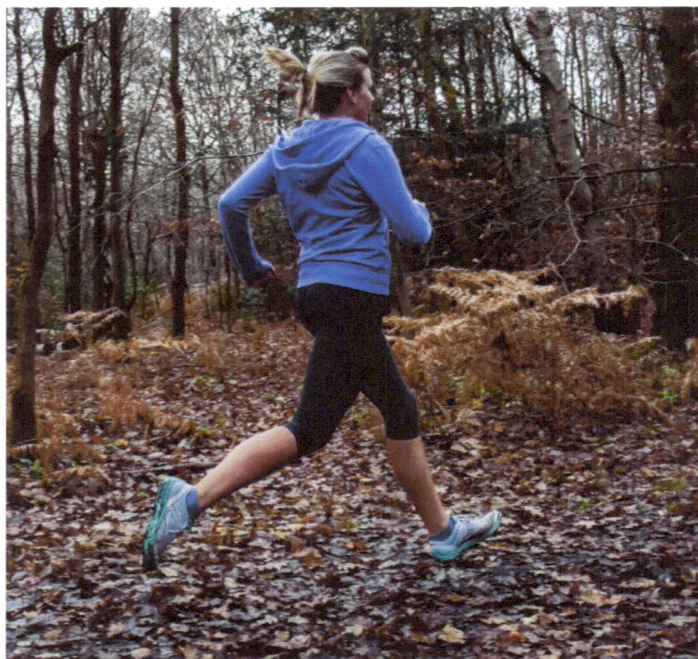

When heel striking, the lead leg will extend ahead of the body's centre of gravity

In our modern day running culture, heel strike running is arguably the most common technique used. A study in 2007 by Hasegawa *et al* observed 74.9% of runners in a half marathon used a heel strike. The mechanism involved is initiated by dorsiflexing the foot and extending the leading leg ahead of the body's centre of gravity (COG). The heel is the first point of contact with the ground, then the foot pronates by rolling across the lateral aspect of the foot and onto the ball, the force is then shifted to the big toe which is used in toe/push off to generate forward momentum.

In theory, this technique is far more energy efficient for a mid to long distance runner. This is because a more evenly distributed working effort is achieved between the musculature of the legs, including the Gluteals, Quadriceps, Hamstrings and Gastroc complex. This even distribution of effort means that the natural braking mechanism of the body, involving the Hip Flexors, Hamstrings and Dorsiflexors, works equally alongside the accelerating mechanism, which includes the Gluteals, Quadriceps and Gastroc complex. The initial strike of the heel being ahead of the centre of gravity (COG) illustrates the use of a braking system. Whereas the constant momentum and forward movement identifies the use of the power dominant acceleration system. This also means that the Gluteals and Quadriceps do not burn as much energy as in other techniques, thus reducing the effects of fatigue, such as lactic acid.

Another consideration with this technique is the natural shock absorbing ability of the body by way of the numerous joints not only in the feet and ankles, but also all through the kinetic chain. It has been suggested that this technique generates a lot of stress through the ankles, knees, hips, and lower back (Morris, 2010). Running in general, in spite of what technique is used, generates a lot of stress – in fact it is estimated the force through the kinetic chain during gait is 3-5 x bodyweight (Lieberman *et al*, 2010). With this in mind, distributing the force and shock, especially over a considerable running distance, should be of primary concern.

Based on the principles considered, this technique is not about speed; it favours the basic values of energy efficiency and equal weight distribution across the joints. This means it would suit any runner considering running a considerable distance such as 10km and further. Changing to a heel strike technique can be rather difficult for any runner employing a different style. This in most part is due to the elongation of the stride, which can take some getting used to. Once it has been adapted to, runners will often find the technique comfortable to use, and may describe the experience as 'bouncing' through the foot strike.

Initially however, runners complain of muscle soreness down the front of the shinbone (tibia), which can also be misinterpreted as shin splints. This soreness is more often than not a result of delayed onset of muscle soreness (DOMS) in the Tibialis Anterior, which runs down the front of the shin. It is used more during this technique compared to the others due to the need to dorsiflex the foot. This prevents any scuffing of the big toe, and thus any potential to trip and fall. A heel strike technique may take some time and re-education to perfect. It will however greatly improve running efficiency over mid to long distances.

Neutral Strike Running

In a similar fashion to the heel strike technique, the foot will dorsiflex during a neutral strike, however the knee joint will not fully extend. This means that the point of contact with the ground is mildly ahead of the centre of gravity (COG). The neutral strike technique concludes similarly to the heel strike technique, as it utilises the generated momentum from the lateral foot, ball of the foot and big toe contact with the ground.

This technique is between the heel strike and forefoot techniques. Although a closer look at this technique, suggests that it has more in common with the forefoot strike technique. This is due in large part to the shock absorption properties of the talar and subtalar joints being substituted for the elastic recoil properties within the muscles of the foot and lower limb. It can prove very difficult during a real-time gait analysis, without the use of a slow motion camera, to appreciate whether the technique is either neutral or forefoot unless the examiner is extremely vigilant.

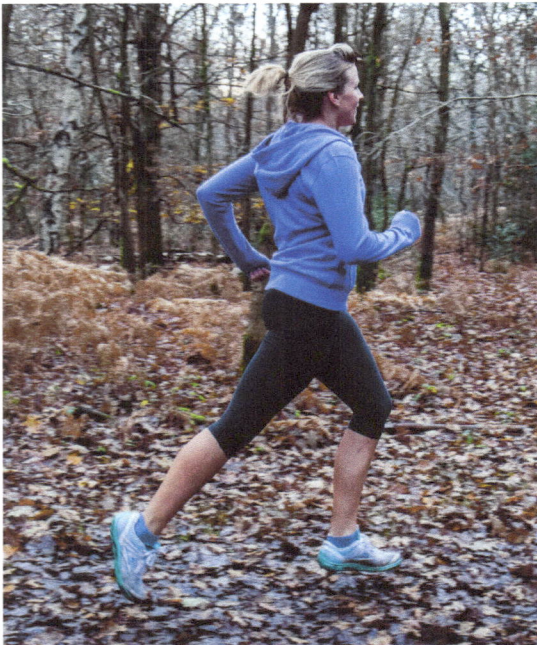

Morris (2010) suggests that this technique uses the pre-stretched position of the calf muscles on impact with the ground, to preserve energy. He identifies the pre-stretched position as the engagement of the calf muscles as the dorsiflexed foot contacts the ground. This in theory is ideal, the calf muscles acting like a springboard – reusing the energy from the impact with the ground to push the body forwards, which results in less force being absorbed by the joints. However, the multiple joints available between the bones of the feet are structurally perfect to absorb shock. This means that the substituted connective tissues are placed under greater demand than just performing muscle contraction and relaxation.

Neutral striking utilises a contact point with the ground closer to the body's centre of gravity

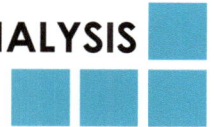

One piece of connective tissue that is placed under increased demand is the plantar fascia. This is a small, tough, web-like piece of tissue that connects the calcaneus to the distal heads of the metatarsals. It acts in a similar fashion to an elastic band, and its primary role is to maintain the arch of the foot.

The plantar fascia will take much of the shock during the neutral foot strike, as it is the first connective tissue to be stretched along the kinetic chain. Due to the plantar fascia's reduced elastic properties in comparison to a normal muscle, an overuse or sudden increased demand on the tissue may result in an injury known as plantar fasciitis, which is similar to a tendonitis injury.

With this in mind, it can be postulated that the neutral foot strike technique will neither provide maximum speed, due to the substantial foot contact with the ground, or maximum energy efficiency, due to the increased demand placed on the muscles to absorb shock. However, it does facilitate a faster running speed potential than the heel strike technique, due to the more dominant muscle activity of the acceleration muscle chain (Gluteals, Quadriceps and Gastoc complex), compared to the deceleration chain. Consequently this technique would suit a fit mid-distance runner, running between 5km and 15km. A moderate level of fitness and experience using this technique is advised for runners running over 10km, this is to reduce the risk of overuse and strain to the connective tissues.

It has been stated in journals and blogs (Morris, 2010; Michaud, 2014; RunningWarehouse, 2014) that the neutral foot strike reduces the risk of injury compared to other techniques. However, there appears to be no significant evidence to support this theory. Each running technique, or sport for that matter, carries a degree of injury risk. This technique in particular places a lot of strain on the connective tissues of the lower limbs, and a considerable amount of anterior stress on the knee joints. This means that running moderation and stretching should be fundamental components when using this technique to best prevent overuse injuries, such as plantar fasciitis and patellofemoral pain syndrome (Runners Knee).

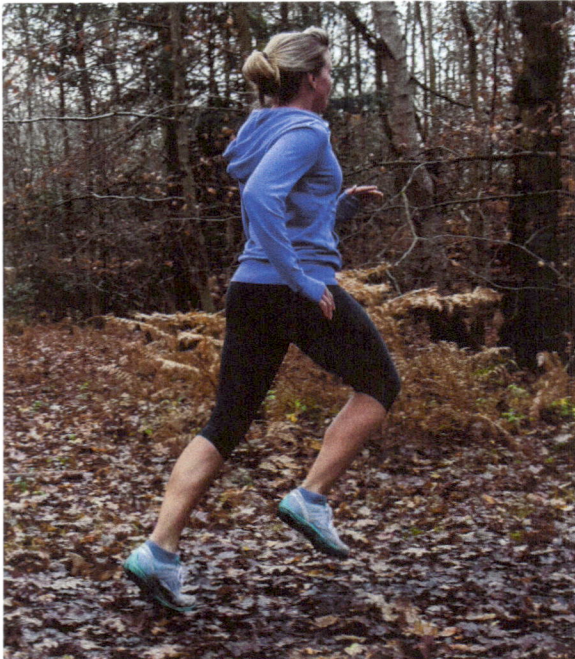

CHAPTER 7.

Forefoot Strike Running

Over the past few years, the phrase on every running club's and running enthusiast's lips has been "barefoot running", and consequently forefoot or toe running. What is it? Is it any good? Does it work?

It is important to first understand that barefoot and forefoot running are two very different things. Barefoot running is the choice to run without trainers or footwear, whereas forefoot running is a technique that can be utilised regardless of footwear. Although, in today's social running clubs the philosophy of barefoot running has led to the fascination in forefoot/toe running and the development of more mainstream minimalist trainers. Professionally however, sprinters have been running on their toes for decades.

Forefoot striking for speed will place the body's centre of gravity ahead of the foots contact point

Striking the ground with the forefoot is very similar in principle to the neutral strike technique, the main difference is that the forefoot strike is usually performed at a greater speed – between 75-100% maximum running speed. The momentum is generated by shifting the weight of the body ahead of the centre of gravity, combined with a strong 'paw-back' of the lower limb and foot. The 'paw-back' was described by Leiberman *et al* (2010), whereby the intense contraction of the Gastroc complex along with the co-contraction of the Quadricep and Gluteal muscles, powerfully drive the flexed leg towards the ground.

At a speed between 75-100% maximum speed the point at which the foot makes contact with the ground should be slightly ahead of the centre of gravity (COG). However during the acceleration phase, especially in sprinting from a block start, the point of contact will be behind the COG as a low, aerodynamic frame is utilised.

A combination of maximal muscle contraction and a high proportional use of the acceleration muscle chain (Gastrocs,

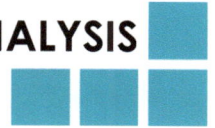

Quadriceps and Gluteals) will result in a quicker onset of fatigue, resulting in tiredness and cramping of the muscles. This is due in large part to the large amounts of energy required to utilise these components of forefoot running. These considerations make this technique ideal for short distance runners covering distances between 100m and 3km. Aerobic capacity may limit a runner's ability to maintain this technique beyond this distance without significant training. Also similarly to the neutral strike technique, the forefoot strike over considerable distance will place excessive anterior stress on the knee joint, as well as an increased strain on the connective tissues of the lower limb.

It is important that when an individual first attempts forefoot running the starting distance is small, thus reducing the effects of fatigue and stress on the kinetic chain.

Barefoot Running

Barefoot running was claimed to enhance the ability to run using a forefoot technique, by reducing the risk of injury compared to other footwear and technique choices. Five-finger trainer manufacturer Vibram, who in early 2014 were sued $3.75million for false health claims in relation to their trainers, supported this ideology (McCue, 2014). In reality, running beyond 400m on a solid surface in either minimalist footwear or barefoot using a forefoot strike technique, is likely to contribute towards injuries such as Morton's Neuroma and the aforementioned plantar fasciitis.

The debate surrounding barefoot running has gained incredible popularity over the past few years, owed in large part to the author Christopher McDougall, the writer of "Born to Run". In which he discovers the tremendous long-distance running ability of hidden Amazonian tribes. This reignited the sporting worlds desire to better understand why we choose to run in supportive trainers over running barefoot.

Some argued that running barefoot is how, long before the invention of trainers, Homo sapiens hunted, and that it is the most naturally intended form of running, which is of course a reasonable point. Firstly however, consideration for the absorption properties of concrete – the surface most commonly run on across the world, is important. Running along a beach, forest floor or even a field will provide some shock absorption to the kinetic chain whilst running, whereas running on concrete provides almost no shock absorption at all. Trainers were originally ergonomically designed to enable humans to comfortably run along the ever more present concrete roads and footpaths. This makes running a more comfortable experience for runners in all environments.

Secondly, when Homo sapiens used to hunt barefoot, they would hunt over short distances rather than trying to outrun their prey. The reason for this was to preserve energy in order to hunt for a longer period of time. Homo sapiens utilised their tact and cunning to hunt rather than sheer endurance, which means that when they ran, they sprinted. They sprinted barefoot over short distances; most likely using a forefoot strike technique. This does not mean that barefoot running is wrong or bad for the sporting world, it just identifies that there should be an individual consideration for the motives to start running barefoot along with the environmental conditions. In the modern world the most ideal place to run barefoot is along the beach or in a field.

Barefoot running can also have some very positive effects. Besides the added sense of freedom that the majority of barefoot runners describe, the constant gripping of the feet and toes on the ground can result in a better activation in the intrinsic muscles of the lower limbs and feet. This has been known to improve pain during running often caused by over-pronation or flat feet.

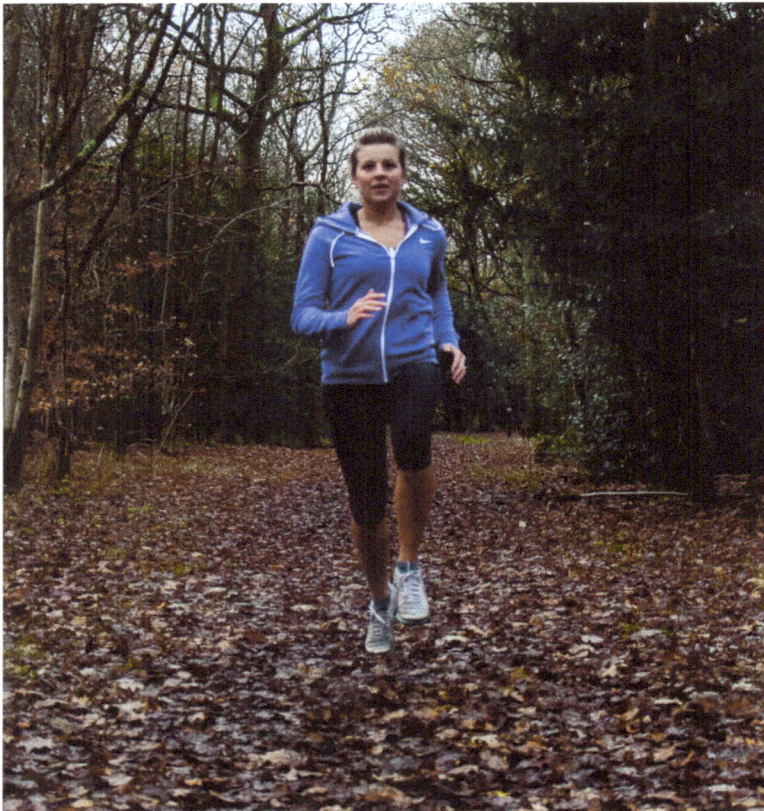

Consider environment, distance and existing injuries when running

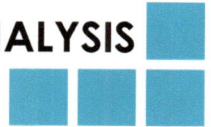

In conclusion, there is no right or wrong way to run, or which type of footwear to use. There is only individual choice, which should be based upon individual's goals. Elite runners vary in their preference as much as the average running community. When trying to decide footwear and technique, there are three things to consider, these include intended distance, environment and existing injuries/weaknesses.

At the end of each chapter, each case study and questions will be relevant to the knowledge acquired in the previous chapter(s).

Case Study 7

A 28-year old professional female triathlete approaches you with regards to her training. She performs well, but wants to push herself on to the next level, which she admits will mean focusing on her weakest discipline, running. It has always been the slowest aspect, even though she feels like she puts the most effort into it. The client/patient does openly admit that she doesn't have the best motivation when it comes to running.

The client/patient does see an Osteopath regularly for general "muscle stiffness", but otherwise is fit and healthy.

You decide the best option is to firstly assess her gait to establish her current style and form. You observe:

- She uses a more neutral/forefoot strike technique
- Her stride looks 'awkwardly' short
- Calcaneal movement appears normal
- There is reduced hip extension bilaterally
- Reduced shoulder swing bilaterally, otherwise normal
- Mild anterior head carriage
- Hypotonic glutes bilaterally

Generally her gait does not look very relaxed, and she appears tense. You also test Talus Neutral, which appears normal with no excess pronation or supination.

1. Consider the distance that this client/patient runs. Do you feel that her technique is the most energy efficient? Using your anatomical and physiological knowledge please explain your answer.

2. Can you identify the origin, insertion and action of the Soleus muscle?

3. How would you address this client/patients motivation towards running? Please explain your answer.

Notes

8. Functional Motor Patterns

Learning Objectives

- To understand the importance and relevance of various motor patterns
- To understand and demonstrate a high level of knowledge and application of motor pattern testing.
- An ability to interpret various findings from upper and/or lower limb motor pattern tests, and apply the results to an individual appropriately.

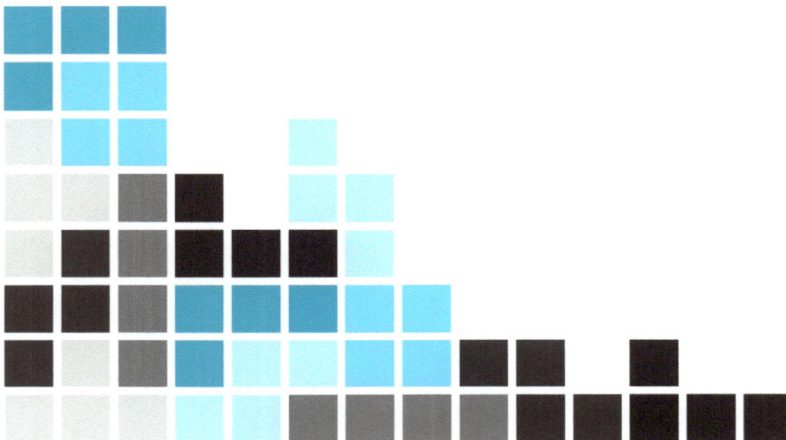

Assessment of certain biomechanical motor patterns is an essential part of any functional analysis. Motor patterns can be either full ranges of motion, such as *Shoulder Range of Motion*, or more specific smaller actions, such as the *Lunge Test*. The majority of fully dynamic movements can be broken down into stages and more isolated actions, which can consequently be assessed, to better understand the biomechanics involved. This allows the assessor to determine any weakness or compensation through the neuromusculoskeletal system during the motor pattern, which once identified can be trained, strengthened and re-educated to improve performance and efficiency.

The motor patterns described in this chapter are considered to be the fundamental tests for generically assessing a client/patient. However, based on the individual client/patients daily or sporting requirements there may be other movements that the assessor will want to assess. Any movement can be broken down into constituent motor patterns. Using both experience as well as anatomical and biomechanical knowledge from the previous chapters, it is encouraged to explore new motor pattern tests that are applicable and individual to a client/patient. Ultimately, the functional motor pattern tests should provide findings individual to a client/patient, enabling an informed decision to be made regarding improved function and performance.

Key Point: Discovering and understanding muscular imbalance, weakness and kinetic compensation should always be the primary concern. This information can be methodically interpreted to understand the strain on the kinetic chain.

8.1 Shoulder Range of Motion

The shoulder complex is arguably the most intricate mechanism in the human body, with four individual joints and eighteen muscles per shoulder; it is easy to appreciate its intricacy. The movements available at the shoulder, along with their normal range of motion can be broken down into:

- Flexion – 180 degrees
- Extension – 45 degrees
- Abduction – 180 degrees
- Adduction – 80 degrees
- Internal Rotation – 90 degrees
- External Rotation – 90 degrees

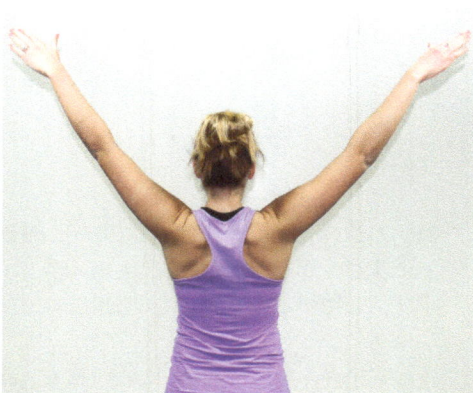

Record all ranges of motion

CHAPTER 8.

Key Point: When assessing Shoulder Range of Motion, it is important to consider movement at all four available joints: Glenohumeral Joint, Acromioclavicular Joint, Sternoclavicular Joint and the Scapulothoracic Joint.

Abduction of the arm primarily occurs at the glenohumeral joint. The initial 30° of abduction in fact occurs entirely at the glenohumeral joint, and from 30°-180° the movement follows a two to one ratio (2:1) between the glenohumeral joint and the scapulothoracic joint; for every 3° of abduction, 2° occurs at the glenohumeral joint, and 1° at the scapulothoracic joint (Hoppenfeld, 1995). Although the scapulothoracic joint is not a 'true' joint, due to its lack of joint capsule, it is relatively important in relation to shoulder range of motion.

The ranges of motion should be synchronous between all of the muscles and joints of the shoulders, displaying fluidity and efficiency.

How to perform examination:

- It is important that the scapula is clearly visible. For this ideally, clients/patients should remove their t-shirt. With women particularly it is important to be considerate and warn them beforehand that this may be the case. Assessing a female in a bra is ideal, however either a sports bra or crop top should be adequate.
- Ask the client/patient to stand with sufficient space either side of them to allow for full range of motion.
- Then ask the client/patient to perform one shoulder range of motion at a time, often in the sequence of:

  1. Abduction
  2. Flexion
  3. Extension
  4. Adduction
  5. Internal Rotation
  6. External Rotation

- Start with the non-painful or non-restricted limb and compare to the opposing shoulder. If neither shoulder is painful or restricted, it is advised to start with the more dominate shoulder.
- Finally, ask the client/patient to perform the ranges of motion with both at the same time and note any differences or

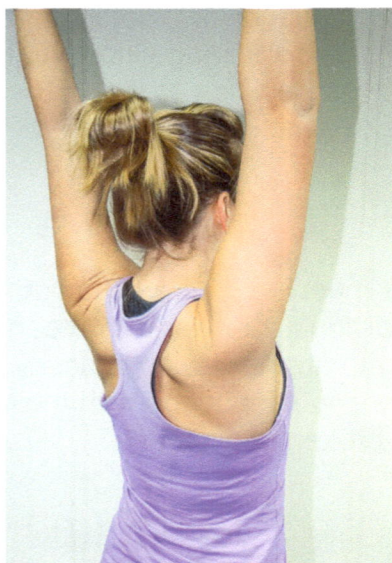

All ranges of shoulder motion should be assessed

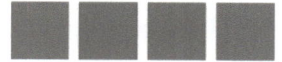

abnormalities.

Test the range of motion of individual shoulders initially, starting with the more fully functional shoulder, before assessing the shoulders together. For each singular movement, observe the range of motion, any production of pain, and any compensatory actions the client/patient may have, such as:

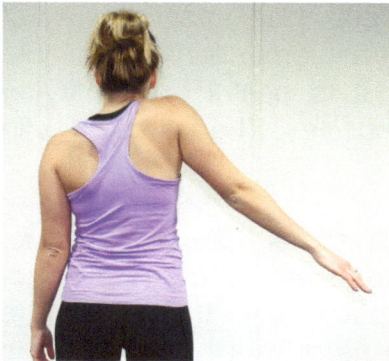

An initial shrug during abduction may indicate a muscle tear or adhesive capsulitis

- **Shoulder Shrug (Muscle Tear)** – If abduction appears to be initiated with the shoulder being shrugged up towards the ear, rather than the arm being raised, it will often be an indication of a tear in either the Supraspinatus or Upper Trapezius. The shrug will be initiated by the Levator Scapulae, at which point the Deltoid will pull the humerus up into the acromion to compensate for the lack of Supraspinatus activity. This coincides with a reduced range of motion during active abduction and flexion.
- **Shoulder Shrug (Frozen Shoulder)** – A shoulder shrug can also be present with Adhesive Capsulitis, more commonly known as Frozen Shoulder. The majority of all ranges of motion at the shoulder will occur at the scapulothoracic joint due to the 'sticky' nature of the capsule surrounding the glenohumeral joint. The restriction at the glenohumeral joint will result an action similar to a shoulder shrug.
- **Winging Scapula** – Throughout most shoulder movements, if the medial border of the scapula appears to be protruding away from the ribcage, this may suggest a weakness of the Serratus Anterior. This is the muscle that anchors the medial border of the scapula to the ribcage. A weakness may also become more apparent as the muscle is fatigued through repetitive action.
- **Painful Arc** – If the client/patient experiences pain between 60°-120° of abduction, it is most commonly associated to Supraspinatus tendonitis, otherwise known as impingement syndrome. This indicates an observation of pain or discomfort within the Painful Arc. Infraspinatus tendonitis and subacromial bursitis can also be other causes of a pain or discomfort within the Painful Arc.
- **Pain in Multiple Ranges** – In disorders concerning the tendons, such as Supraspinatus or Biceps tendonitis, there

is often pain in one specific movement (abduction, flexion, internal rotation, etc.), which is due to the load placed upon a specific tendon. However, if there is pain in all ranges, it is likely that either the glenohumeral capsule or the subacromial bursa is inflamed.

8.2 Apley Scratch Test

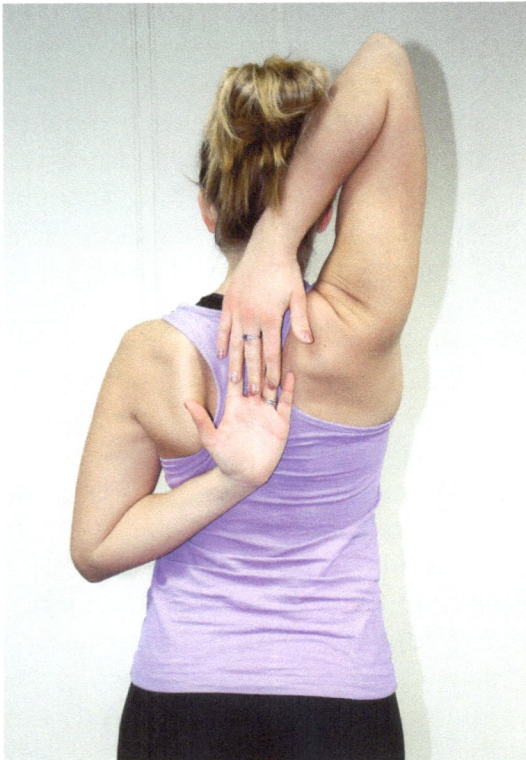

Using the Apley Scratch Test is an effective way of assessing a combination of movements only available at the shoulder complex. It is useful in identifying restricted joints and tight muscles. The test itself is in two parts:

1. Flexion, Abduction and External Rotation – Instruct the client/patient to raise one arm above the head, bending at the elbow to reach down the spine. The client/patient should reach as far down the spine as they can without any pain. The level should then be marked, enabling it to be compared with the other side.

2. Extension, Adduction and Internal Rotation – The client/patient should reach their arm behind their back, bending at the elbow with the posterior surface of their hand against their back. As they reach as far as they can up their spine, mark the farthest point so that it can be compared with the other arm.

The Apley Scratch test assesses the extreme ranges of shoulder motion

Key Point: It is common to observe greater restriction on a client/patients dominant side, which is due to the increased muscle mass.

Observe any differences between the left and right arms during the motor pattern. If a client/patient displays an inability to perform this test, it will often be an indication of tightness within the rotator cuff muscles, otherwise known as the SITS muscles (Supraspinatus, Infraspinatus, Teres Minor and Subscapularis). The Apley Scratch Test can also assess the integrity of the joints related to the shoulder complex. Unfortunately, it is not extremely easy to distinguish which structure is limiting the range of motion, making interpretation rather difficult from this test alone. Functionally however, it will offer an understanding of the shoulder's muscular performance.

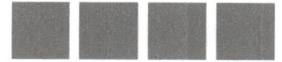

8.3 Push Up Test

With this test, several aspects of the neuromusculoskeletal system can be observed, including scapula winging and general upper body strength and endurance. Encourage the client/patient to perform a full body Push Up, as it will give the truest indication of muscular control. A half Push Up will often accompany poor form, as it is a lot easier to cheat – clients/patients will often drop their chest to the floor, rather than lower their body weight.

How to perform:

- The client/patient should set their palms on the floor directly under the shoulders.
- Extend the legs with feet together – the feet can be set wider apart if the client/patient appears unstable.
- The body is then raised off of the floor, whilst maintaining a neutral spine to the starting position.
- Instruct the client/patient to place their shoulders directly above their hands, and to lower their body down towards the floor with control until a 90° angle is achieved at the elbow joints.
- They should then raise their body up, extending at the elbow joints, to the starting position.
- This is then repeated.

> **Key Point**: The spine should be neutrally maintained throughout. The test should be stopped the moment neutral spine is lost, as this indicates a weakness along the kinetic chain.

Certain points should be observed during the Push Up, which will add to the general functional impression of the client/patient:

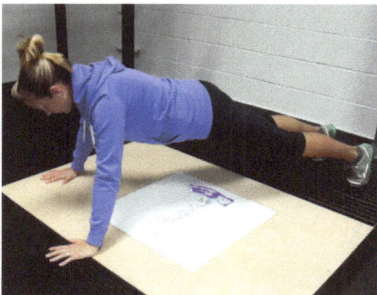

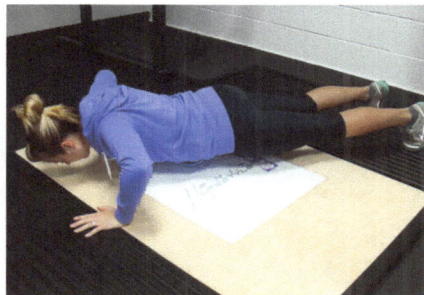

Push-Up test should demonstrate controlled movement

- Stable lowering of the body to an angle of 90° at the elbow joint. If the movement appears to be juddering or not fluent, it could suggest a lack of upper body strength, generally or in specific muscles – most commonly the Pectorals or Rhomboids. Observe closely as these muscles may appear to excessively twitch as a result, which can often indicate weakness.
- The lumbar spine should be neutrally maintained throughout

the concentric and eccentric part of the movement – note any lifting of the bum or hyperextension of the lower back. If the client/patient lifts their bum, it may indicate a weakness across the abdomen. Alternatively, a hyperextension of the lower back may suggest a weakness in the Paraspinals or posterior trunk muscles. These would also be observed during a plank.

- Head position should be neutral, without any anterior head carriage. A failure to hold the head in a neutral position may indicate deep neck flexor weakness or neck extensor hypertonicity. An increase in the prevalence of sedentary postures means that weakness is often observed in the muscles of the neck.

- Smooth, controlled scapulo-thoracic movement without any winging of the scapulae should be observed. Winging of the scapula may suggest weakness of the Serratus Anterior – the muscle fixing the scapula to the ribcage.

- An ability to raise the body from the 90° elbow position. Similar to the lowering phase, it demonstrates strength. If wanting to test the upper body endurance of the client/patient, instruct them to perform as many Push Ups as they can. Below is the endurance score chart as suggested by McArdle *et al* (2006):

Men	Age: 20-29	Age: 30-39	Age: 40-49	Age: 50-59	Age: 60+
Excellent	54 or more	44 or more	39 or more	34 or more	29 or more
Good	45-54	35-44	30-39	25-34	20-29
Average	35-44	24-34	20-29	15-24	10-19
Poor	20-34	15-24	12-19	8-14	5-9
Very Poor	20 or fewer	15 or fewer	12 or fewer	8 or fewer	5 or fewer
Women	Age: 20-29	Age: 30-39	Age: 40-49	Age: 50-59	Age: 60+
Excellent	48 or more	39 or more	34 or more	29 or more	19 or more
Good	34-48	25-39	20-34	15-29	5-19
Average	17-33	12-24	8-19	6-14	3-4
Poor	6-16	4-11	3-7	2-5	1-2
Very Poor	6 or fewer	4 or fewer	3 or fewer	2 or fewer	1 or fewer

Table 8: McArdle et al's push up score chart

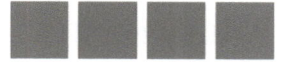

8.4 Wall Angel Test

Various musculoskeletal discrepancies can be observed during the Wall Angel Test. The primary objective is to assess thoracic rigidity, however, tightness in the Pectorals and rotator cuff muscles, as well as stiffness in the lumbar spine can also be assessed. Men generally display a greater amount of tightness compared to women, especially men who regularly weight train without adequate stretching.

How to perform:

- The client/patient should stand with their back to the wall — buttocks and head touching the wall.
- Feet should be approximately 20cm from the wall
- Arms should be abducted to 90°, and elbows bent 90° so that the forearm and back of the hand along with all five fingers are flat to the wall.
- The client/patient should then attempt to flatten their wrists against the wall, maintaining contact with all five fingers and the elbows.
- They then should also attempt to flatten the entire spine against the wall.

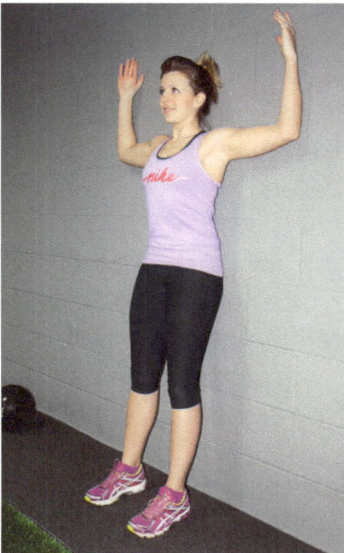

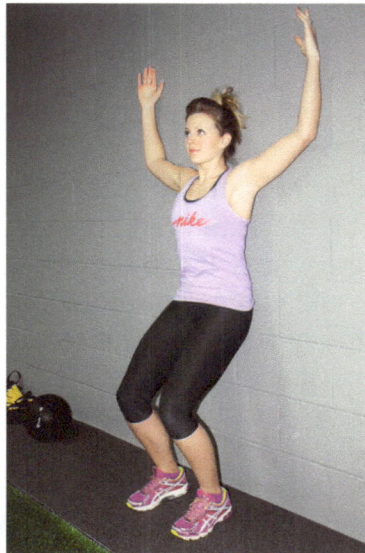

Certain findings may indicate specific functional issues along the client/patients kinetic chain. These include:

• An inability to bring the posterior aspect of the shoulder in contact with the wall may suggest a tightness of the Pectoral muscles. This can be correlated to any potential indications of an upper-crossed posture.

• The client/patient should be able to maintain contact with the wall at the elbow and wrist without the posterior shoulder coming away. If contact is lost, the internal rotator muscles of the shoulder, such as the Pectorals and Subscapularis may be excessively tight.

Wall Angel test assesses thoracic rigidity

- The spine should stay in full contact with the wall, including the head and lower back. Generally this can be quite tasking for most people, and is often not achieved. From this finding it is possible to assume that the client/patient has difficulty extending through their thoracic spine. This may be in relation to a structural or muscular issue, such as either Scheuermann's disease or muscular hypertonicity, respectively.

The Wall Angel Test should be fundamentally used to assess a client/patient's general shoulder and thoracic movement and mobility, rather than being used to isolate a specific muscle or movement.

8.5 Parallel Squat Test

An essential part of the many sporting and daily movements, whether through a sagittal plane or not, is a Squat. Being able to Squat with perfect form and control is the foundation to enhancing every day function, as well as reducing the risk of placing key weight-bearing joints under avoidable stress. Contrary to general use, the Squat can be used not only as an exercise, but also to assess a client/patient's muscular function and joint flexibility.

Key Point: The Squat is important to numerous functional movements and exercises. However, it is essential to correct form and control before progressing to a lunge. This is because the control required to stabilise the lunge, due to its unstable base, is greater than with a Squat.

How to perform:

- The client/patient should stand with their feet shoulder width apart and turned out 5° – this is due to the natural position of the hip joint being mildly externally rotated.
- Arms should be extended out in front of the body.
- Keeping the chest up and head facing forwards, the client/patient should slowly squat as low as possible, keeping both heels on the ground whilst also maintaining neutral spine.
- The client/patient should be able to wiggle their toes at the lowest part of the squat – indicating their weight is appropriately distributed.
- Knees should remain behind the toes, thus minimising the stress placed on the anterior structures of the knee.
- During the ascent, the lumbar spine and pelvis should remain neutral, without any posterior or anterior tilting.

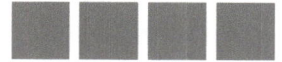

The assessor should be observing functional mobility, form, balance, speed and control, and making note of any pain or discomfort throughout the test. Functionally, the Squat Test will assess:

- **Hip Flexion** – Often hip flexion can be compensated for with lumbar flexion, indicating either tightness through the glutes, hamstrings or even the adductors. Hip flexion can also be restricted by stiffness or restriction of the lumbar spine and sacrum.
- **Pelvic Stability** – Hips should also stay in the midline of the body throughout the Squat Test. An unsmooth motion or drop/rotation of the hips or pelvis could indicate a muscular imbalance, weakness or inhibition through the kinetic chain. The commonest contributing factor towards this is often stiffness throughout the joints of the lumbar spine.
- **Knee Flexion** – If hip and knee mobility allow, it may be possible to assume a deep Squat position. If this is forced it may result in a dislocation type force being placed upon the anterior structures of the knee, potentially damaging the anterior cruciate ligament and meniscus. The knee should be able to achieve a normal position of at least 90° of flexion.

Observe the knees during the squat test

- **Knee Alignment** – Knees should also remain facing the same direction as the toes throughout the entire test. A drifting, or a lack of control, could indicate an injury to a structure at the knee, or muscular weakness or inhibition, resulting in poor muscular control. One of the most common problems often observed during this test is poor muscular control between the Vastus Medialis Oblique (VMO) and Vastus Lateralis, which is demonstrated by the knees buckling inwards during the test (knee valgus).
- **Ankle Dorsiflexion** – Clients/patients with restricted ankle dorsiflexion will demonstrate a heel raise as they descend through the Squat Test. This can also be due to poor form – The client/patient may shift their weight towards the forefoot

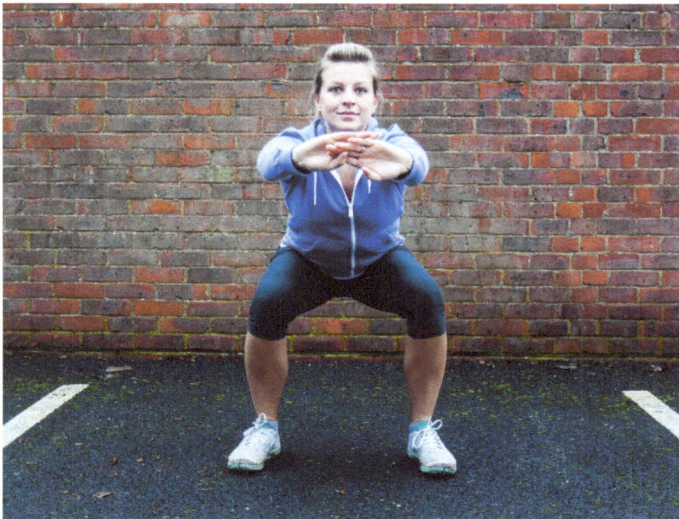

CHAPTER 8.

as opposed to the hind foot.

- If there is restricted dorsiflexion, the knee may internally rotate towards the end-range to allow a lower Squat position to be achieved. This may be initially mistakenly observed as over-pronation.
- A reduced dorsiflexion also may be caused by the soleus or gastroc complex being tight.

A deep Squat is the progression to the parallel squat test. It tests the client/patient's pelvic, hip and knee flexibility to its maximum. Its use is recommended to assess clients/patients involved in activity or sport from an intermediate up to elite level that require maximum strength and joint stability through as full range of motion as possible e.g. an Olympic weightlifter. Otherwise a Parallel Squat is sufficient for the majority of functional requirements.

Key Point: Too much flexibility can also be detrimental in some sports and activities. For example, a rugby player with too much flexibility may be under increased risk of injury due to the nature of impact at some of the joints during the game.

Flexibility may be limited by muscular tightness, joint restriction or the girth of individual body parts, such as the pelvis or femurs. However, Squat flexibility may improve under load. This phenomenon is known as Dynamic Muscle Loading (Kisner & Colby, 2012). It identifies the muscles' ability to stretch farther when placed under an increased load, such as a barbell, compared to the muscles' normal flexibility against gravity.

The Squat Test can be used to assess endurance as well as movement patterns. By performing the test repetitively until the muscles fatigue, the muscles' ability to work aerobically can be examined. Importantly, the Squats should have good form throughout, and as soon as the form is compromised the test is stopped and the result recorded. This is because it identifies the muscles are fatiguing.

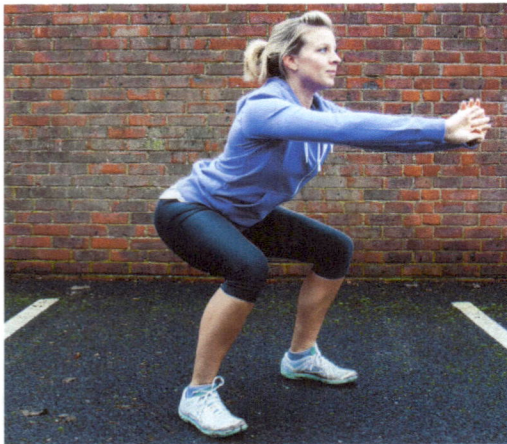

Correct form and control is important when assessing endurance

Research in 2007 by Hoffman *et al*, supported previous investigations into the squat not only being a valid test, but also contributing to immediate enhancement of sporting performance, such as increase in jump height and an enhanced sprint cycle performance (Chiu *et al*, 2003; French *et al*, 2003). It is believed that a maximal or near-maximal activity before testing increases the neural signal that activates

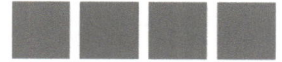

the muscle, known as muscle post-activation potentiation (Hamada *et al*, 2000). Although these investigations identify an increase in immediate performance, it is not specified how long a duration the effects are sustained. This makes application for endurance or fartlek sports, such as football, rugby, hockey etc. rather difficult. It would not be appropriate to bring a player off at intervals during a game to perform maximal squat repetitions, and then send them back onto the pitch to continue playing.

8.6 Lunge Test

A variation of the Lunge Test that is often described within some literature, is more comparable to a Soleus stretch test (Pope *et al*, 1998; Gabbe *et al*, 2004), however it does not provide enough dynamic range of motion in order to assess function and stability at the key joints such as hip, knee and ankle.

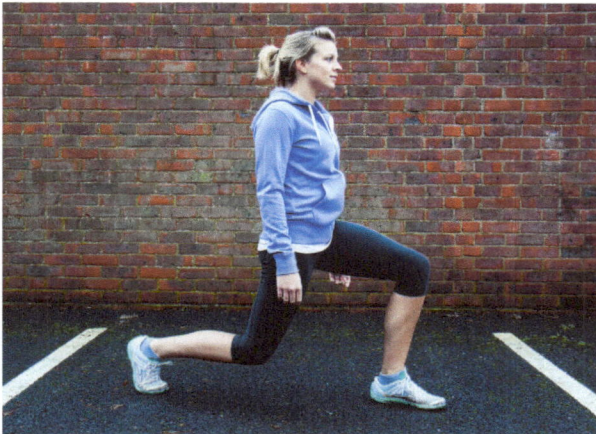

The lunge test assesses stability across numerous joints

The Lunge motor pattern is a component of decelerating actions, as well as changes in direction, which are frequently found in various sporting movements. The Lunge Test is intended to place the stress of rotation, deceleration and lateral movement on the body in a simulated, controlled manner. Stability across the lower back, shoulders and pelvic girdle is as important as the control through the ankle and knee joints.

How to perform:

Key Point: There should be very minimal movement at the lower back throughout the test, as there should be adequate extension available at the hip joints.

*   The client/patient should stand with their feet facing forwards and positioned shoulder width apart.
*   With their hands placed on their hips, they should lunge forwards – dominant or non-painful leg first.
*   The feet should maintain a shoulder width position rather than an in-line Lunge position.
*   As the lead leg lands and descends, the trailing leg should descend also, demonstrating a smooth pattern.
*   The lead leg should land heel first without the knee travelling ahead of the toe.

CHAPTER 8.

- Pushing off from the lead leg, the client/patient should ascend, returning back to the starting position with feet still shoulder width apart.
- This is then repeated on the opposite leg.

The assessor should be observing form, control and stability throughout the test, and recording any discrepancies. The Lunge Test will assess key aspects of functional movement such as:

- **Hip Flexion** – the lead leg should be able to achieve enough hip flexion to perform a test fully (approximately 90°). Restricted mobility may be due to tight Adductors or Gluteal muscles, often Gluteus Maximus.
- **Hip Extension** – the trailing hip should extend as far as possible to allow the lowest position to be achieved. The client/patient may purposefully limit their stride length, or they may appear to not be maximally extending the hip on their trailing leg as they descend into the Lunge. This could indicate tightness in the Rectus Femoris or Iliopsoas. Hyperextension of the lumbar spine may also be observed to accommodate for the reduced extension at the hip joint.
- **Pelvic Stability** – the pelvis should remain level throughout the test. The pelvis may demonstrate a hip drop (Trendelenburg sign), in a similar fashion that may be observed during gait. Be sure to correctly observe which hip is truly 'dropping', as it can be difficult at first glance to determine. This is most commonly associated with weak hip abductors, namely the Gluteus Medius and Minimus.
- **Knee Alignment** – the knees should remain aligned with the feet and hips, as well as the trailing knee descending close to the floor. The knee may appear unstable or demonstrate a valgus deformity, which may indicate a weakness or an imbalance in strength between the knee stabilising muscles, such as the Vastus Medialis Oblique and Vastus Lateralis.
- **Ankle Dorsiflexion** – a reduction in dorsiflexion will often result in either a shortened Lunge or a dramatic heel raise in the trailing leg. This is often due a displaced subtalar joint,

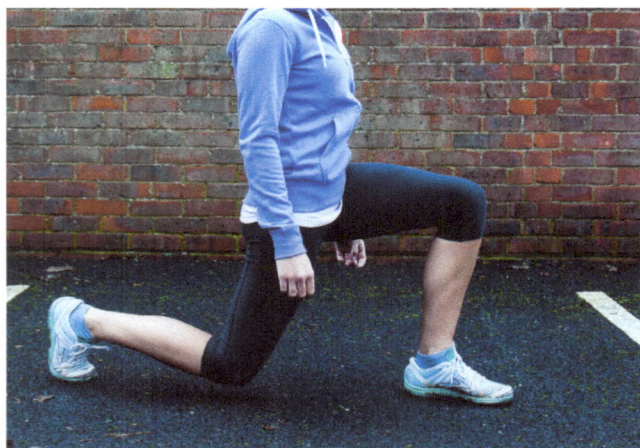

Observe the front and back leg, as both will move differently

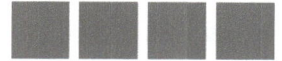

which commonly occurs following an inversion sprain of the ankle. It may also indicate tightness of the soleus or gastroc complex.

The Lunge Test is better performed with the client/patient wearing shorts ideally, so that the knees are in full view.

8.7 Active & Passive Straight Leg Raise

The Straight Leg Raise as a test can be performed either actively or passively. When testing actively, it can be used to assess lumbopelvic stability (Mens *et al*, 1999) as well as the muscular control involved with flexing the hip. The test allows the activation of the limbs individually in an unloaded position whilst continually engaging the trunk musculature. Being able to perform this test passively allows for the assessment of the body's biomechanics without the engagement of the muscles. This allows appreciation of how much the musculature is contributing towards the dysfunction and mechanical stress the client/patient may be experiencing.

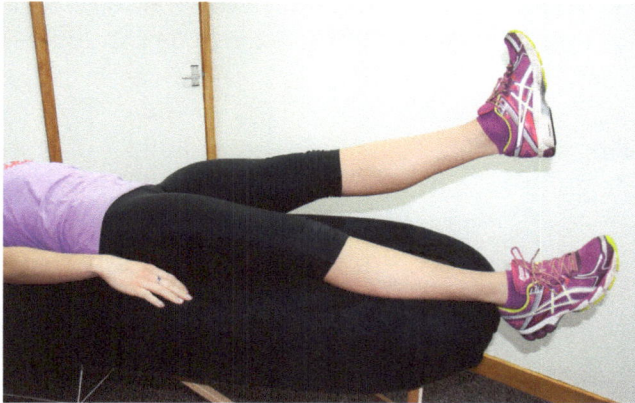

The active leg raise has been used in research for many years

Liebenson *et al* (2009) proved that the Active Single Leg Raise test was reasonable for testing lumbar spine stiffness. They also were able to support other research findings by Grenier & McGill (2007), which suggested an abdominal brace reduced lumbar axial rotation. These findings reinforce the concept that the abdominal brace may be an appropriate preventer who pain as a result of excessive movement of the lumbar spine and pelvis.

How to perform:

- **Active Straight Leg Raise** – With the client/patient lying on their back with both legs extended, they should be instructed to slowly raise one leg as high as they can, keeping the leg straight. This should be either the non-painful or dominant leg first.
- They should then slowly lower the leg down, ask the client/

patient to hold it briefly at 20°.

- At this point, the assessor should apply a small overpressure at the ankle, watching for any rotation at the pelvis.
- They should then lower the leg completely and repeat with the opposite leg.

- **Passive Straight Leg Raise** – The client/patient should then be instructed to allow both legs to relax the leg completely.
- The assessor then, keeping the leg straight, raises one leg (non-painful or dominant leg first) as far as they can until the range of motion feels tight or the client/patient experiences discomfort
- Gently lower the leg, and repeat with the opposite leg.
- Throughout the test the client/patient should inform the assessor of any pain or discomfort. If there is any lower back pain during either Active or Passive Leg Raise, instruct the client/patient to apply a moderate pressure either side of their lower abdominals, approximately over the Iliopsoas muscles.
- Then repeat the test.

The orientation of Iliopsoas, if tight, could potentially pull the lumbar vertebrae into lumbar extension. This will result in the Quadratus Lumborum being stretched, and consequently will reduce the flexibility of the hamstrings due to the immobility of the pelvis. Applying pressure to the Iliopsoas will partially restrict the muscle from firing. If the flexibility of the hamstring increases with Iliopsoas pressure, it can be assumed that any hamstring tightness is partly due to lumbopelvic rigidity created by tight trunk muscles.

The test is useful at identifying numerous components of lower limb muscle activation and motion, and will assess aspects such as:

- **Hip Flexion** – the initial stage of flexing the hip is activated by the lower Abdominals and then facilitated by the Iliopsoas and Rectus Femoris muscles. The pelvis should remain neutral without any rotation. If rotation is observed, it may indicate a weakness at either of the aforementioned muscles, which is compensated for by trunk rotation to enable the leg to be

raised.

- **Hamstring Flexibility** – the angle of flexion achieved at the hip joint should be recorded. It is difficult to propose a normal range, as there are many variables that will predispose a person's flexibility such as sex, level of activity, height etc. However, ideally the client/patient should be able to achieve at least 80°. Observe whether one leg appears tighter than the other, or feels tighter than the other during the Passive Straight Leg Raise.

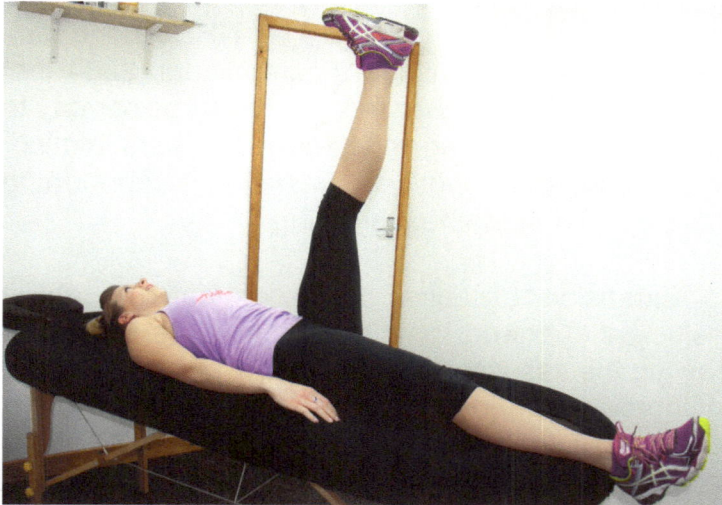

A passive straight leg raise reduces the muscle activity present during an active straight leg raise

- **Active Control** – lowering the leg is an important phase of the test – smooth, equal control should be observed. If the client/patient experiences painful or discomfort, it may indicate instability of the lumbar spine or pelvis, or excessive activation of some of the trunk muscles, such as the Quadratus Lumborum. During the lowering phase, there should be minimal Gluteal involvement as there is no extension of the hip. All of the control required to lower the leg is achieved by a co-contraction of the trunk muscles.

- **Lumbopelvic Stability** – as the overpressure is applied to the client/patient's leg at 20°, observe for any shifting of load to the lumbopelvic joints, which will be evidenced by the pelvis lifting off of the ground, resulting in rotation occurring at the lumbar spine. The strain should be on the hip flexors, particularly the Iliopsoas, thus meaning any rotation might indicate a weakness of the hip flexors.

The passive aspect of this test is to eliminate the active muscular control involved with raising a straight leg. If the client/patient experiences pain or discomfort with the Active Straight Leg Raise, which diminishes with the Passive Straight Leg Raise, it can be assumed that the pain or discomfort is of a mechanical origin.

If the client/patient experiences any tingling or pins and needles into the leg or foot, advice them to see a medical professional to investigate the symptoms further.

8.8 Hip Extension

This motor pattern is a significant pattern to everyone, as throughout the day it is thought that the average sedentary person will initiate hip extension between 1,000–3,000 times per day when walking. The NHS and British Heart Foundation launched a campaign in 2004 that encouraged the public to walk 10,000 steps per day to promote healthier living. With those numbers in mind, it is understandable why Hip Extension is important to daily living, let alone healthy living.

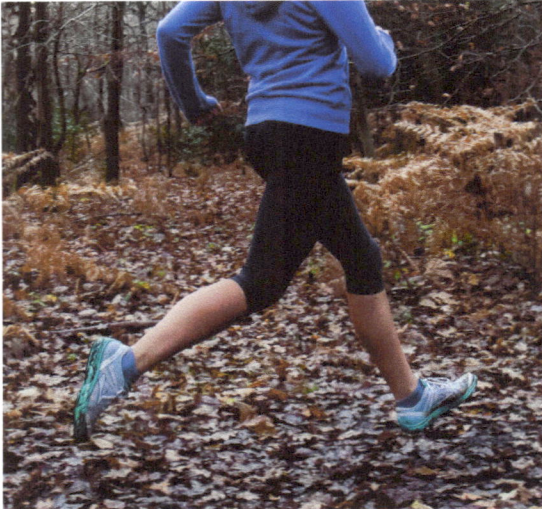

Hip extension is a fundamental motor pattern during gait

Hip Extension assesses the client/patients ability to efficiently extend their hip against gravity, whilst enabling the assessor to observe muscular activation, lumbopelvic extension, and any compensatory mechanisms such as pelvic rotation. In practice, there is often a correlation between chronic lower back pain and an inefficient Hip Extension motor pattern, thus making it a fundamental component in preserving a pain-free state.

How to perform:

Key Point: Palpation is a skill, which can initially make this test difficult for an assessor to evaluate. This test should be practiced on numerous subjects to improve the assessor's palpation skills.

- With the client/patient lying face down (supine), the assessor should place their thumb and little finger on the client/patients Gluteus Maximus and Hamstring, respectively of the leg being tested. Then place the thumb and little finger of the opposite hand on each Quadratus Lumborum.
- The client/patient should then be instructed to slowly raise one leg off of the floor/bench as high as they can. This should be the non-painful or dominant leg first.
- As the client/patient performs this, the assessor should be, through palpation, monitoring the muscle-firing pattern under their respective thumbs and little fingers. The result, along with any pain or limitation should be recorded.
- The assessor should then swap their hands to the opposite leg, and then instruct the client/patient to repeat the test on the opposite leg. Again the muscle-firing pattern, pain or limitation should be recorded.

Janda (1987) suggested that correct Hip Extension is initiated by the activation of specific muscles in a certain order:

1.   Hamstrings
2.   Gluteus Maximus
3.   Contralateral Erectus Spinae/Quadratus Lumborum
4.   Ipsilateral Erectus Spinae/Quadratus Lumborum

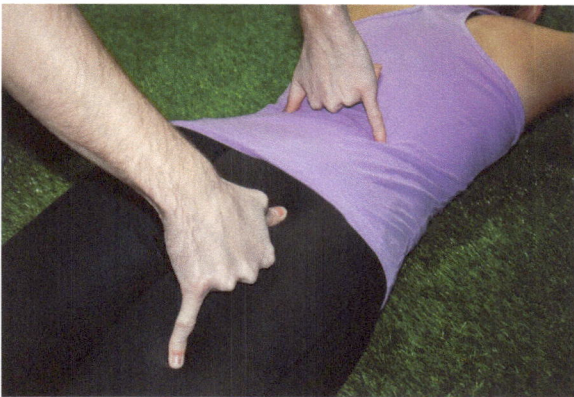

Having different points of contact can help identify which muscles are activating at which time

However, it is still unknown whether activation patterns dissimilar to what Janda suggested have a greater predisposition to injury, especially lower back pain. This identifies a need for more research on this test. Although, in addition to what Janda suggested, it is also important to consider that the lumbar spine should be stabilised before and during any functional motor test, which is initiated by the trunk muscles via an abdominal brace. This may be confused with palpation of the Erectus Spinae and Quadratus Lumborum activation.

Liebenson (1996) proposed utilising the Hip Extension motor pattern to analyse what occurs during the midstance phase of gait. However, although the findings may often appear interesting, they should not be taken on face value. This is because the test may not be an accurate interpretation of what occurs during the gait cycle. Performing this test prone, results in the body working against gravity, compared to true hip extension during gait, where gravity acts as a neutral force.

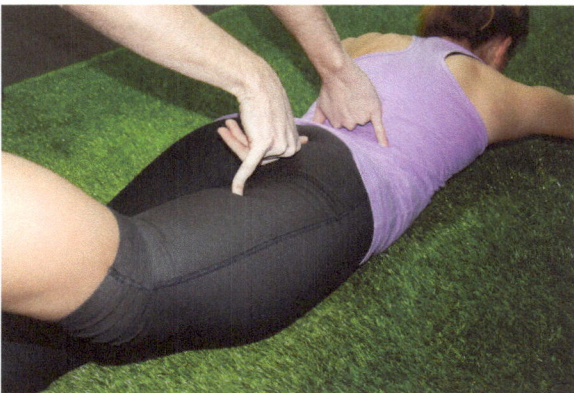

Testing hip extension is best performed with the client/patient prone

The findings from the Hip Extension test along with other tests such as the parallel squat, lunge etc. and gait combined can provide an overall appreciation for lumbopelvic and lower limb activation and control. During the Hip Extension pattern, observe for:

•   **Muscle Activation** – An abnormal pattern of muscle activation between Janda's suggested muscles (Hamstring, Gluteus Maximus, Quadratus Lumborum and Erectus Spinae), may

CHAPTER 8.

indicate an under or an overactive muscle group.

- Over activity firstly by the hamstrings and then secondly by the lower back muscles, may suggest a weakness or poor control of the Gluteus Maximus.
- An over active Gluteus Maximus, may result in the lower back muscles not adequately stabilising the lumbar spine and pelvis.

- **Anterior Pelvic Tilt/Lumbar Extension** – If the lower back muscles (Quadratus Lumborum & Erectus Spinae) contract without an abdominal brace, the lumbar spine may be pulled into extension resulting in the pelvis tilting anteriorly. This may cause pain at the lower lumbar spine.

8.9 Hip Hinge

Another fundamental motor pattern, the Hip Hinge, is utilised not only during sport, but also in everyday life. For example, getting out of a chair, brushing teeth and even lifting an object. In training, exercises such as deadlifts and squats rely heavily on a fully functioning Hip Hinge that is both strong and flexible.

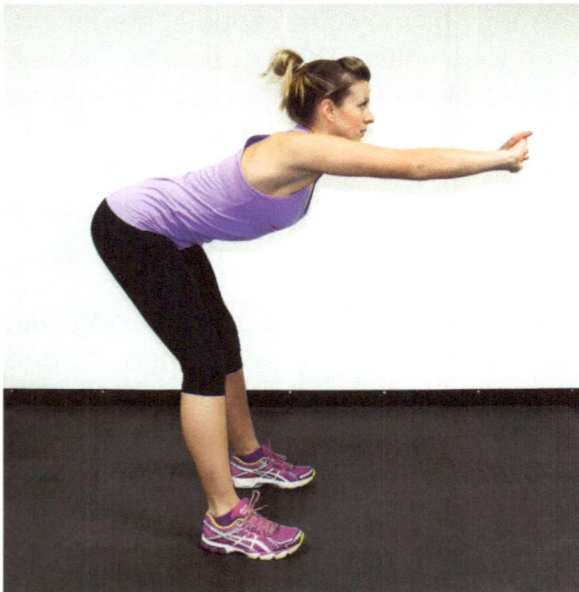

Postural muscles, particularly of the lower back are often subject to tightness and shortening, unlike phasic muscles that are more likely develop a weakness or inhibition (Janda, 1968). The strain placed upon the postural muscles of the lower back during sedentary work can greatly affect the ability of the muscles to perform adequately during exerting tasks often required with activity. Prolonged increased flexion at the lumbar and lower thoracic spine, commonly associated with sedentary posture, may result in the Quadratus Lumborum and Erectus Spinae muscles becoming overworked. This will often result in the muscles becoming tight, which inevitably places strain on the muscles attachment points (vertebrae and facet joints).

The hip hinge an important movement in everyday life

211

FUNCTIONAL MOTOR PATTERNS

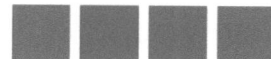

A common problem with the Hip Hinge is that people display a roll or flexion of the lumbar spine rather than hinging at the hip. This causes the thoracic spine to excessively flex – in a similar way to slumping in a chair. Collins (2011) suggested that the body will take the path of least resistance to adapt, and that the least stiff part of the body will compensate for the part(s) that are stiff. Sahrmann in 2002 expanded on this by proposing repetitive daily activities, along with sporting demands place an increase risk of permanent change along the kinematic chain. Due to the numerous times the Hip Hinge is performed on a daily basis, it is important that it is performed correctly in order to prevent stress being placed on other compensatory mechanisms.

How to perform:

- With the client/patient stood with their feet shoulder width apart and facing forwards, they should be instructed with an abdominal brace and slight bend at the knees, to flex at the hips, reaching as far forwards as possible.
- The assessor should be observing for any flexing at the lumbar and/or thoracic spine, and any compensatory bending of the knees.
- The client/patient should be instructed to reach forward only go as far as they can whilst maintaining a neutral spine and adequate weight distribution.
- The angle of hip flexion should be recorded for future comparison, along with any experienced pain or discomfort.

The Hip Hinge is a well utilised movement in activities of daily living, such as reaching for something on a shelf, or even with additional load, such as picking up a child. This makes the test generically relevant to the majority of people. The findings from this test can be useful in understanding lumbopelvic and hip control:

- **Hamstring Flexibility** – A reduced angle of hip flexion may indicate tight hamstrings either bilaterally or unilaterally – hamstring length should then be tested using the Straight Leg Raise and Hamstring Stretch Test.
- **Balance & Proprioception** – Another reason for a reduced

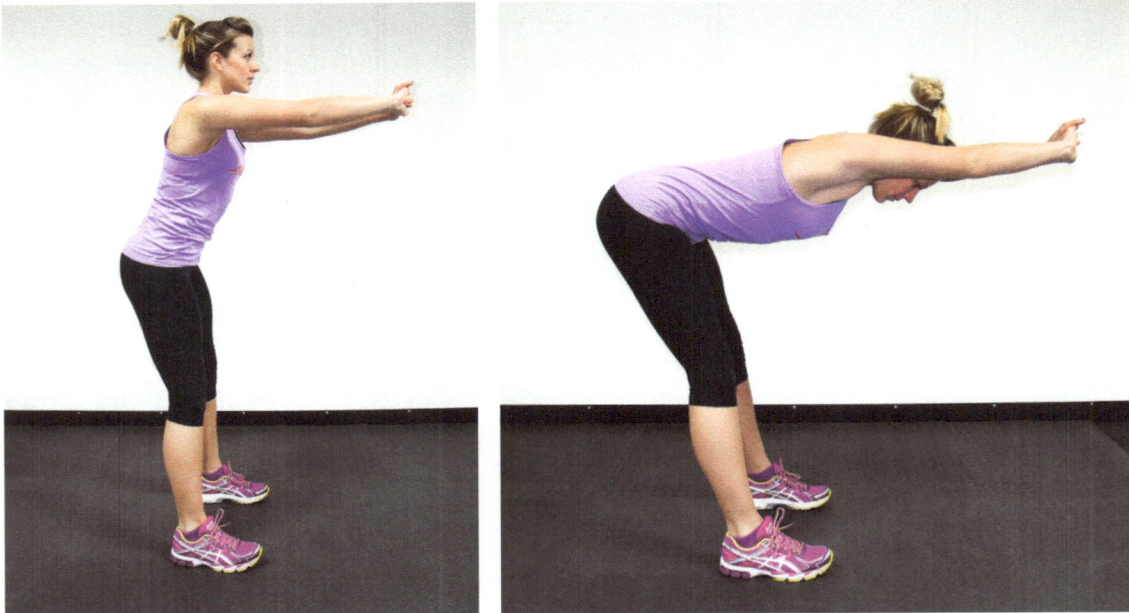

Assessing the hip hinge relies on good instruction and observation by the assessor

hip angle may be a poor sense of balance or proprioception. This can often be the case if the client/patient has suffered an injury such as a sprained ankle, which has consequently damaged the ligaments and tendons. Ask the client/patient about previous injuries to either the knees or ankles if they appear unbalanced. This could also be age related, as well as a problem with the ears such as an infection.

- **Lumbar Flexion** – Flexing at the lumbar spine may indicate an abnormal muscular balance between the lower back and abdominal muscles, which would result in poor control of the lumbar spine during the Hip Hinge.

- **Lumbar Extension** – Extension in the lumbar spine may also be observed during this test, particularly in women. This due to the increased flexibility women often have compared to men. It is important to remember that neutral is not a position of extension – the lumbar spine has a natural lordotic curve.

8.10 Step-Down Test

The step-down test is arguably the most accurate and reliable test for assessing the ankle mobility and stiffness (Loudon *et al*, 2002). As it is unilaterally loaded, it also offers scope to assess knee and hip stability. The ankle joint should have an unrestricted range of motion through dorsiflexion with an elastic end to the range, which is due to the normal properties found in the gastroc complex.

As well as being an important feature of running and jumping, the dorsiflexion assessed during this test is found in some of the most basic movements, such as getting out of a chair, picking something up off the floor and even walking. Having this range of motion functioning efficient is paramount, as it is often one of the first mechanisms utilised along the kinetic chain. It is also worth noting that a restricted range of motion may not be something that can be rectified with exercise, it may need manual treatment such as Chiropractic, Osteopathy or some forms of Physiotherapy.

The step-down test is performed on a raised platform, roughly 7-8" high. This will allow for full range and control to be tested.

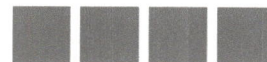

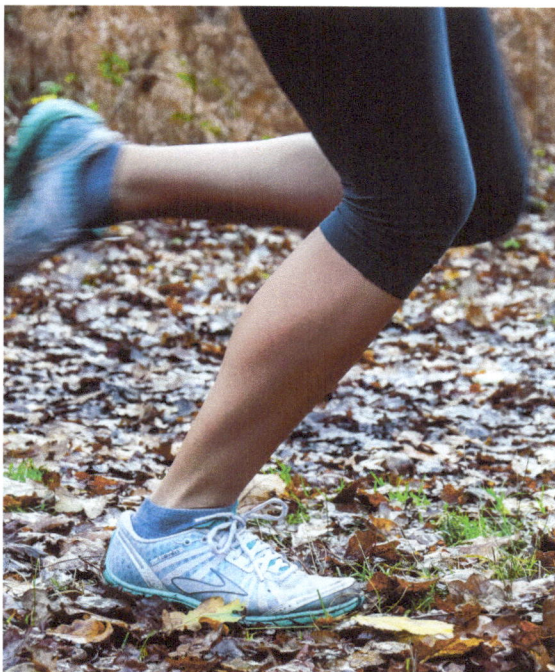

Adequate ankle dorsiflexion is important during running and walking

How to perform:

- The client/patient is instructed to stand (without shoes on) close to the edge of the platform, it is important that their toes are not gripping the edge, as this adds additional stability, which is not accurate.
- They should then, whilst standing on one leg, extend the other leg out in front of them, as if stepping off the platform.
- The standing leg's heel should stay in contact with the platform.
- They should take the extended leg's heel down towards the ground as far as they can. If they are able to get their heel to the ground, it should only briefly touch the before the client/patient returns to the start position, not rest on the ground.
- They should then repeat the test on the opposite leg, repeating multiple times if necessary. Any differences, pain or discomfort should be recorded.

The Step-Down Test can provide information regarding both the standing and reaching leg, so it is important to be vigilant when assessing this test.

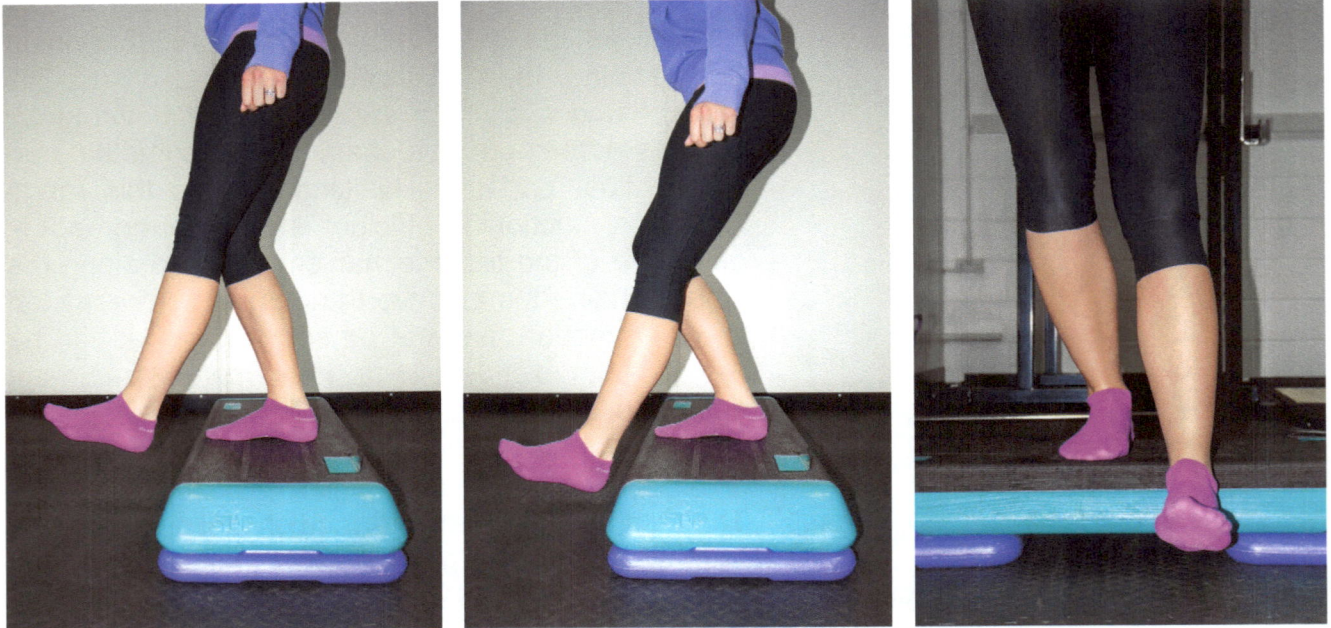

There are several aspects to observe during the step-down test

When observing the standing leg:

- **Lumbar Flexion** – the lumbar spine should be neutral as well as the trunk muscles remaining engaged throughout. An increase in lumbar flexion could indicate either a tightness of the Iliopsoas or weakness of lower back postural muscles.
- **Pelvic Drop** – much like during gait, the non-standing hip may appear to drop (Trendelenburg Sign), this could be due to a weakness of Gluteus Medius on the standing hip. It may also be a compensatory movement to accommodate restricted dorsiflexion, thus also not allowing the heel to reach the ground.
- **Genu Valgus** – the knee may appear to manoeuvre into a valgus deformity, again possibly to accommodate restricted dorsiflexion at the ankle. The external rotators of the hip might also be weak or inhibited, resulting in a similar finding.
  - **Knee Control** – if the knee appears to lack control through the descent, then the muscles of the Quadriceps,

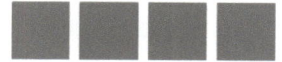

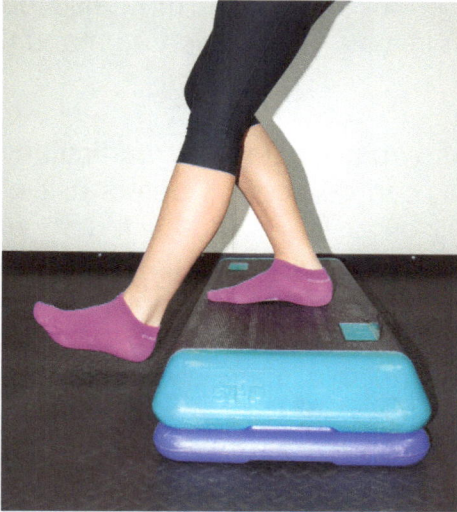

Ankle dorsiflexion and control can be easily assessed

particularly the relationship between the Vastus Lateralis and the Vastus Medialis Oblique (VMO), should be considered. This could also predispose to a knee injury such as patellofemoral pain syndrome.
- **Ankle Dorsiflexion** – the client/patient may feel that dorsiflexion is restricted, which may cause them to raise their hell as they descend. This may indicate a structural restriction of the talar or sub-talar joint, however it may also indicate tightness of the Gastroc complex.
- **Ankle Control** – the client/patient may feel unbalanced or like they lack control at the ankle. Enquire as to any ankle sprains or injuries where there may have been ligament damage. The ankle joints and ligaments may have poor proprioception that could need rehabilitation and proprioceptive training.

When observing the stepping leg:

- **Pelvic Rotation** – a client/patient with a unilateral weakness across the pelvis, may demonstrate a shifting of weight and control over the standing leg. This rotation through the hips and pelvis will enable the client/patient to incorrectly to touch the ground with their heel. They are quite possibly compensating for a weakness or restriction that is preventing them from touching their heel on the ground.
- **Hip Flexion** – the hip should be flexed as the leg should be extended. If the hip struggles to maintain hip flexion, the flexors may be weak, or if the test is taking too long they may also be fatigued.

8.11 Single-leg Squat

This is one of the more advanced motor pattern tests, which will understandably not be needed for the general population. Only use this when the assessor deems it a potentially useful test, based upon lifestyle and activity, should it be used. For example, this test may provide useful information regarding the control of a single leg's kinetic chain for the majority of clients/patients participating in competitive sport. The results may offer insight into potential weaknesses or areas for improvement that can be

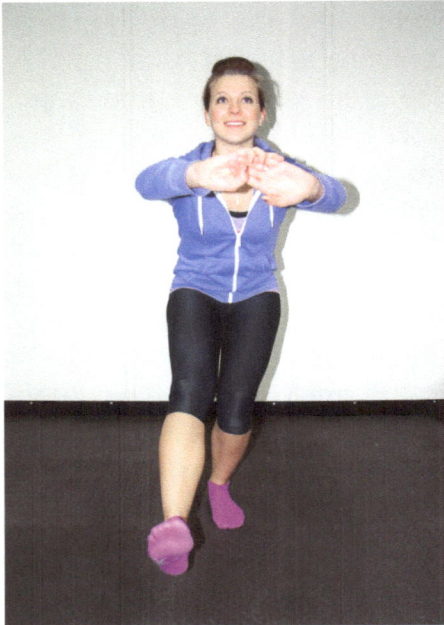

Single-leg squat test is often used to detect risk of injury

focused upon to enhance performance. This may also be the case for professions that involve lifting, such as manual labourers.

Research suggests that motor pattern testing, particularly tests involving the knee joint, can be used to detect risk of injury to the lower limb (Willson & Davis, 2008; Munro *et al*, 2012). The single-leg squat test isolates the standing leg's function and mobility through a very challenging range of motion. A study by Crossley *et al* (2011) suggests that the single-leg squat test is a reliable method of detecting individuals with hip muscle dysfunction.

How to perform:

- The test is performed with the client/patient standing facing forwards, feet together – unlike the Squat Test, the centre of gravity will be unilateral, meaning the standing leg will have to remain close to the midline of the body.
- They should then be instructed to raise one foot out in front of them, flexing at the hip. This should be the painful or non-dominant leg first. Allow them a few seconds to establish their balance.
- With a neutral spine and an abdominal brace, they should then in a slow, controlled manner, descend through the squat as far as possible.
- They should then return to a single leg standing position.
- The test is then repeated on the other leg, with observations and comparisons between the two legs being recorded. This particular squat can also be utilised as an exercise, otherwise known as a pistol squat.

Due to the challenging nature of the Single-Leg Squat Test, there may be numerous minor discrepancies during the test. It is important that the assessor remains objective, by keeping in mind the reason for using the test. Ultimately, the findings should be significant to the individual or asymmetrical when compared to the opposing leg. Observe for:

- **Knee Angle** – an angle of at least 60° should be achieved

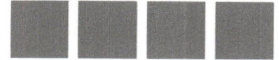

with good speed and control. An inability to achieve this could be due to poor hip flexibility, often associated with Gluteal tightness, or muscle control. Restricted talar or sub-talar joints can also reduce the knees maximum range.

- **Trunk Stability** – the trunk should remain neutral, without any lateral deviation or excessive lumbar flexion. There may be a degree of lumbar flexion, as this will allow for the hip to achieve its maximum range of motion. This is due to anatomical orientation of the hip joint being mildly internally rotated, rather than the neutral position accommodated in a parallel squat, to facilitate the unilateral weight distribution. A lateral deviation may indicate poor balance, impaired proprioception, or it may be a compensatory mechanism in response to joint restriction.

- **Pelvic Drop** – the pelvis should remain level without any rotation or dropping of the hip (Trendelenburg sign). Any evidence of this could indicate a muscular weakness or inhibition, possibly at the Gluteus Medius.

- **Internal Rotation** – the hip joint should not appear to excessively internally rotate or adduct. If there is it may indicate a weakness in the external rotators of the hips, such as the Gluteal muscles. This position will place excessive stress on the hip capsule, including the surrounding ligaments.

- **Knee Tracking** – the knee position should stay in-line with the foot position, with minimal knee valgus. This could indicate poor muscle control between the muscles of the Quadriceps, in particular the Vastus Lateralis and Vastus Medialis Oblique (VMO), or a excessive pronation that the foot and ankle.

Single-leg squat is a difficult movement pattern to perform

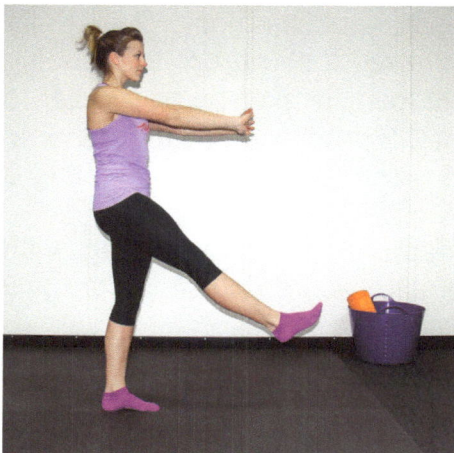

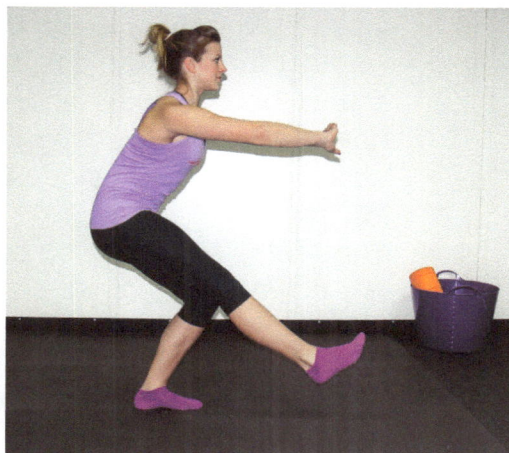

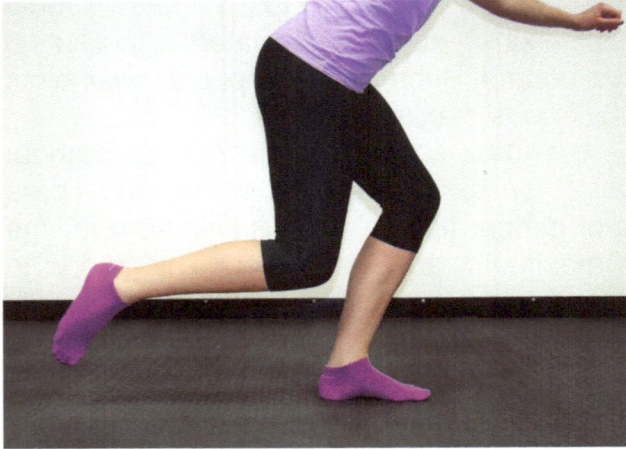

It is advisable to record the standing hop test, as it happens very quickly

8.12 Standing Hop Test

This test is often used to measure performance and recovery, to justify when an athlete can participate in sport following an injury. It assesses lower limb strength and stability, as well as neuromuscular control (Reid *et al*, 2007). The purpose of this test in a rehabilitative setting is to assess the performance of the combined muscle groups working to perform and control a movement often used throughout numerous sporting activities.

The test may happen very quickly, making it very difficult to assess. For this reason it be more beneficial to record the test, so that it can be played back. Recording the test will also enable the assessor to play it back to the client/patient. It may be useful to ask the client/patient to wear shorts so that as much of the lower limb is in view.

How to perform:

- The client/patient should be instructed to stand on one leg without wearing shoes, allow them a few seconds to establish their balance. This should be the non-painful or dominant leg first.
- They should then jump off the ground as high as they can. They are allowed to use recoil, meaning they are allowed to squat down on the single leg before pushing off.
- As they land on the same leg they took off on, the landing should be controlled and balanced. It may be beneficial to have the client/patient perform 2-3 practice hops beforehand, although this may fatigue the muscles if they are exerting a lot of power.
- The test should then be repeated on the opposite leg, with any differences, pain or discomfort recorded. Also record any obvious findings from witnessing the test.

The Standing Hop Test has two elements to observe, the take-off and the landing. For this reason it is important the client/

patient leaves the ground during the test, this ensures that an adequate amount of joint control can be assessed. However, the main objective is to observe the muscular control under stress and load, particularly during the landing. The specific height that the client/patient achieves is also irrelevant during this motor pattern. Findings may be similar to those found during a Single-Leg Squat, including:

*   **Pelvic Drop** – the pelvis should remain level without any rotation or dropping of the hip (Trendelenburg sign). Any evidence of this could indicate a muscular weakness or inhibition, possibly at the Gluteus Medius. If this is observed during in the descent before the take-off, the client/patient may be more Quadricep dominant through an acceleration phase of movement.
*   **Internal Rotation** – the hip joint should not appear to excessively internally rotate or adduct on the landing. If there is it may indicate a weakness in the external rotators of the hips, such as the Gluteal muscles. This position will place excessive stress on the hip capsule, including the surrounding ligaments.
*   **Knee Tracking** – during both the take-off and landing, the

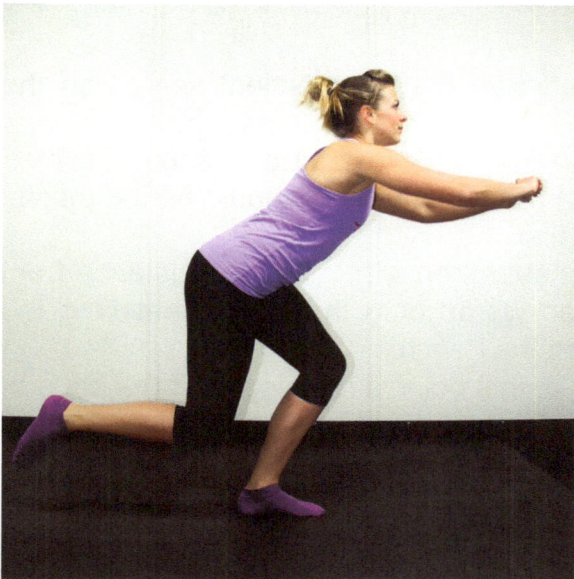

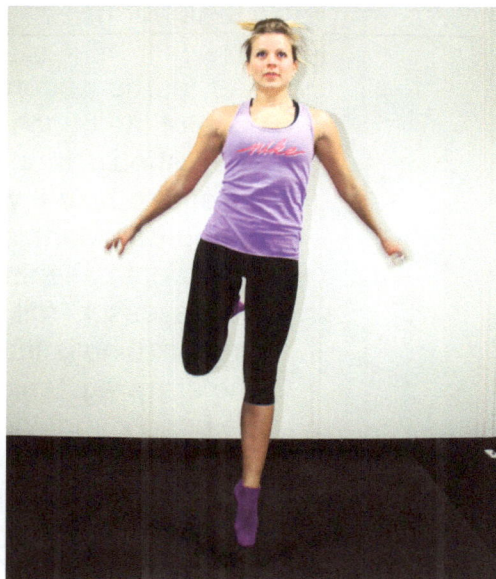

It is important that the client/patient leaves the ground

knee position should stay in-line with the foot position, with minimal knee valgus. This could indicate poor muscle control between the muscles of the Quadriceps, in particular the Vastus Lateralis and Vastus Medialis Oblique (VMO), or a excessive pronation that the foot and ankle. It is unlikely that any varus deformity will be observed in the knee due to the unilateral weight distribution.

8.13 Modified Thomas Test

This test over the years has been used to assess hip flexibility, more specifically the flexibility of the Iliopsoas and the Rectus Femoris. The test was named after Dr Hugh Owen Thomas (1834-1891), and since then its application has been adapted. More recently in 1998, Harvey used a Modified Thomas Test to assess the flexibility in elite athletes. It involved the client/patient initially starting the test sitting at the very edge of the bench as opposed to lying on the entire length of the table. Since then it has become the gold standard test for assessing the flexibility available at the hip.

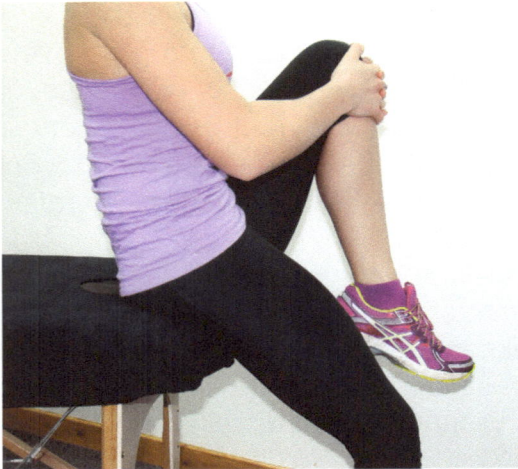

The modified Thomas test involves starting in a seated position

How to perform:

- The test is performed with the client/patient seated on the edge of the bench.
- They should then be instructed to pull one knee into their chest and hold it with both hands. This should be the painful or non-dominant leg first.
- The client/patients should then with guided assistance from the assessor, roll backwards onto the bench, ensuring the lumbar spine is flat on the bench.
- The stray leg, which at this point is hanging over the edge of the bench, should be completely relaxed and allowed to drop as far as it can.
- Two angles can then be measured, the first is the angle of hip flexion/extension, and the second is the angle of flexion at the knee.
- The assessor may apply a slight overpressure to the upper thigh to challenge the flexibility of the hip, and then a slight

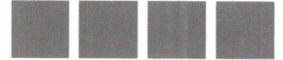

overpressure to the tibia to challenge the flexibility of the Rectus Femoris.

- The test is then repeated on the opposite leg, with any pain, discomfort and differences in flexibility being recorded.

As with the majority of flexibility tests, the findings are often very specific to an area, such as:

- **Hip Angle** – if the angle at the hip is noticeably flexed, it could indicate a tightness in the Iliopsoas. If this is the case, an overpressure on the upper thigh will feel similar to pulling an already tight elastic band.
- **Hip Abduction** – if the hip abducts away from the midline of the body, it may suggest a tightness in the leg abductors, such as the Tensor Fascia Latae or Gluteus Medius.
- **Knee Angle** – if the angle of flexion appears reduced at the knee, it may indicate tightness of the Quadriceps, more specifically the Rectus Femoris.

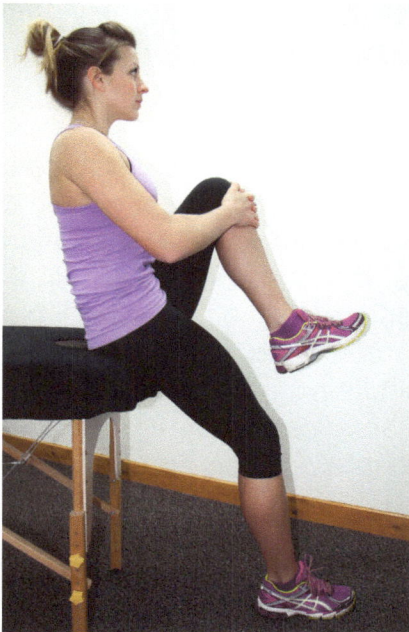

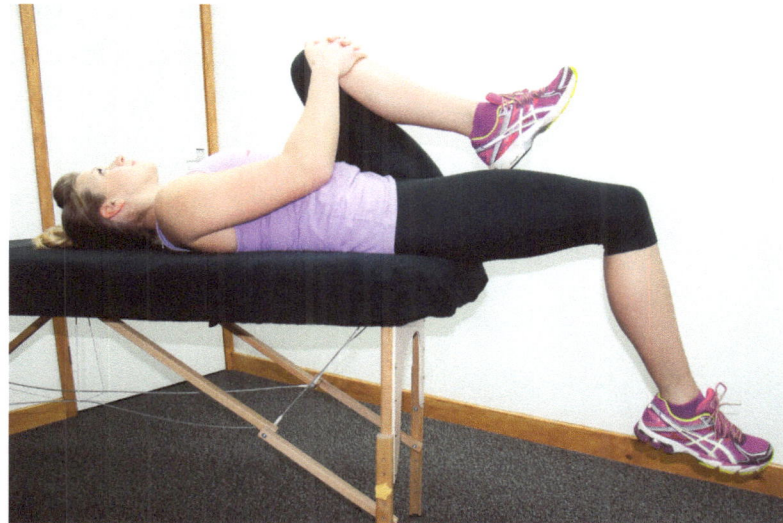

Modified Thomas test assesses hip flexor and quadricep tightness

8.14 Soleus Stretch Test

Often mistakenly referred to as a 'Lunge Test' in some research (Pope *et al*, 1998; Gabbe *et al*, 2004), it more accurately assesses the flexibility of the soleus and ankle joint. This test can prove a valuable tool in assessing whether a client/patient's reduced dorsiflexion is in response to muscle tightness, or in fact due to restrictive biomechanics at the talar or other joints of the ankle. Bojsen-Møller *et al* (2004) explained that the gastrocnemius provided the greater contraction when the knee was in full extension, compared to when the knee was maximally flexed, which resulted in a greater contraction at the soleus. Thus identifying the need to involve knee flexion when assessing the flexibility of the soleus.

How to perform:

- The test is performed with the client/patient stood, facing a wall.
- They should place the toes of the leg being tested 10cm away from the wall. This should be non-painful or dominant leg first.
  - They should then be instructed to bend the knee whilst keeping their heel on the ground.
  - The test is then repeated on the opposite leg, with any pain or discomfort recorded, along with the distance the knee is away from the wall.

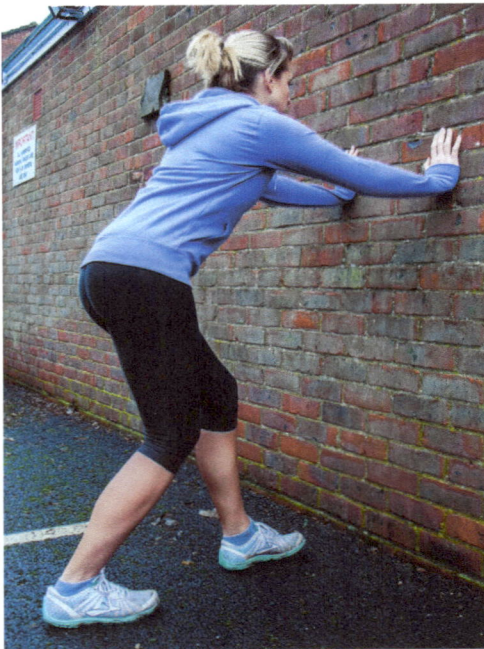

An inability to reach the wall with their knee may indicate a restriction in the talar or subtalar joint, or tightness in the soleus muscle. This will be better identified by the sensation the client/patient experiences. If they experience a tight, stiff sensation along the posterior aspect of the lower limb, it would suggest that the Soleus muscle is generating the sensation. If the client/patient describes a restricted or pinching sensation along the anterior aspect of the ankle, it would suggest that a joint is in a position that is limiting movement.

Stretching the soleus can help relieve tightness in the muscle

8.15 Hamstring Stretch Test

The flexibility of the Hamstrings is relatively easy to measure, although there appears to be some confusion in the literature as to which is the most accurate. Jackson & Baker (1986) used the "Sit and Reach Test" to examine Hamstring flexibility. However, due to the flexion occurring at the mid and lower back to reach

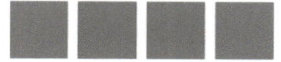

forwards, it does not specifically isolate Hamstring flexibility. This is because the range of motion achieved could also be limited by tightness in the Erectus Spinae or Latissimus Dorsi muscles for example. In a more recent study, the authors used a "Passive Straight-Leg Raise" to determine Hamstring flexibility (Lopez-Minarro & Alacid, 2010). This may be a reasonable application of this test, however, clinically, clients/patients will often experience tension at the posterior aspect of the knee. Anatomically, the Hamstrings diverge towards their insertion points, on the medial and lateral aspects of the lower limb, approximately 2-3 inches superior to the knee joint. Thus suggesting, the structure that is felt to be under tension at the posterior aspect of the knee is more likely to be the sciatic nerve or Popliteus muscle rather than the Hamstrings. A more accurate way of assessing the Hamstrings is to eliminate any spinal flexion and potential sciatic tension.

How to perform:

- This test is performed with the client/patient lying supine.
- As the true flexibility of the Hamstrings is being tested rather than the active flexibility, the assessor will perform the test.
- The hip of the leg being tested should be flexed to 90°. The assessor should then slowly extend the knee keeping hip flexion at 90°. This should be the non-painful or dominant leg first.
- The leg not being tested should be fully extended and flat to the ground/bench.
- As tension is felt in the hamstrings the assessor should then record the angle achieved, along with any pain or discomfort.
- The test is then repeated on the opposite leg.

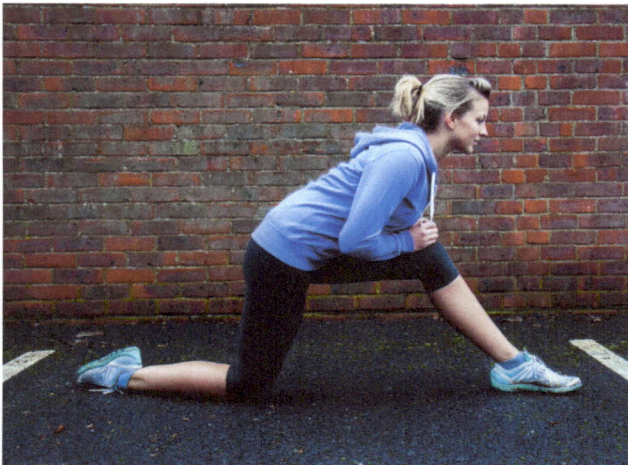

An active hamstring stretch is similar to the stretch test

With the hip at 90°, adequate Hamstring flexibility is achieved when the knee reaches full extension. An inability to achieve this would suggest tightness in the hamstring. However, bilateral tightness as an independent finding may not be functionally significant. This should coincide with a specific dysfunction or further test findings.

224

8.16 Quad Stretch Test

The assessment for Quadricep flexibility is reasonably standardised, with very little argument among research studies. It is important that this test is done passively, as the contraction of the hamstrings will prevent the full range of motion available at knee. Thus giving an inaccurate measure of Quadricep flexibility.

How to perform:

*   With the client/patient lying prone with both legs extended.
*   The assessor should bring one legs heel towards the buttock of the same leg, whilst ensuring the pelvis remains neutral with no rotation. This should be the non-painful or dominant leg first.
*   A measurement is then taken between heel and buttock and recorded, along with any pain or discomfort.
*   The test is then repeated on the opposite side.

If the client/patient is able to achieve full range of motion by managing to get their heel to their buttocks, then they are considered to have a adequate Quadricep flexibility. Due to muscle mass and joint integrity, the specific angle achieved at the knee joint among individuals may differ greatly. For that reason, it is difficult to compare an individual person's Quadricep flexibility to another's.

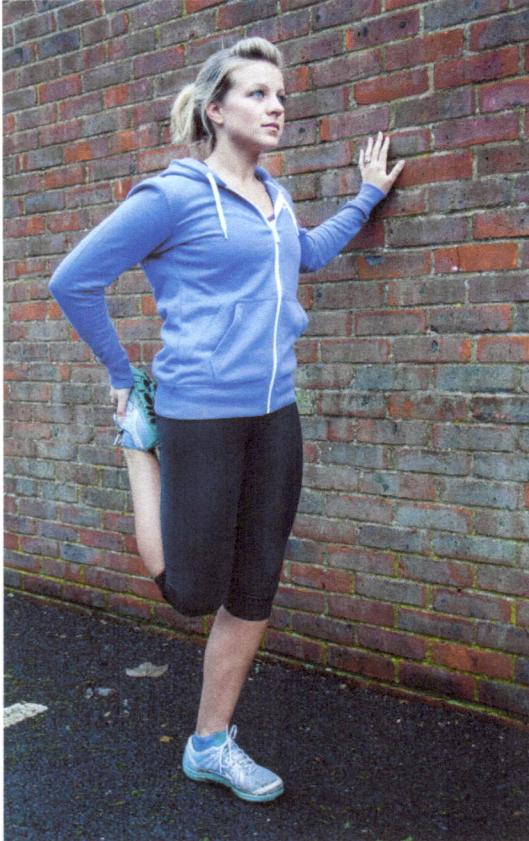

A quadricep stretch can be used to reduce quadricep tightness

At the end of each chapter, each case study and questions will be relevant to the knowledge acquired in the previous chapter(s).

Case Study 8

A 49-year old, 6'0", 80kg male accountant presented to a Chiropractor with a chronic history of lower-back discomfort. He described it as more of a dull ache, which was more left sided than right. It generally gets worse throughout the day, but it is occasionally stiff in the morning.

Work is mostly sedentary, however the client/patient owns the firm and tries to encourage a relaxed atmosphere. There are various styles of chairs scattered around the office, but he admits he will often sit for hours at a time once he's "found a good'en".

After some successful manipulative treatment, including some soft tissue work, they are referred to you. The basic instructions that have been passed on from the Chiropractor include:

Tight hamstrings, hip flexors, and QLs. Weak glutes, trunk muscles. Poor posture

You decide on a number of functional motor tests. You observe and record:

- Parallel Squat – lumbar flexion, mild shift of weight to the right on ascent, bilateral knee instability, heels off of the floor.
- Lunge – short stride bilaterally, more unbalanced on the left leg, mild hip drop bilaterally.
- Passive Straight Leg Raise – no lower-back pain, right leg 45° hip flexion, left leg 60° hip flexion
- Hip Extension – very little gluteal activation bilaterally, tight QL's – left more than right.

1. Based on the given information, what areas/muscles do you feel you would like to target with functional rehab, and how?

2. Using your knowledge, please suggest a training routine specifically for this client/patient lasting a maximum of 30-minutes? Include information regarding reps and sets.

3. Are there any tests other than the ones above that you would have liked to perform for this client/patient? Why?

CHAPTER 8.

Notes

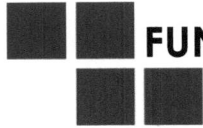

References

ALARANTA, H., HURRI, H., HELIÖVAARA, M., SOUKKA, A. & HARJU, R. 1994. Non-dynamometric trunk performance tests: reliability and normative data. *Scandinavian Journal of Rehabilitation Medicine*. 26 (4), p211-5.

ALFREDSON, H., PIETILÄ, T., JONSSON, P. & LORENTZON, R. 1998. Heavy-load eccentric calf muscle training for the treatment of chronic Achilles tendinosis. *American Journal of Sports Medicine*. 26 (3), p360–6.

ALLPORT, G. W. & POSTMAN, L. 1947. *The Psychology of Rumour*. New York: Holt, Rinehart & Winston.

AMERICAN HEART ASSOCIATION. 2013. *The Price of Inactivity* [Online]. Available from: http://www.heart.org/HEARTORG/GettingHealthy/PhysicalActivity/StartWalking/The-Price-of-Inactivity_UCM_307974_Article.jsp [Accessed: 07/11/2013].

ANDERSSON, E. A., ODDSSON, L. I., GRUNDSTRÖM, H., NILSSON, J. & THORSTENSSON, A. 1996. EMG activities of the quadratus lumborum and erector spinae muscles during flexion-relaxation and other motor tasks. *Clinical Biomechanics*. 11 (7), p392-400.

ANDERSSON, G. B. J. 1997. *The epidemiology of spinal disorders*. In: Frymoyer, J. W., Ducker, T. B., Hadler, N. M., Kostuik, J. P., Weinstein, J. N. & Whitecloud, T. S. The Adult Spine: Principles and Practice. Philadelphia, PA: Lippincott-Raven. p93–141.

ARDITO, R. B. & RABELLINO, D. 2011. Therapeutic Alliance and Outcome of Psychotherapy: Historical Excursus, Measurements, and Prospects for Research. *Frontiers of Psychology*. 2: 270.

AUSTIN, W. M. 1994. What about supination? *Orthopedic Notes*. (12), p1-2.

BAECHLE, T. R., EARLE, R. W & WATHEN, D. 2000. *Essentials of Strength Training and Conditioning* (2nd Edition). Champaign, Illinois: Human Kinetics.

BANDURA, A. & CERVONE, D. 1983. Self-evaluativeand self-efficacy mechanisms governing the motivational effects of goal systems. *Journal of Personality and Social Psychology*. 45 (5), p1017-1028.

BANDURA, A. 1977. *Social Learning Theory*. Englewood Cliffs, New Jersey: Prentice Hall.

BANTON, R. A. 2012. Biomechanics of the Spine. *Journal of The Spinal Research Foundation*. 7 (2), p12-20.

BARTLETT, F. C. 1932. *Remembering*. Cambridge University Press.

BIERING-SORENSEN, F. 1984. Physical measurements as risk factors for low-back trouble over a one-year period. *Spine*. 9, p106-119.

BOJSEN-MOLLER, J., HANSEN, P., AAGAARD, P., SVANTESSON, U., KJAER, M. & MAGNUSSON, S. P. 2004. Differential displacement of the human soleus and medial gastrocnemius aponeuroses during isometric plantar flexor contractions in vivo. *Journal of Applied Physiology*. 97, p1908–1914.

BOUCHER, M. 2013. *Proprioception and Aesthetic Sense* [Online]. Available from: http://www.archipel.uqam.ca/5343/1/proprio-and-aestheticARCHI.pdf [Accessed 09/07/2013].

BRZYCKI, M. 1998. *A Practical Approach to Strength Training*. New York: McGraw-Hill.

CAMBIO, T. M. 2013. *Planks cause back pain* [Online]. Available from: http://www.toddcambio.com/planks-cause-back-pain [Accessed: 14/01/2014].

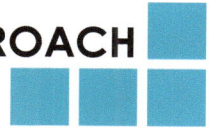

CHOLEWICKI, J., PANJABI, M. M. & KHACHATRYAN, A. 1997. Stabilizing function of trunk flexor-extensor muscles around a neutral spine posture. *Spine*. 22 (19), p2207-12.

CHIU, L. Z. E., FRY, A. C., WEISS, L. W., SCHILLING, B. K., BROWN, L. E. & SMITH, S. L. 2003. Postactivation potentiation response in athletic and recreationally trained individuals. *Journal of Strength and Conditioning Research*. 17, p671-677.

COHEN, L. A. & COHEN, M. L. 1956. Arthrokinetic Reflex of the Knee. *American Journal of Physiology*. 18, p433-437.

COLLINS, D. F., REFSHAUGE, K. M., TODD, G. & GANDEVIA S. C. 2005. Cutaneous Receptors Contribute to Kinesthesia at the Index Finger, Elbow, and Knee. *Journal of Neurophysiology*. 94 (3), p1699-1706.

COLLINS, S. 2011. *Hip Hinge! Your Body Wants You To* [Online]. Available from: http://lostinfitness. blogspot.co.uk/2011/02/hip-hinge-youre-body-wants-you-to.html [Accessed 16/07/2013].

CORBIN, C. B., LINDSEY, R. & WELK, G. 2000. *Concepts of Physical Fitness* (10th Edition). New York: McGraw-Hill.

CORPUS, J. H., MCCLINTIC-GILBERT, M. S. & HAYENGA, A. O. 2009. Within-year changes in children's intrinsic and extrinsic motivational orientations: Contextual predictors and academic outcomes. *Contemporary Educational Psychology*. 34, p154-166.

CROSSLEY, K. M., ZHANG, W. J., SCHACHE, A. G., BRYANT, A. & COWAN, S. M. 2011. Performance on the single-leg squat task indicates hip abductor muscle function. *American Journal for Sports Medicine*. 30 (4), p866-873.

DAINOFF, M. J. 1999. *Ergonomics of seating and chairs*. In: Salvendy, C. Handbook of human factors and ergonomics. CRC Press, Boca Raton.

DAY, R. H. 1969. *Human Perception*. New York. Wiley. p15.

DECHANT, Z. 2010. *Training Rotational Movement Patterns* [Online]. Available from: http://articles. elitefts.com/training-articles/training-rotational-movement-patterns/ [Accessed 25/03/2014].

DE HOUWER, J., THOMAS, S. & BAEYENS, F. 2001. Associative learning of likes and dislikes: A review of 25 years of research on human evaluative conditioning. *Psychological Bulletin*. 127, p853–869.

DELORME, T. L. 1945. Restoration of muscle power by heavy-resistance exercises. *Journal of Bone and Joint Surgery*. 27, p265-647.

DI FABIO, R. P. 1992. Making Jargon from Kinetic and Kinematic Chains. *Journal of Orthopaedic and Sports Physical Therapy*. 29 (3). p142-143.

DIENER, E. 1984. Subjective well-being. *Psychological Bulletin*. 95, p542-575.

DOS REMEDIOS, R. 2007. *Men's Health Power Training*. Rodale Inc. 23.

DRAKE, R. L., MITCHELL. A. W. M. & VOGL, W. 2005. *Gray's Anatomy for Students*. Philadelphia: Elsevier.

ERHARD, R. E., DELITTO, A. & CIBULKA, M. T. 1994. Relative Effectiveness of an Extension Program and a Combined Program of Manipulation and Flexion and Extension Exercises in Patients With Acute Low Back Syndrome. *Physical Therapy Journal*. 74 (12), 1093-1100.

FAULKNER, J. A. 2003. Terminology for contractions of muscles during shortening, while isometric, and during lengthening. *Journal of Applied Physiology*. 95 (2), p455–459.

FISHBEIN, M. & AJZEN, I. 1975. *Belief, attitude, intention, and behavior: An introduction to theory and research.* Reading, Massachusetts: Addison-Wesley.

FRENCH, D. N., KRAEMER, W. J. & COOKE, J. B. 2003. Changes in dynamic exercise performance following a sequence of preconditioning isometric muscle actions. *Journal of Strength and Conditioning Research.* 17, p678-685.

GABBE, B. J., FINCH, C. F., WAJSWELNER, H., & BENNELL, K. L. 2004. Predictors of lower extremity injuries at the community level of Australian football. *Clinical Journal of Sports Medicine.* 14 (2), p56-63.

GAFFNEY, K., WILLIAMS, R. B., JOLLIFFE, V. A. & BLAKE, D. R. 1995. Intra-articular Pressure Changes in Rheumatoid and Normal Peripheral Joints. *Annals of the Rheumatic Diseases.* 54, p670-673.

GILLET H, LIEKENS M. 1969. A further study of joint fixations. *Annual Swiss Chiropractic Association.* 4, p41–46.

GOTO, K., NAGASAWA, M., YANAGISAWA, O., KIZUKA, T., ISHII, N. & TAKAMATSU, K. 2004. Muscular Adaptations to Combinations of High and Low-Intensity Resistance Exercises. *Journal of Strength & Conditioning Research.* 18 (4), p730-737.

GRENIER, S. G. & MCGILL, S. M. 2007. Quantification of lumbar lumbar stability using two different abdominal activation strategies. *Archives of Physical Medicine and Rehabilitation.* 88, p54-62.

GROSS, R. & MCILVEEN, R. 2004. *Psychology a New Introduction.* London. Hodder & Stoughton. p250-251.

HALL-FLAVIN, D. K. 2013. *Is there a link between pain and depression? Can depression cause physical pain?* [Online]. Available from: http://www.mayoclinic.com/health/pain-and-depression/AN01449 [Accessed: 03/09/2013].

HAMADA, T., SALE, D. G. & MCDOUGALL, J.D. 2000. Postactivation potentiation in endurance trained male athletes. *Medicine and Science in Sports and Exercises.* 32, p403-411.

HARVEY, D. 1998. Assessment of the Flexibility of elite athletes using the modified Thomas test. *British Journal of Sports Medicine.* 32, p68-70.

HASEGAWA, H., YAMAUCHI, T. & KRAEMER, W. J. 2007. Foot strike patterns of runners at the 15-km point during an elite-level half marathon. *Journal of Strength & Conditioning Research.* 21 (3), p888-893.

HEATH, B. H. J. E. & CARTER, J. E. L. 1967. A modified somatotype method. *American Journal of Physical Anthropology.* 27 (1), p57-74.

HEDGE, A. 2013. *Ergonomic Seating? Lecture Notes.* [Online] Cornell University. p1. Available from: http://ergo.human.cornell.edu/studentdownloads/DEA3250pdfs/ErgoChair.pdf [Accessed: 28/11/2014].

HENNEMAN, E. 1957. Relation between size of neurons and their susceptibility to discharge. *Science.* 126, p1345–1347.

HODGES, P. W. & RICHARDSON, C.A. 1998. Delayed postural contraction of transversus abdominis in low back pain associated with movement of the lower limb. *Journal of Spinal Disorders.* 11(1): p46-56.

HODGES, P.W. and RICHARDSON, C.A. 1997. Contraction of the abdominal muscles associated with movement of the lower limb. *Physical therapy.* p77.

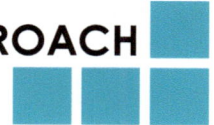

HOFFMAN, J. R., RATAMESS, N. A., FAIGENBAUM, A. D., MANGINE, G. T. & KANG, J. 2007. Effects of maximal squat exercise testing on vertical jump performance in American college football players. *Journal of Sports Science and Medicine*. 6, p149-150.

HOLM, L., REISTELSEDER, S., PEDERSEN, T. G., DOESSING, S., PETERSEN, S. G., FLYVBJERG, A., ANDERSEN, J. L., AAGAARD, P. & KJAER, M. 2008. Changes in muscle size and MHC composition in response to resistance exercise with heavy and light loading intensity, *Journal of Applied Physiology*. 105, p1454-1461.

HONEYBOURNE, J., HILL, M & MOORS H. 2000. *Advanced Physical Education & Sport for A-Level*. Cheltenham. Nelson Thornes Ltd.

Hoppenfeld, S. 1995. *Physical Examination of the Spine & Extremities*. New Jersey: Pearson Education.

JACKSON, A. W. & BAKER, A. A. 1986. The relationship of the sit and reach test to criterion measures of hamstring and back flexibility in young females. *Research Quarterly for Exercise and Sport*. 57 (3), p183-186.

JANDA, V. 1968. *Postural and phasic muscles in the pathogenesis of low back pain*. Proceedings of the 11th Congress of International Society of Rehabilitation of the Disabled. Dublin, Ireland. p553-554.

JANDA, V. 1987. Muscles and motor control in low back pain: Assessment and management. In: Twomey, L. T. *Physical therapy of the low back*. Churchill Livingstone: New York. p253-278.

JANDA, V. 1988. *Muscles and Cervicogenic Pain Syndromes*. In: Grand, R. Physical Therapy of the Cervical and Thoracic Spine. New York: Churchill Livingstone.

KANDEL, E. R., SCHWARTZ, J. H. & JESSEL, T. M. 2000. *Principles of Neural Science* (4th Edition). New York. McGraw-Hill.

KENDAL, F. P., MCCREARY, E. K., PROVANCE, P. G., RODGERS, M. M. & ROMANI, W. A. 2005. *Muscle Testing and Function with Posture and Pain* (5th Edition). Baltimore, Maryland: Lippincott Williams & Williams. p49-65.

KIBLER, W. B., PRESS, J., & SCIASCIA, A. 2006. The role of core stability in athletic function. *Sports Medicine*. 36 (3), p189-198.

KISNER, C. & COLBY, L. A. 2012. *Therapeutic Exercise: Foundations and Techniques* (6th Edition). Philadelphia: F. A. Davis.

KONRADSEN, L. 2002. Factors Contributing to Chronic Ankle Instability: Kinesthesia and Joint Position Sense. *Journal of Athletic Training*. 37 (4), p381–385.

LANG, A. R. 1983. *"Addictive Personality: A Viable Construct?"* In: Commonalities in Substance Abuse and Habitual Behaviour. Lexington, Mass. Lexington Books. p157-235.

LEDERMAN, E. 2009. The myth of core stability. *Journal of Bodywork and Movement Therapies*.

LEPHART, S. M., PINCIVERO, D. M., GIRAIDO, J. L. & FU, F. H. 1997. The Role of Proprioception in the Management and Rehabilitation of Athletic Injuries. *American Journal of Sports Medicine*. 25 (1), p130-137.

LEIBENSON, C. 1996. *Rehabilitation of the Spine*. Baltimore: Williams & Wilkins.

LIEBENSON, C., KARPOWICZ, A. M., BROWN, S. H. M., HOWARTH. S. J. & MCGILL, S. M. 2009. The active straight leg raise test and lumbar spine stability. *American Academy of Physical Medicine and Rehabilitation*. 1, p530-535.

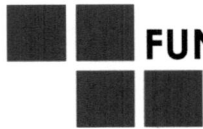

LIEBERMAN, D. E., VENKADESAN, M., DAOUD, A. I. & WERBEL, W. A. 2010. *Biomechanical Differences Between Different Foot Strikes* [Online]. Available from: http://www.barefootrunning.fas.harvard.edu/4BiomechanicsofFootStrike.html. [Accessed 08/08/2014].

LINDSAY, K. W. & BONE, I. 1998. *Neurology and Neurosurgery Illustrated* (3rd Edition). Edinburgh. Churchill Livingstone. p168.

LOPEZ-MINARRO, P. A. & ALACID, A. 2010. Influence of hamstring extensibility on spinal curvatures in young athletes. *Science & Sports*. 25 (4), p188-193.

LOUDON, J. K., WIESNERT, D., GOIST-FOLEY, H. L., ASJEST, C. & LOUDON, K. L. 2002. Intrarater reliability of functional performance test for subjects with patellofemoral pain syndrome. *Journal of Athletic Training*. 37 (3), p256-261.

MACKENZIE, B. 1997. *Conditioning* [Online]. Available from: http://www.brianmac.co.uk/conditon.htm. [Accessed 2/7/2013].

MACKENZIE, B. 2002 *Core Muscle Strength and Stability Test* [Online]. Available from: http://www.brianmac.co.uk/coretest.htm [Accessed 15/01/2014].

MACKENZIE, B. 2003. *Core Stability* [Online]. Available from: http://www.brianmac.co.uk/corestab.htm [Accessed 09/12/2013].

MAEO, S., TAKAHASHI, T., TAKAI, T. & KANEHISA, H. 2013. Trunk Muscle Activities during Abdominal Bracing: Comparison among Muscles and Exercises. *Journal of Sports Science and Medicine*. 12 (3), p467-74.

MAGILL, R. A. & SCHOENFELDER-ZOHDI, B. 1996. A visual model and knowledge of performance as sources of information for learning a rhythmic gymnastics skill. *International Journal of Sport Psychology*. 27 (1), p7-22.

MARTIN, R. C. & DAHLEN, E. R. 2005. Cognitive emotion regulation in the prediction of depression, anxiety, stress, and anger. *Science Direct*. p1249–1260.

MATSEN, F. A., LIPPETT, S. B., BIRTLESEN, A., ROCKWOOD, C. A. & WIRTH, M. A. 2009. *Glenohumeral Instability. In: The Shoulder*. Philadelphia. Elsevier.

MCCARDLE, W. D., KATCH, F. I. & KATCH, V. L. 2006. *Essentials of Exercise Physiology: Energy, Nutrition and Human Performance*. Baltimore, Pennsylvania: Lippincott Williams & Wilkins.

MCCUE, M. 2014. *Vibram Agrees to Settle Class Action Lawsuit* [Online]. Available from: http://www.runnersworld.com/general-interest/vibram-agrees-to-settle-class-action-lawsuit [Accessed 24/08/2014].

MELDRUM, C. 2012. *The effect of chiropractic manipulation and/or a combination of abdominal strengthening exercises on the feed-forward reaction of the deep abdominal muscles in people with chronic mechanical low back pain*. MSc Dissertation, Johannesburg University.

MENS, J. M., VLEEMING, A., SNIJDERS, C. J., STAM, H. J. & GINAI, A. Z. 1999. The active straight leg raising test and mobility of the pelvic joints. *European Spine Journal*. 8, p468-473.

MENS, J., HOEK VAN DIJKE, G., POOL-GOUDZWAARD, A., VAN DER HULST, V. & STAM, H. 2006. Possible harmful effects of high intra-abdominal pressure on the pelvic girdle. *Journal of Biomechanics*. 39 (4), p627-635.

MERGENER, T., HLAVACKA, F. & SCHWEIGART, G. 1993. Interaction of vestibular and proprioceptive inputs. *Journal Vestibular Research*. 3, p41–57.

MICHAUD, T. 2014. *Is It Harmful To Heel Strike When Running?* [Online]. Available from: http://running.competitor.com/2014/02/injury-prevention/is-it-harmful-to-heel-strike-when-

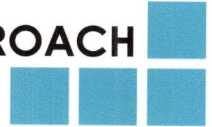

running_95678 [Accessed: 18/08/2014].

MILLER, J. 2013. *Definitive guide to reps, sets, rest, and tempo* [Online]. Available from: http://www.limitless365.com/2012/01/31/definitive-guide-to-reps-sets-rest-and-tempo-oh-my [Accessed: 14/10/2013].

MUNRO, A., HERRINGTON, L. & COMFORT, P. 2012. Comparison of landing knee valgus angle between female basketball and football athletes: possible implications for Anterior Cruciate ligament and Patellofemoral joint injury rates. *Physical Therapy in Sport.* 13 (4), p.259-265.

MUNSON, M. 2013. My body: *Why your muscles hurt 48 hours later* [Online]. Available from: http://www.americanathletemag.com/ArticleView/tabid/156/ArticleID/22/MY-BODY-Why-Your-Muscles-Hurt-48-Hours-Later.aspx [Accessed: 15/10/2013].

NATIONAL INSTITUTES OF HEALTH, UNITED STATES DEPARTMENT OF HEALTH AND HUMAN SERVICES. 2005. *An Update of NIH Pain Research and Related Program Initiatives* [Online]. Available from: http://www.hhs.gov/asl/testify/t051208a.html [Accessed: 18/09/2013].

NATIONAL SCOLIOSIS FOUNDATION. 2013. *Information and Support* [Online]. Available from: http://www.scoliosis.org/info.php [Accessed: 19/11/2013].

NHS. 2013. *Causes of back pain* [Online]. Available from: http://www.nhs.uk/Conditions/Back-pain/Pages/Causes.aspx [Accessed: 10/12/2013].

NHS. 2012. *Walking for Health* [Online]. Available from: http://www.nhs.uk/Livewell/getting-started-guides/Pages/getting-started-walking.aspx [Accessed: 25/05/2014].

OXFORD DICTIONARY. 2013. *Function* [Online]. Available from: http://oxforddictionaries.com/definition/english/function. [Accessed 02/07/2013].

PANJABI, M. M. 1992. The Stabilising System of the Spine. Part I. Function, Dysfunction, Adaptation, and Enhancement. *Journal of Spinal Disorders & Techniques.* 5 (4). p383-389.

PANJABI, M. M. 1992. The Stabilising System of the Spine. Part II. Neutral Zone and Instability Hypothesis. *Journal of Spinal Disorders & Techniques.* 5 (4). p390-396.

PAVLOV, I. P. 1927. *Conditioned Reflexes: An Investigation of the Physiological Activity of the Cerebral Cortex.* Translated and Edited by G. V. Anrep. London: Oxford University Press.

PETTMAN, E. 2006. *Manipulative Thrust Techniques. An Evidence-based Approach.* Abbotsford, Canada: Apherna Publishing.

PICARD, A. 2013. *Why the Sedentary Life is Killing us* [Online]. Available from: http://www.theglobeandmail.com/life/health-and-fitness/health/why-the-sedentary-life-is-killing-us/article4613704/ [Accessed: 07/11/2013].

PLOWMAN, S. 1992. *Physical activity, physical fitness, and low back pain.* In: Holloszy, J. O. Exercise and Sport Sciences Reviews. Baltimore: Williams & Wilkins. p221-242.

POPE, R., HERBERT, R., & AND KIRWAN, J. 1998. Effect of ankle dorsiflexion range and pre-exercise calf muscle stretching on injury risk in Army recruits. *Australian Physiotherapy.* 44 (3), p165-172.

PROSKE, U. & MORGAN, D. L. 2001. Muscle damage from eccentric exercise: mechanism, mechanical signs, adaptation and clinical applications. *The Journal of Physiology.* 537, p333-345.

PRYOR, R. R., SFORZO, G. A. & KING, D. L. 2011. Optimizing power output by varying repetition tempo. *Journal of Strength and Conditioning Research.* 25 (11), p3029-3034.

RADEBOLD, A., CHOLEWICKI, J., PANJABI, M. M. & PATEL, T. C. 2000. Muscle response pattern to sudden trunk loading in healthy individuals and in patients with chronic low back pain. *Spine.* 25 (8), p947-54.

RAFFLE, C. 2012. *Eccentric Exercise. Bigger. Stronger. More Powerfuller. Resistant to Injury* [Online]. Available from: http://www.caryraffle.com/2012/08/eccentric-exercise-bigger-stronger-more.html [Accessed 03/07/2013].

REID, A., BIRMINGHAM, T. B., STRATFORD, P. W., ALCOCK, G. K. & GIFFIN, J. R. 2007. Hop testing provides a reliable and valid outcome measure during rehabilitation after anterior cruciate ligament reconstruction. *Physical Therapy.* 87 (3), p337-349.

REULEAUX, F. 1876. *The Kinematics of Machinery: Outlines of a Theory of Machines.* London, UK: Macmillan and Co.

ROOTS, M. 2013. *Fitness Buzzword Explained: Eccentric Training* [Online]. Available from: http://www.core-condition.com/quick-tips/fitness-buzzword-explained-eccentric-training/ [Accessed 03/07/2013].

RUNNING WAREHOUSE. 2014. *Shoes 101* [Online]. Available from: http://www.runningwarehouse.com/learningcenter/shoes101.html [Accessed 18/08/2014].

SAGE, G. 1977. *Introduction to Motor Behaviour: A neuropsychological approach* (2nd Edition). Reading, Massachusetts: Addison-Wesley.

SAHRMANN, S. 2002. *Diagnosis and Treatment of Movement Impairment Syndromes.* New York. Elsevier. p13.

SANDOZ R. 1976. Some physical mechanisms and effects of spinal adjustments. *Annual Swiss Chiropractic Association.* 6, p91–142.

SATYENDRA, L. & BYL, N. 2006. Effectiveness of physical therapy for Achilles tendinopathy: An evidence based review of eccentric exercises. *Isokinetics and Exercise Science.* 14 (1), p71-80.

SCHOBERTH, H. 1962. *Sitzhaltung, Sitzschaden, Sitzmobel.* Berlin, Springer-Verlag.

SCHULTZ, S. J., SCHULTZ, J. J. & PERRIN, D. H. 2005. *Examination of Musculoskeletal Injuries* (2nd Edition). North Carolina: Human Kinetics. p55-60.

SELIGMAN, M. E. P. 1975. *Helplessness: On Depression, Development, and Death.* San Francisco: W. H. Freeman.

SHERRINGTON, C. S. 1907. On the proprioceptive system, especially in its reflex aspect. *Brain.* 29 (4), p467–85.

SKINNER, B. F. 1938. *The Behavior of Organisms: An Experimental Analysis.* New York: Appleton-Century.

SKINNER, B. F. 1948. 'Superstition' in the pigeon. *Journal of Experimental Psychology,* 38, p168-172.

SMETACEK, V. & MECHSNER, F. 2004. Making sense. *Nature.* 432, p21.

STEINDLER, A. 1955. *Kinesiology of the Human Body Under Normal and Pathological Conditions.* Springfield, Illinois: Charles C Thomas Publisher.

STERNBERG, R. J. & STERNBERG, K. 2012. *Cognitive Psychology* (6th Edition). Belmont. California: Wadsworth.

STONE, W. J. & COULTER, S. P. 1994. Strength/endurance effects from three resistance training protocols with women. *Journal of Strength and Conditioning Research.* 8, p231-234.

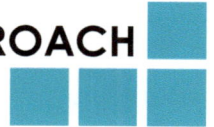

SULLIVAN, M. 2004. Exaggerated pain behaviour: by what standard? *The Clinical Journal of Pain.* 20 (6), p433-439.

THORNDIKE, E. L. 1898. Animal intelligence: An experimental study of the associative processes in animals. *Psychological Monographs: General and Applied.* 2 (4), pi-109.

TWOMEY, L. & TAYLOR, J. 1995. Exercise and Spinal Manipulation in the Treatment of Low Back. *Spine.* 20 (5), 615-9.

UK BEAM TRIAL TEAM, 2004. United Kingdom back pain exercise and manipulation (UK BEAM) randomised trial: effectiveness of physical treatments for back pain in primary care. *British Medical Journal.* 329 (7479), p1377.

VERA-GARCIA, F. J., ELVIRA, J. L., BROWN, S. H. & MCGILL, S. M. 2007. Effects of abdominal stabilization maneuvers on the control of spine motion and stability against sudden trunk perturbations. *Journal of Electromyography Kinesiology.* 17 (5), p556-67.

VERNON, H. & MROZEK, J. 2005. A Revised Definition of Manipulation. *Journal of Manipulative and Physiological Therapeutics.* 28 (1), p68-72.

WANDEL, J. A. 2000. *Position and Handling.* In: Solomon, J. W. Pediatric Skills for Occupational Therapists. London: Mosby.

WATSON, J. B. & RAYNER, R. 1920. Conditioned emotional reactions. *Journal of Experimental Psychology.* 3 (1), p1-14.

WEST, D. W., KUJBIDA, G. W., MOORE, D. R., ATHERTON, P., BURD, N. A., PADZIK, J. P., DE LISIO, M., TANG, J. E., PARISE, G., RENNIE, M. J., BAKER, S. K. & PHILLIPS, S. M. 2009. Resistance exercise-induced increases in putative anabolic hormones do not enhance muscle protein synthesis or intracellular signaling in young men. *Journal of Physiology.* 587 (21), p5239-47.

WHITE, S. G. & MCNAIR, P. J. 2002. Abdominal and erector spinae muscle activity during gait: the use of cluster analysis to identify patterns of activity. *Clinical Biomechanics.* 17 (3), p.177-84.

WILLSON, J. D. & DAVIS, I. S. 2008. Utility of the frontal plane projection angle in females with patellofemoral pain. *Journal of Orthopaedic Sports Physical Therapy.* 38, p606-615.

WILMOT, E. G., EDWARDSON, C. L., ACHANA, F. A., DAVIES, M. J., GORELY, T., GRAY, L. J., KHUNTI, K. YATES, T. & BIDDLE, S. J. H. 2012. Sedentary time in adults and the association with diabetes, cardiovascular disease and death: systematic review and meta-analysis. *Diabetologia.* 55 (11), p2895-2905.

WOLFF, J. 1986. *"The Law of Bone Remodeling".* Berlin, Heidelberg, New York: Springer.

WOOLFOLK, A. 2013. *Educational Psychology.* New Jersey. Pearson.

FUNCTIONAL REHABILITATIVE TRAINING

Index

A

Abdominal · 95
    Brace · 104, 106, **113-114,** 132, 206, 210, 211, 212, 217
    Intra-abdominal Pressure · 101
    Hollowing · 115
Active Subsystem · 89-90
Addictive Personality · 12
Anatomy · 13
Anterior · **4**, 22, 83, 92, 96, 106, 121, 130, 178, 186, 188, 201-202, 223
Anterior Head Carriage · 83, 94, 171, 199
Apley Scratch Test · 197
Arthrokinetic Reflex · 104
Avulsion · 178

B

Barefoot Running · **187-189**,
Behaviour · **56-58**, 61, 67, 103
    Fear-avoidance · 58
    Pain · 68
Biceps · 5, 7, 26, 129
Breakdown Sets · 161
Burn-out Sets · 164

C

Calcaneal Eversion · 177
Calcaneal Inversion · 177
Cavitation · 26
Central Nervous System · **17**, 89, 103
Cerebrotonic · 11
Cervical · **22**, 23, 25
Chronic Pain · 70
Classical Conditioning · **59-60**
Closed Kinetic Chain · 76

Coccyx · 22, **24**
Congenital Hip Dysplasia · 175
Contractibility · 5
Contraction
    Concentric · **7**, 147, 150, 199
    Eccentric · **7**, 125, 147-148, 150, 160, 199
    Isometric · **8**

Core Stability · **101-103**, 116, 120
Coupled Motion · 25
Coupling Principle · 173
Cutaneous Receptors
    Free Nerve Endings · 21
    Hair Follicle Receptors · 21
    Krause Corpuscles · 21
    Meissner's Corpuscles · 21
    Merkel Cells · 21
    Pacinian Corpuscles · 21
    Ruffini Corpuscles · 21

D

Deep · **4**, 51, 106
Deltoid · 35, 82, 130, 196
Dermatome · 17
Distal · **4**, 5, 26, 76, 92, 186
Drehmann Sign · 175
Drop Sets · 152
Dynamic Muscle Loading · 203
Dysfunction · 2, 5, 27, 39, 59, 89, 92, 129, 178, 206, 217, 224

E

Ectomorph · 10-11
Elastic Barrier · 5
Elasticity · 5
Endomorph · 10-11
Endurance · 143

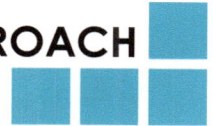

Absolute · 144
Relative · 144
Erectus Spinae · **37**, 75, 84-85, 95, 96, 101, 127, 132, 174, 210-211, 224
Ergonomic · 77, 87
Excitability · 5
Excitation-Contraction · 148
Explosive Strength · 140, 149, 154
Extensibility · 5
Exteropceptors · 18

F

Facet · 23, **24-25**, 39, 76, 96, 101, 113, 128, 173, 211
Failure · 140
Fast Oxidative Glycolytic Fibres (type IIa) · 141
Fatigue
Dynamic · 108
Isometric · 108
Feedback
Continuous · 63
External/extrinsic · 64
Internal/intrinsic · 64
Knowledge of Performance · 63
Knowledge of Results · 63
Negative · 64
Positive · 64
Terminal · 63
Fixation · 5, 180
Force · 120
Forefoot Strike Running · 187
Free Nerve Endings · 21
Frozen Shoulder · 82
Functional Assessment · 79, 110

G

Gait · **165**
Foot Flat · 167

Heel Off · 167
Heel Strike · 167
Midstance · 167
Midswing · 167
Toe Off · 167
Gait Analysis Form · 168
Genu Recurvatum · 84, **176**
Genu Valgum · **175**
Genu Varum · 83, **175**
Giant Sets · 158
Glenohumeral Joint · 4, 31, 94, 195, 196
Gluteus Maximus · 95, 96, 174
Gluteus Medius · **43-44**, 82, 95, 173, 174, 205, 215, 218, 220, 222
Goal Setting · **65-66**, 70-71

H

Hallux Rigidus · 180
Hamstring Flexibility · 208-209
Hamstrings · **45**, 174-175, 183, 210, 223-224
Heavy Singles · 154
Heel Strike Running · 183
Helical · 129-130
High-Steppage Gait · 174-175, 178
Hip Hinge · 211
Hypertrophy · 143
Myofibril · 143-145
Sarcoplasmic · 143-145
Hypomobility · 5

I

Iliopsoas · **41**, 95-96, 205, 207-208, 215, 221, 222
Individual Pain Scale · 68
Inferior · **4**, 14, 82, 121
Infraspinatus · 82, 94, 196-197
Insertion · 5, 7, 20, **26**, 175, 224
Intensity · 139

Internal Oblique · 106-107, 113
Interoceptors · 18
Intra-abdominal Pressure · 101
Intra-articular Pressure · 25

K

Kinematic Chain · **76**, 212
Kinesthesia · 19-21
Kinetic Chain · **76-77**, 92, 120, 166, 172-173,
      176-179, 184, 186, 188-189, 200, 202,
      214
Knee Tracking · 218
Kyphosis · 76, 78, 83, 90, 92, 94, 96, 171

L

Lactic Acid · 142, 156, 159, 184
Lateral · **4**, 15, 25, 47, 91, 94, 130, 178, 181,
      183, 185, 204, 218, 224
Latissimus Dorsi · 127, 224
Law of Acceleration · 124
Law of Inertia · 124
Law of Reaction · 125
Learned Helplessness · 70-71
Levator Scapulae · **29**, 81, 93, 94, 121, 196
Locus of Causality · 63
Lordosis · 39, 76, 83, 90, 94-96, 115
Lower Trapezius · 31, 93
Lower-crossed Posture · 94-96
Lumbar · **22-25**, 37, 39, 41, 83, 211, 213, 215

M

Manipulation · 5
Medial · **4**, 14, 15, 29, 47, 82, 181, 196, 224,
      228
Mesomorph · 9-11
Metabolic Rate · 159
Morton's Neuroma · 188

Motivation · 62
      Extrinsic · 63
      Intrinsic · 62
Motor Neurone · 18, 141
Motor Patterns · 127, 194
Motor Skill · 64, 151
Multifidus · **101-102**, 104
Muscle Fibres · 141
      Fast Glycolytic Fibres (type IIb) · 142
      Fast Oxidative Glycolytic Fibres (type
      IIa) · 142
      Slow Oxidative Fibres (type I) · 141
Muscle Memory · 151
Myotome · 18

N

Negative Sets · 160
Neutral Spine · **88-91**, 115, 130, 198, 201,
      212, 217, 229
Neutral Strike Running · 185
Neutral Zone · 89-90

O

Open Kinetic Chain · 76
Operant Conditioning · **59-61**, 151
Origin · **4-5**, 7, 20, 26, 67, 103, 208
Orthotics · 170
Otolith Crystals · 19
Over-pronation · 83, 179-181, 189
Over-supination · 179
Oxygenated Blood · 142, 153, 157

P

Pacinian Corpuscles · 21
Pain Behaviour · 69
Painful Arc · 196
Paraphysiological Space · 5

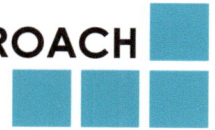

Paraspinals · 95
Passive Subsystem · 89-91
Patellofemoral Pain Syndrome · 47, 91, 186, 216
Pectoral · 33, 83, 92-94, 130, 200
Peripheral Nervous System · 17
Peroneus Longus · 49
Pes Cavus · 180
Plane
    Coronal · 4
    Horizontal · 4
    Sagittal · 4
    Transverse · 4
Plank · 110, 199
Plantar Fascia · 186
Plantar Fasciitis · 186, 188
Plumb Line · **81**, 83, 171-172
Popliteus · 224
Posterior · **4**, 22, 24, 27, 43, 45, 49, 81, 90-92, 95-96, 121, 130, 132, 174, 197, 200-201, 223-234
Postural Triggers · 87
Posture · 27, 29, 33, 35, 37, 45, 66, **74-79**, 81-82, 84-85, 87-93, 96, 97, 114, 170, 171-172, 211
    Assessment · 79
    Lower-Crossed Posture · 94
    Seated · 84-85
    Standing · 78
    Upper-Crossed Posture · 27, 29, 31, 83, 87, 92-94, 96, 171, 200
Proprioception · **18-20**, 22, 49, 63, 130, 177, 213, 216, 218
Proximal · **4-5**, 37, 188
Pyramid Sets · 153

Q

Quadratus Lumborum · 37, **39-40**, 43, 45, 82, 83, 85, 95-96, 101, 132, 207, 208-211

Quadriceps · 25, 37, 183, 186, 215, 218, 221

R

Rectus Abdominus · 101
Rectus Femoris · 95-96, 205, 207, 221, 222
Rhomboids · **33**, 81-83, 93, 172, 198
Ruffini Corpuscles · 21
Running Techniques · 182

S

Sacrum · 22, **24**, 37
Scalene · 81
Scapula Winging · 198
Schemas · 11, **56-58**, 67, 68
Scheuermann's · 83, 201
Scoliosis · 82, 173
Self-esteem · 67
Sensory Receptors
    Golgi Tendon Organs · 20
    Muscle Spindles · 20
Serratus Anterior · 82, 93, 96, 199
Size Principle · 141, 145, 152, 153, 155, 160
Slipped Upper Femoral Epiphysis · 174
Slow Oxidative Fibres (type I) · 141
Social Learning Theory · 66
Soleus · **51**, 222
Somatic · 5, 17-18
Somatic Dysfunction · 5
Somatotonic · 11
Somatotypes
    Ectomorphy · 8
    Endomorphy · 8
    Mesomorphy · 8
Splenius Capitus · **27**, 29
Squat Test · **201-203**, 217
Step-down Test · 213-214
Sternocleidomastoid · 81, 193
Strain · 122

Strength · 56, 71, 101, 105, 120-122, 143, 144
    Absolute · 121
    Maximum · 121
    Relative · 122
Strength-endurance Continuum · 139, 146
Stress · 122
Stretch Reflex · 20, 103-104, 148-150
Strip Sets · 152
Subluxation · 5
Subscapularis · 94, 200
Subsystem
    Active · 89
    Neural · 89
    Passive · 89
Superficial · **4**, 21, 107, 127
Superior · **4**, 14, 27, 35, 94, 224
Supersets · 155
Supraspinatus · **35**, 82, 94, 131, 196-197

T

Talus Neutral · 181
Tempo · 147
Tensor Fascia Latae · 82, 222
Teres Minor · 94
Therapeutic Alliance · 67, 69
Thoracic · 22-25, 83, 171
Tibial Torsion · 83, 176
Tibialis Anterior · 184
Torque · 126
Torsion · 83, 120, **126-128**
Torsional Assistance · 129
Torsional Control · 120, **128-131**
    Exercise · 129
    Isolating · 129
    Training · 131
Torticollis · 81, 171
Transverse Plane · 40
Transversus Abdominis · **101-103**, 106
Trapezius · 29, **31**, 35, 81, 131, 196

Trendelenburg · 82, **173**, 205, 215, 218, 220
Triceps · 7, 130, 158
Tri-sets · 157
Trunk Endurance · 110
Trunk Musculature · 105, 108, 113-114, 129-130, 206
Trunk Strength · 108

U

Upper Trapezius · 82, 93-94, 121

V

Vastus Lateralis · 47, 91, 202, 205, 216, 218, 221
Vastus Medialis Oblique · **47**, 91, 202, 205, 216, 218, 221
Vestibular System · 19
Vibram · 188
Visceral · 17
Viscerotonic · 11

W

Wall Angel Test · 200
Winging Scapula · 196
Withdrawal Reflex · 104
Wolff's Law · 145, 151

www.ingramcontent.com/pod-product-compliance
Lightning Source LLC
Chambersburg PA
CBHW060831270326
41932CB00005B/40